Nursing Ethics
through the Life Span
FOURTH EDITION

Nursing Ethics
through the Life Span
FOURTH EDITION

Elsie L. Bandman, RN, EdD
Professor of Nursing, Emeritus
Hunter College–Bellevue School of Nursing
Hunter College of the City University of New York
New York, New York

Bertram Bandman, Phd
Professor of Philosophy
Brooklyn Campus of Long Island University
Brooklyn, New York

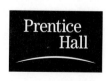

Upper Saddle River, New Jersey

Library of Congress Cataloging-in-Publication Data

Bandman, Elsie L.
  Nursing ethics through the life span/Elsie L. Bandman, Bertram Bandman.—4th ed.
    p. ; cm.
  Includes bibliographical references and index.
  ISBN 0-8385-6976-5
    1. Nursing ethics. I. Bandman, Bertram. II. Title.
    [DNLM: 1. Ethics, Nursing. WY 85 B214n 2002]
  RT85 .B33 2002
  174′.2—dc21

                                                                    00-068465

Publisher: *Julie Alexander*
Executive Editor: *Maura Connor*
Acquisitions Editor: *Nancy Anselment*
Director of Production and Manufacturing: *Bruce Johnson*
Managing Production Editor: *Patrick Walsh*
Manufacturing Manager: *Ilene Sanford*
Production Liaison: *Julie Boddorf*
Production Editor: *Emily Autumn*
Creative Director: *Marianne Frasco*
Cover Design Coordinator: *Maria Guglielmo*
Cover Designer: *Amy Rosen*
Director of Marketing: *Leslie Cavaliere*
Marketing Coordinator: *Rachele Triano*
Editorial Assistant: *Beth Romph*
Composition: *The Clarinda Company*
Printing and Binding: *R.R. Donnelley & Sons*

Prentice-Hall International (UK) Limited, *London*
Prentice-Hall of Australia Pty: Limited, *Sydney*
Prentice-Hall Canada, Inc., *Toronto*
Prentice-Hall Hispanoamericana, S.A., *Mexico*
Prentice-Hall of India Private Limited, *New Delhi*
Prentice-Hall of Japan, Inc., *Tokyo*
Prentice-Hall Singapore Pte, Ltd., *Singapore*
Editora Prentice-Hall do Brasil, Ltda., *Rio de Janeiro*

---

10 9 8 7 6 5 4 3 2

ISBN 0-8385-6976-5

We dedicate this effort to the significant people in our lives:
Nancy Bandman-Boyle, Thomas Boyle, and
Samuel Phillip Boyle—our grandson,
who is a source of our continuing joy—
for their steadfast support, love,
graciousness, and good humor.

Contents

Preface   xi

Part One   Moral Pathways in Nursing   1

Chapter 1   The Moral Significance of Nursing   1

The Meaning of Nursing in the History of Humankind /
Ethics and Science / The Function of Nursing Ethics /
What Is Ethics? What Is Nursing Ethics? / What Is Good
or Harm? / What Is the Good Life? / Health as a Goal
of the Good Life / Important Ethical Issues in Nursing /
Methods of Moral Reasoning / The Role of Care in
Nursing Ethics / The Role of the Nurse in Ethics / The
Interdisciplinary Role of the Nurse in Ethics

Chapter 2   Models of Professional Relationships   19

Models of Physician-Patient Relationships: Emanuel and
Emanuel / Nursing Models / The Role of the Nurse
as Patient Advocate / The Importance of Advocacy /
Three Models of Patient Advocacy / Arguments For
and Against the Nurse as Patient Advocate / Moral
Implications in Codes of Ethics / The American Nurses
Association (ANA) *Code for Nurses* / The International
Council for Nurses Code of Ethics / The Functions of a
Code for Nurses / The American Medical Association
Code of Ethics / Evaluation of Professional Codes

Chapter 3   Self-Interest Morality   40

Perennial Issues in Nursing: Self-Interest Ethics in Relation
to Alternative Theories / Three Views of the Social
Contract / Individualism in Relation to Collectivism,
Existentialism, and Phenomenology / Nursing Dilemmas
in Deciding What to Do

Chapter 4   Virtue Ethics in Nursing   53

Four Views of the Social Contract: Altruism, Objectivism,
Skepticism, and Nihilism / The Use of the Socratic
Method in Nursing Ethics / Plato's Response to Perennial
Issues and to Self-Interest Ethics: Rational

Paternalism / Aristotle's Conception of Ethics Applied to Nursing: Happiness through Self-Realization / Aquinas's View of Ethics: Life as a Gift

Chapter 5   **Consequentialist or Utilitarian Ethics**   66

Utilitarianism / Classical Utilitarianism in Nursing Ethics / Recent Utilitarian Formulations and Applications

Chapter 6   **Duty-Based Ethics: Universal Moral Principles**   74

Kant's Principles of Universality / Strengths of Kant's Ethics / Some Difficulties of Kantian Ethics / Voluntarism: Individual and Social / W. D. Ross's Attempted Solution: Prima Facie Values / A Further Attempted Solution: Kohlberg's Stages of Morality

Chapter 7   **Rights-Based Ethics**   84

Ethics Based on Justice: Rawls / Responses to Rawls's Social Contract View: Libertarianism and Equality / Values in Conflict / Post-Rawlsian Rights-Based Ethics / The Role of Rights and Virtues in Nursing Ethics / Rights and Virtues

Chapter 8   **Ethical Decision Making in Nursing**   96

Values Supportive of Shared Health Care Decisions / The Patient Self-Determination Act / Assessment of Patient Capacities and Competence / Guidelines for Shared Decision Making / Pitfalls of Reasoning: Fallacies

Part Two   Nursing Ethics through the Life Span   117

Chapter 9   **Nursing Ethics in the Procreative Family**   117

Family Functions, Dynamics, and Values / Three Models of Family and Marriage / Family Dynamics and Values / The Nurse's Role in Family Ethical Issues / Ethical Issues in Reproductive Technology / Genetics / The Ethical Issues of Genetic Screening: Mandatory Versus Voluntary / The Nurse's Role in Genetic Counseling

Chapter 10   **Ethics and the Problem of Abortion**   141

Legal Status of Abortion / Reproductive Technology and Abortion / Ethical and Religious Issues in Abortion / The Nurse's Role in Abortion

Chapter 11   **Ethical Issues in the Nursing Care of Infants**   160

Overview: Developmental Highlights / Arguments For and Against Saving Premature and Deformed Infants / Newborn HIV Testing / Ethical Considerations in the Nursing Care of Infants / Ethical and Philosophical Considerations

Chapter 12   **Ethical Issues in the Nursing Care of Children**   176

Overview: Developmental Highlights / Ethical Issues Related to Children With Relevant Cases / Ethical Issues in the Care of Children with HIV/AIDS / Moral Implications in the Nursing Care of Children / Ethical-Philosophical Approaches to Nurse-Child-Parent Relationships: Rights, Dependency, Paternalism, and Freedom

Chapter 13   **Ethical Issues in the Nursing Care of Adolescents**   194

Developmental Highlights: Early, Middle, and Late Adolescence / Adolescent Health Care Issues / Ethical Issues in the Life and Death of Adolescents / Ethical Issues in Quality-of-Life Cases of Adolescents / The Nurse's Role in Adolescent Care / Ethical Considerations in the Adolescent-Nurse-Parent Relationship / The Biological/Biographical/Social/Cognitive Distinction Applied to Adolescents

Chapter 14   **Ethical Issues in the Nursing Care of Adults**   208

Adult Development / The Application of Ethical Principles to Selected Cases / Moral-Philosophical Considerations / Ethical and Philosophical Considerations of Personhood / Rights in and to Health Care / The Nurse's Role / American Hospital Association: *A Patient's Bill of Rights*

Chapter 15   **Ethical Issues in the Nursing Care of the Elderly**   233

Developmental Highlights: Retirement, Advanced Old Age, the Frail Elderly, Dementia / Problems and Prospects for the Elderly / Selected Cases and Principles / Ethical-Philosophical Considerations in the Nursing Care of the Elderly: Five Methods of Allocating Health Care / A Trilogy of Elderly Patients' Rights / Competence and the Rights of Elderly Patients / Justice Between Generations / Nursing Implications / The Sanctity of Life Versus the Quality of Life

Chapter 16   **Ethical Issues in the Nursing Care of the Dying**   **260**
Meanings and Definitions of Death   /   Selected Cases
and Principles Involving Nursing Judgments and Actions   /
Related Ethical Issues   /   Ethical Principles in the Care
of the Dying   /   Voluntary and Involuntary Euthanasia   /
Religious Aspects of the Nursing Care of the Dying   /
The Role of the Nurse in the Care of the Dying Patient

Glossary of Selected Terms   291

Appendix   297
Code for Nurses With Interpretive Statements   /
American Medical Association: *Code of Medical Ethics*   /
American Hospital Association: *A Patient's Bill of Rights*   /
Choice In Dying Living Will

Index   317

Preface

Far reaching changes have occurred in the health care delivery system that decisively affect the practice of nursing. The managed care sector attempts to justify its practices as cost containment with no loss in the quality of care. The incompatibility of these two objectives is obvious. Moves to cut costs have resulted in the restructuring of nursing staff, with reductions in the numbers and qualifications of professional nurses along with increases in nonlicensed assistive personnel. Consequently, the role of the nurse as patient advocate has never been more important to the safety of patients and the protection of their rights.

Nurses have invoked the principles of the American Nurses Association (ANA) *Code for Nurses* of respect for patients and safeguarding them from unsafe, incompetent, and inadequate nursing care. Nurses have successfully demonstrated and struck against hospitals, winning contracts for improved staffing and working conditions. In this way, nurses have achieved two goals: the direct improvement of conditions of patient care, and the improvement of organization ethics. Protesting nurses have forced organizations to publicly defend their stated mission and the role of moral reasoning in providing quality health care services. Demonstrating nurses have provoked positive media coverage as well as public interest, sympathy, and support. Although organizational mechanisms, such as ethics committees and patient representatives, may be broadened to address ethical health care concerns at all levels of the organization and even the community, no mechanism is as valuable or as effective as the practicing nurse who is trusted by patients to advise them regarding their rights to respect, to informed consent, and to receive and to refuse care in accordance with their values. We intend to strengthen and support nurses' determination to provide curative and preventive care to persons, to relieve their pain and suffering, and to promote public health and welfare measures. These are the goals of this text.

In this edition, we have reorganized the chapters. For the chapter on models, we applied the Emmanuel's model to nursing. In Part 1, we use a topical approach to ethics based on a philosophical examination of self-interest ethics, virtue ethics, consequentialist (utilitarian) ethics, duty-based ethics, and rights-based ethics; each is discussed in context of its historical development as well as its strengths and difficulties. Sharpening fundamental principles of each theory increases its applicability and usefulness to the student. The presentation includes the foundation of early Greek and Christian moral philosophy, including natural law, altruism, double effect, and its moral and religious impact on nursing. Consequentialist (utilitarian) ethics, with its emphasis on majority happiness and current health care delivery, is explored extensively. Kant's duty-based ethics emphasizes duty and responsibility, truth-telling, and promise keeping, and in treating humans as ends in themselves and not solely as means for other people's advantages. We then analyze rights-based ethics and its current implications for the nursing care of patients.

Part 2 examines and applies ethics to the life span of patients, beginning with the procreative family, then proceeding through abortion, infants, children, adolescents, adults, the elderly, and the dying. Cases are distributed throughout the chapters. Problems of HIV/AIDS are included in the cases and text. Chapters on the elderly and the dying deal extensively with issues of allocation, restraint, abuse, active and passive euthanasia, and assisted suicide. Nurses play a central role in the compassionate care of dying patients, helping them to maintain their humanity, often to the last breath. We support nurses' obligations to respect and support patients' religious beliefs regardless of the content of their own beliefs.

The intent of this text is to serve a variety of uses. It can be used as the primary text for a course of ethics, either at the undergraduate or graduate level. The format of the text also lends itself to use in successive courses, based on developmental levels, as the student moves through the curriculum. Our conception is that of applied ethics "from the womb to the tomb" correlated with most nursing curricula.

We are grateful to the Board of Trustees, and to the Research and Released Time Committee of Long Island University, Brooklyn Campus, for the grant of released time to write for this fourth edition. We appreciate the help of Nancy Anselment, nursing editor of Prentice Hall Health, for her support in this effort, and also her staff. We especially thank Emily Autumn, Senior Production Editor at Clarinda Publication Services. We gained a great deal from the monthly bioethics seminars at Montefiore Hospital conducted by Nancy Dubler and Jeffrey Blustein. We are also appreciative of several computer monitors at the Holyoke Community College, especially Ms. Florence Rice, Ms. Kelly Trombley, Ms. Milly Claudio, Mr. Chuck Schumer, and Mrs. Melissa Latour. We also gained considerable computer help from Mr. Devebrata Mondale, director of the Long Island University Faculty Resource Center and to his highly capable staff members. Lastly, we wish to acknowledge, with our gratitude, three nurses whom we believe epitomize the moral ideals of nursing in their practice; Cheryl D. Smith, RN, family practitioner and nurse diabetic educator, whose generosity of heart and mind touches each of her patients; and Susan Maher, RN, President of District 1 of the Massachussetts Nurses Association, and Bonnie Pierce, RN, for their professionalism, patient advocacy and dedication. These women give meaning to the notion that ethics is practical.

Elsie L. Bandman
Bertram Bandman

Nursing Ethics
through the Life Span
FOURTH EDITION

PART ONE

Moral Pathways in Nursing

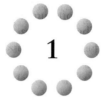

1

The Moral Significance
of Nursing

Study of this chapter enables the learner to:

1. Give reasons for the importance of the moral development of nurses.
2. Distinguish ethics and science.
3. Justify the participation of nurses in moral decisions affecting individuals, groups, families, and health care delivery.
4. Evaluate the relation of nursing to the goals and processes of a good life.
5. Use the four methods of moral reasoning to analyze ethical issues, problems, and dilemmas.
6. Apply the ethics of caring to everyday nursing practice.
7. Implement nursing participation in ethical decision making.

OVERVIEW: THE MEANING OF NURSING IN THE HISTORY OF HUMANKIND

In the history of human events, nurses have made a special and extraordinary contribution. They have helped to alleviate suffering and to protect, promote, sustain, and restore health. Nursing has been and is essential to patient health care needs and interests. The persistent thread that runs throughout nursing history is the continuity of care and nurture of human beings regardless of socioeconomic status, race, religion, culture, or the nature of the health problem. Thus, nurses have cared for the diseased and wounded, such as lepers and other outcasts of society, for the sake of doing good and preventing harm, which is so essential to ethics and to ethically justifiable behavior.

With the advent of secular nursing in the 19th century, nurses became educated and responsive to rational standards of conduct requiring highly disciplined, scientific, technological, and professionally effective judgments. In this century, professional nurses with advanced degrees continue to respond to the health care needs and interests of the sick, the diseased, the wounded, the disabled, and the homeless in a society that is rapidly oriented by scientific and technologic processes and values. For most nurses, the belief in "doing good" continues to be a powerful motive for performing the often arduous, demanding, and complex work of nursing. In the course of their daily and nightly practice, nurses are often faced with choices that may significantly affect their patients' lives that give rise to such questions as, "Did I do the right thing?", "Would it have been better to do X instead of Y?" "Did I help my patients to understand their choices and the consequences of each?" Every dedicated, caring nurse has at some time been tormented by such doubts. The purpose of this work is to clarify these issues and thereby facilitate the decision-making processes in nursing.

In return for the nursing profession's dedication to patients', families', and the community's well-being, society recognizes the profession's authority and expects nurses to act responsibly. Self-regulation is a characteristic of an accountable, and therefore mature, profession.[1] (Whether any profession measures up to this standard is debatable. Two further difficulties are contained in the effort to define a profession as accountable and mature, and to identify a mature profession as therefore good.) The nurse's interaction with the patient is guided by moral principles of "respect for human dignity and the uniqueness of the client."[2] The nurse is expected to meet the patient's health care needs keeping concerns for the client's safety and best interests uppermost. The nurse's diagnosis of the patient's health needs is based on assessment processes of physical, psychological, and social responses of the client as well as perception of the individual as a whole human being who values life.

ETHICS AND SCIENCE

There is no single science of moral values. Rather, there are alternative theories of ethics and dialogue between these values. Alternative theories of morality orient the role of nursing in the care of patients. These models of moral values are like overlapping circles (Fig. 1–1). Each theory describes its values with an attempted justification to some decision-making aspect of nursing. St. Thomas Aquinas (1225–1274 AD), for example, held that human life is a gift that is never to be taken by any human. He used certain principles of Christianity, known as Agapism, to justify his view of the sacredness of life. The principle that life is a gift is then used to "justify" or help justify a nurse's decision to save life at all costs, even the life of an underweight, preterm infant.

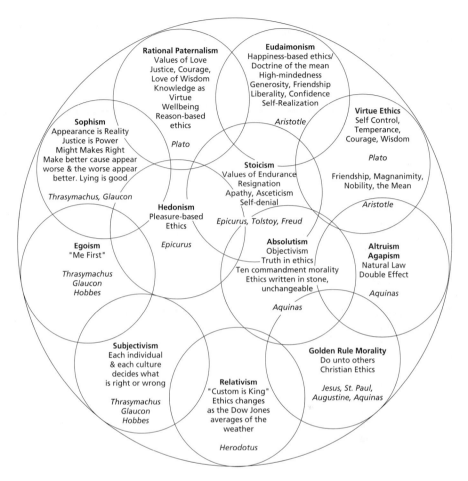

Figure 1–1. Models of moral values.

Major Differences Between an Ethical Theory and a Scientific Theory

Although there are similarities between a scientific and an ethical theory (for example, both seek to explain what is good for people), there are also vast differences. Three key differences between a scientific and an ethical theory are: (1) a scientific theory aims to explain phenomena, whereas an ethical theory aims to justify human action; (2) a scientific theory is true or false, whereas an ethical theory generally is not regarded as such and may be right, wrong, or neither, depending on one's justifiable acceptance of the theory; (3) a scientific theory presents explanations, descriptions, and predictions, whereas an ethical theory presents obligations or "ought" statements along with justifications.

An ethical theory may be formal, empirical, dialectical, or intuitive (distinctions discussed later), and makes use of moral principles as well as factual premises aimed at justifying a particular action. An ethical theory includes a practical action

---

Scientific Theories and Laws

A scientific theory or law expresses a universal, invariant, and demonstrable relation between two phenomena, such as the force of gravitation between the earth and the sun.

For example, the law of gravitation states that any two particles in the solar system move toward each other in proportion to the product of their masses and inversely to the square of the distance between them.

An Ethical Theory

An ethical theory includes one or more value premises (or end-state premises) and several factual means-ends premises. A scientific theory is descriptive, verifiable, and predictive, whereas a value theory is prescriptive and evaluative. A value theory, however, following Aristotle's practical syllogism (discussed in Chapter 4) has both factual, means-ends, and value premises.

For example, a value premise is to promote the quality of a patient's life. The factual means-ends premises are that Mr. Hill, age 87, is recovering from a hip operation. The quality of Mr. Hill's life is improved by turning him every hour.

Evaluative-Directive Conclusion: Therefore, turn Mr. Hill every hour.

---

that guides a principle or principles, such as Judeo-Christian ethics with its Ten Commandments, and instrumental means-ends statements or factual statements that set forth ways of achieving one's goal or principle.

The boxes above are syllogistic examples that may help to clarify the difference between a scientific theory and an ethical theory. In an ethical theory, one may start with a major evaluative premise, such as "Do no harm," (nonmaleficence) which contributes to the nursing principle: Promote the quality of your patient's life (beneficence). One then supplies means-ends factual premises, which give particular application to a general moral principle. A requirement about the minor premise is that it is consistent with the major evaluative premise. Part of an expert nurse's role is to apply the best means for promoting the quality of a patient's life. Because the value and factual premises go together in a means-ends continuum and do not exist in isolation, value questions are a continuous concern of an expert nurse. Hence, nursing ethics is value-laden. In scientific theories, value premises do not have the same insistent, continuous role.

THE FUNCTION OF NURSING ETHICS

Through advances in medical technology, the opportunities for intervening in patient destiny by restoring heartbeat, respiration, and other vital functions are many. The future promises even more ways of controlling vital functions and altering body parts. Nurses are part of these interventions. At the primary level of prevention and care, patients and families look to "their" nurses for information, advice, and support when facing difficult decisions of this nature. At the secondary level of curative care, nurses are actively involved in monitoring and sustaining treatment modalities such as life-support systems. At the tertiary level, nurses practice advanced levels of clinical competence and shared decision making. At a societal level, nurses are or are expected to be actively involved in policy formulation within the health organization, in professional societies, and in legislative bodies.

Thus, nursing is an indispensable part of the health care delivery system. More than in any other discipline, the practitioner of nursing is in continuous contact with the patient and the family. This position offers unique privileges and responsibilities. Nurses are privy to the patient's most intimate fears, hopes, and regrets. The family's relationship with the patient becomes vividly clear as the illness strips interactions of superficiality. The depth of the family's care or lack of concern and respect for the patient is revealed as illness progresses. By word and by deed, the nurse manifests to the family a sense of caring and fundamental human dignity, thereby contributing to a positive change in the immediate family relations with the patient and with other members of the interdisciplinary healthcare team. What makes the contribution of nursing even more spectacular is that nurses cope admirably and heroically with the economic and health care challenges of "managed care." Costs and profits occasionally place serious burdens in the way of health care providers' interests and efforts to give adequate patient care.

Nurses strive to meet universal human needs for care in illness, promotion of health, and prevention of disease. Expert nurses seek to conserve that which is of value to every individual: the optimum functioning of all body systems and of the body as an integrated unit. Above all, nursing is a human health service that has the quality of mercy and the potential for ennobling both the provider and the recipient. The practice of nursing "is concerned with humans and is humanizing."[3] A central concern of this practice is to enhance the personhood and the humanity of all involved in care.[4]

Indeed, we identify the nursing of both the well and the sick with doing good. But why is nursing good? It is good because it aims at doing good in common-sense terms. For example, when we say "Nurse Smith is giving nursing care to Mr. Jones," we mean that Nurse Smith is doing good by providing whatever nursing assistance is of value to Mr. Jones in gaining health. In fact, we habitually identify nursing with the good that it becomes both a contradiction and morally reprehensible to say, "Nurse Smith aims to harm Mr. Jones."

If nurses intend to do good, why do we need nursing ethics? Good intentions are not enough, because knowledge or ignorance of alternatives can also be a cause of good or harm. Reasons for choosing one alternative over another, or refusing treatment altogether, need to be critically examined in relation to other possibilities. Moreover, nurses do not wish to impose their treatment choices on other persons whose autonomy is to be supported. The nurse's beliefs concerning the good life may differ from those of the patient. It is precisely this difference that needs to be acknowledged and respected as a mark of personhood and separateness. Therefore, knowledge of the views that support the reasons for one choice over another are indispensable to the nurse in daily practice and in everyday life. Thus, the function of nursing ethics is to guide the activity of nursing on behalf of the presumed good.

WHAT IS ETHICS? WHAT IS NURSING ETHICS?

A preliminary but useful definition of ethics is that it is concerned with doing good and avoiding harm. Nursing decisions affect people. Thus, nurses have the power to do good or harm to their patients. The potential for doing good or harm depends partly on factual knowledge and partly on values. Both facts and values may aptly be consciously and critically evaluated for their potential for good or harm to human beings, whether well or sick.

An example of a presumed good is educating the patient to continue taking medication and to follow a prescribed diet, if doing so is rationally demonstrable. An example of doing harm is to avoid and thus deny the nursing needs of a difficult patient, such as a patient with acquired immunodeficiency syndrome (AIDS) or a patient who does not conform to the nurse's values. Another example of a nurse doing harm is to withhold information and necessary counseling which would enable the patient to make a decision with which the nurse disagrees, such as an elderly primipara's decision to abort a fetus.

WHAT IS GOOD OR HARM?

One must ask: What is good and what is harmful? Good for whom? Harmful to whom? The nurse, for example, may inadvertently cause pain to a patient in the process of passing tubes, injecting fluids and drugs, and irrigating openings, all of which may be essential to the patient's survival. Sometimes it is impossible to do good to someone without also doing them harm. A nurse who acts to benefit clients by relieving suffering, restoring and promoting health, or preventing diseases is doing good. The good accrues primarily to the patient. The nurse who consciously practices competently and intelligently is also doing good and is receiving benefit from the professional and financial recognition from self, colleagues, clients, and families.

But dilemmas about how to do good and avoid harm arise. A dilemma is defined as a problem with no satisfactory solution. For example, a 38-year-old primipara undergoes amniocentesis, which reveals her fetus has Down syndrome. The woman wants very much to give birth. Insofar as "good" and "harm" are not always easily defined, we can find a clue to the good in the example of what the pregnant woman wants, namely, to give birth. The dilemma involves her thwarted will: She cannot give birth to a normal child from this pregnancy. In her thwarted will, we also find a clue to the meaning of the harmful and bad. The woman considers the destruction of the fetus as a harmful act that destroys a life. The woman's husband rejects the possibility of raising a retarded child and feels that the marriage will be suffer as a consequence. This example gives added insight into the problem of defining good and bad.

WHAT IS THE GOOD LIFE?

The good life is a composite, a complex tapestry of many things—caring relationships, a satisfying occupation, a sense of physical well-being, health and safety, goals pursued and achieved, obstacles removed—all without harm to anyone. We have seen that one of the necessary conditions of a good life is health. A means to health is achieved through nursing.

HEALTH AS A GOAL OF THE GOOD LIFE

The practice of nursing is concerned with doing good. One aspect of doing good, and one of the highest values of nursing, is the concern for the goals of the good life. Health is conducive to and part of the good life. On this, Aristotle[5] seems to have had a far better argument than did Kant, who held that even good health may inspire pride and thus detract from a person's "good will," which, he argued, is the only unconditional good.[6] Aristotle believed that health is a necessary condition of a completely happy life, and that the good life for humans, which consists of "living well," depends on the full use of one's limbs and the five senses. One would appreciate this insight if left with broken or missing limbs, or if one became blind or deaf.

IMPORTANT ETHICAL ISSUES IN NURSING

Quantity Versus Quality of Life

The first of these ethical issues concerns quantity versus quality of life. Quantity may mean either the time a patient lives or the number of people affected. An example of the first is when a parent asks the nurse to "pull the plug" on her 14-year-old son, who has been comatose for 8 months. Nurses are in a position to influence questions concerning the quality of life versus its quantity because families often turn first to the nurse providing direct care to their loved one. The question is: What is the morally justifiable position of the nurse?

The importance of this issue became evident in the results of a 1994 survey conducted by *The American Nurse*, the official journal of the American Nurses Association (ANA). Two-hundred seven members were asked what ethical issues they believed to be most critical in the 1990s. Forty-two percent cited decisions regarding the end of life as the second most pressing ethical issue that nurses face.[7] (Health care rationing was the first most pressing issue). Respondents gave such reasons as "Millions of dollars (probably billions) are spent each year in this country prolonging death. We need to come full circle and realize death is natural and 'pull the plug' on all that could be invested elsewhere." (Staff nurse).[8] Fifty-seven percent of respondents said that "physician-assisted suicide should be legalized."[9] Paradoxically, 49.3% said that they did not want to see euthanasia legalized, even though both assisted suicide and voluntary euthanasia are decisions made by a competent adult receiving the assistance of another to die. Other opinions included:

> "Who lives? Who dies? Who decides? There is a fine line between euthanasia and murder. I fear that there would be abuse of this option." (Advanced practice nurse).[10]

> "*I* do not feel that euthanasia should be decided by a physician, but rather by a collaborative team that would take into account the whole picture—family, religion, social worker, the physician, the nurse." (Nurse educator).[11]

> "*I* believe that a patient should be allowed to be comfortable while dying without fear of prolongation (CPR, tube feeding, respirator). But it is not ethical to end that life purposefully. That's God's decision—not mine or anybody else's." (Self-employed nurse).[12]

There appears to be a lack of clarity related to the patient's right to die and the provider's right to refuse assistance in exercising that right, as well as in the distinctions among passive and active, voluntary and involuntary euthanasia and assisted suicide. These issues will be further explored in Chapter 14.

Pro-choice Versus Pro-life

Thirty-three percent of the 207 nurse respondents defined abortion as the third most pressing ethical issue of the 1990s.[13] This topic is often headline news as the media covers demonstrations, marches on the US Capitol, and the killings of one physician in 1993 and another in 1994, all in the name of saving fetal lives. Each year the US Supreme Court is faced with cases seeking to limit or abolish the right to abortion, which is protected by the 1973 *Roe v. Wade* decision. In Congress, the debate on abortion is an annual event as its opponents seek to abolish it through federal budget constraints. Even after the FDA approval of the early abortion pill, RU-486 (mifepristone), the debate may continue at the same intense level of commitment.

Freedom Versus Control

Yet another ethical issue nurses face concerns freedom versus control and prevention of harm. One such example on an individual level is that of a frail, elderly patient who wishes not to have a locking waistbelt, but wants to walk about freely. This freedom is in conflict with the health care team's effort to prevent harm to this patient. Another example is forced feeding of a patient who refuses to eat on grounds of individual rights and freedom. The 1981 film *Whose Life is it Anyway?* further illustrates the issue of freedom versus prevention of harm. Ken Harrison, a hospitalized paraplegic patient, argues for the right to die while the hospital administrator argues for the conflicting principle of trying to prevent harm to him. A further example is a nurse's freedom to strike for better working conditions and quality care versus the hospital's efforts to prevent harm to patients.

Truth-telling Versus Deception

A fourth issue that critical thinking illuminates is veracity (truth-telling) versus deception or lying. Some reasons for deception and lying are to get one's way, to avoid harm by withholding bad news, or to conceal an abuse pattern, such as alcoholism or narcotic addiction. For example, a dilemma exists for someone whose colleague has an abuse problem and he must decide whether to join in the concealment effort or "blow the whistle" by telling the truth. Another dilemma exists if the substance abuser threatens to reveal something that is of a vital professional or personal interest to the would-be whistle blower. What should be done in the case of a formerly dedicated and highly qualified health professional who is a substance abuser and thus in a position to cause serious harm to patients? Another example of the issue of veracity versus deception is the proverbial "sink test" for urine specimens: a laboratory technician takes a specimen to be analyzed, pours it down the sink, and lies about the findings. Or a nurse records treatments, blood pressures levels, temperatures readings, or urine outputs that were not assessed.

Distribution of Limited Resources

A fifth ethical issue concerns the just allocation of limited resources. In *The American Nurse* survey, 56% of the respondents cited health care rationing as the most pressing ethical issue faced by nurses.[14] Health care reform assumed national priority in the Clinton administration's effort to provide universal access to basic health care. Proposals ranging from a single-payer program modeled on the Canadian system to employer- and state-subsidized health insurance to health care as a purchasable commodity in a free market system are the objects of intense debate, political activity, and media attention.

Nurses who practice in inner city hospitals or in poor rural areas are familiar with the consequences of inadequate health care resources for the health of their clients. There are accounts of women in active labor who were refused admission to nonpublic hospitals because of lack of health insurance, and patients who are unable to afford the fee of a surgeon who is unwilling to accept Medicare or Medicaid reimbursement. Expensive, state-of-the-art medications may be beyond the financial means of underinsured patients. Many hospitals are in precarious economic straits because of rising costs, whereas occupancy rates, reimbursement schedules from third-party payers, and operational margins are declining. The number of small hospitals has decreased, and the large medical centers with affiliated medical schools and research programs are claiming serious financial deficits.

Paul Hoffman, Chair of the American Hospital Association's Technical Panel on Biomedical Ethics, cites the growth of intensive care unit beds from 1,000 in 1960 to 70,000 in 1992, at a cost of $14 billion to $20 billion annually, which accounts for 14% to 20% of the US hospital budget.[15] Hoffman reported that in 1992, over 10,000 patients in a persistent vegetative state were hospitalized at an annual cost of $1.3 billion.[16] The "survival" record of a patient in a persistent vegetative state is more than 39 years "achieved" by Rita Greene, a 23-year-old nurse who suffered cardiac arrest the day before discharge, following treatment for tuberculosis that she had contracted as a staff nurse. In 1992, she was 62 years old and still "living" at the District of Columbia General Hospital in Washington, DC.[17] These are but a few of the ethical issues related to the allocation of limited resources.

Empirical Knowledge Versus Personal Belief

A sixth ethical issue is the conflict between empirical knowledge based on science and alternatives based on ideologic, religious, cultural, or economic beliefs. Society poorly rewards research, as investigation often raises disturbing questions about the status quo. Research about the harmful effects of smoking or drinking alcohol may provide evidence that conflicts with economic interests. Research related to commercial and military interests are funded far more extensively than is research related to health care or environmental safety. Women's health issues have been similarly neglected.

The preference of religious beliefs of some groups is evident in the decision to teach Creationism, a literal belief in the Biblical explanation of creation that opposes the theory of evolution. The faith-healing practices of some groups, such as Christian Scientists, is another example of the preference of a religious belief to empirical, scientific evidence. An example of belief in alternative therapies is shown by the nurse who advocated laetrile (amygdalin), by the parents of Chad Greene, a 3-year-old with leukemia, and by various celebrities who rejected chemotherapy for cancer in favor of laetrile, a synthetic derivative of a natural substance whose cancer-fighting properties have not been confirmed.

Nursing conflicts generally occur within the six kinds of issues discussed herein, with variations owing to developmental status; age; physical, cultural, and socioeconomic circumstances; ethical values; and principles.

METHODS OF MORAL REASONING

Various efforts and approaches have been developed to help resolve these and related ethical issues. To clarify the meaning of ethics, we consider four methods of moral reasoning.

Formal Deductivist Aspect

One method of reasoning in ethics is formal, which may be expressed through a professional code. According to the ANA's *Code for Nurses*, a code of ethics makes explicit the primary goals and values of the profession. When individuals become nurses, they make a moral commitment to uphold the values and special moral obligations expressed in their code.[18] The *Code for Nurses* states universal moral principles that "prescribe and justify nursing actions. The most fundamental of these principles is respect for persons, autonomy, beneficence (doing good), nonmaleficence (avoiding harm), veracity (truth-telling), confidentiality (respecting privileged information), fidelity (keeping promises), and justice (treating people fairly)."[19]

The formal mode of ethics deduces what decisions to make based on previously agreed upon principles of ethics. An example of the formal approach to ethics is an ethical system derived from a religion that has a creed, code, and cult that implies moral rules, such as the Ten Commandments. Benner and Wrubel[20] cite formal beliefs as long-term change agents for health; for example, most Americans now have the formal belief that cigarette smoking is harmful. This formalized belief becomes a force for change and the basis for rules that prohibit smoking in public places.

The formal method of reasoning in nursing has several advantages and drawbacks. A major advantage is that if one accepts a moral principle (i.e., doing good) and one notices a health professional harming a patient, one knows that person to be wrong. However, a serious drawback of the formal method of considering nursing ethics is that it is too inflexible to be useful. A second drawback is that there may be conflicting interpretations of a given value that cannot all be implemented. A third problem is that nurses do not always feel motivated to implement moral principles of care.

Conventional (Empirical, Inductivist, or Sociological) Approach to Ethics

A second approach in moral reasoning is a conventional method that is identified as empirical, inductive, or sociological, in which one elicits moral conduct from an empirical study of one's culture or customs. Nurses in the 1920s, for example, stood up when a physician entered a room and "obeyed" medical orders without question. A strength of the conventional approach to moral reasoning is that "custom is king."[21] Herodotus' saying supports behavior that most resembles the majority. Conventional moral principles such as doing good, avoiding harm, truth-telling, and promise-keeping, gain their appeal by being frequently practiced. These principles identify murder, rape, theft, and abuse as morally impermissible. Conventional ethics provide us with what is sometimes publicly accepted as the core of morality.

A disadvantage of conventional reasoning is the possibility of its becoming static and preventing progressive social changes. If nurses obeyed physicians' orders in the 1920s, that does not imply that nurses *should* do so now or at any time in the future nor that they should even ever have "obeyed" those orders. There are, after all, well-known instances, past and present, of physician errors. This is known as the "is-ought" fallacy. One cannot justify an "ought" judgment on the basis of what is. Independent nursing judgment may augment a physician's clinical judgment. Decisions may be made jointly and be better as a result.

Conventional ethics can be helpful for understanding and acting on some core problems of ethics. They do not, however, always help one to understand or justify acting on problems that fall outside the publicly accepted core. On the fringes of ethics, one finds puzzles, dilemmas, and controversial questions that cannot be easily decided, such as euthanasia and assisted suicide. One looks beyond conventional ethics to justify the acceptance of these practices.

Intuition In Moral Reasoning

According to a third approach to ethics, one may use ethics in its everyday intuitive role. In this sense, ethics may be revealed through a figure in literature, such as Platon Karataef, a wise peasant in Tolstoy's *War and Peace,* or Huck in Twain's *The Adventures of Huckleberry Finn,* or through the insight of St. Augustine, who felt that a society without justice is a "band of robbers," or Martin Luther King, Jr., who had a dream that a racially integrated society is morally preferable to a segregated one. These are examples of everyday common sense of the person in the street who expresses moral views.

An attempt to provide an ethical justification may make reference to all four methods of moral reasoning. A model of morality usually emphasizes one or more, but not all, of these approaches. Thus, ethics has objective aspects, as well as subjective and relativistic ones. Some people mistakenly consider ethics in nursing or any other field to be exclusively formal, scientific, philosophical, or a matter of everyday intuition. Instead, philosophical ethics is a composite of all four methods.

Dialectical Reasoning

The difficulties of the formal and conventional methods of reasoning lead one to consider a fourth approach to morality, which occurs when one identifies ethics with some philosophical theory of ethics and shows the interplay and dialogue between such theories. In this sense, ethics is more akin to an art or the ongoing practice of law than an algorithmic or rule-bound, formal or factual science.

Arguing by analogy is one method of moral reasoning, for example, comparing a fetus to a child by calling it an unborn child, or comparing a pregnant woman to a landlady. The first analogy implies that a fetus is a person, and the second implies that a pregnant woman is like a landlady who may evict her "tenant" at will.

Another method of moral reasoning is to refute an argument. One example of refutation is showing that a moral principle is inconsistent. Socrates accomplished this when his contemporary, Cephalus, stated that the key to a good life is to always return what one has borrowed. Socrates countered, "What if a man lent you a weapon, then went mad and asked for the weapon to be returned?"[22] The clear implication is that one does not return a weapon to a madman; thus, he refuted the principle "Always return what is lent."

Dialectal ethics addresses the justification of feelings, principles, and methods of moral reasoning. Unexamined values alone are insufficient grounds for ethical choices for both patients and nurses. Judgments concerning what is good are so important in their effect on human life that they warrant critical examination. Generally, there are eight to fourteen viable philosophical theories of morality. Everyone who is in search of the meaning of good and its relevance to nursing is involved in philosophical discourse and argues for or against one or more of these models of morality. For example, such an argument may occur when trying to answer the question, Should an elderly patient have a locking waistbelt for his or her protection, or should the patient's refusal of a waistbelt to prevent falls be supported?

A strength in appealing to philosophical theories of ethics is that one does not have to agree to unquestioning authority to settle ethical problems. One is quite free to argue against any or almost all existing ethical models. The pro-euthanasia nurse may say, "To me, killing that poor, old, suffering patient is morally permissible." A difficulty with appealing to philosophical theories of morality is that one is stripped of a centralized bureau of standards, or an umpire, to whom disputable cases can be appealed.

THE ROLE OF CARE IN NURSING ETHICS

One example of a theory of morality is the caring model, oriented by an older Agapistic or altruistic theory developed by medieval Christian philosophers such as St. Thomas Aquinas. Caring is a form of doing good and avoiding harm and thus is central to both ethics and nursing ethics. Caring in nursing is such a powerful concept that it is a contradiction to say with approval, "Nurse White didn't care for her patients"; to say this is to condemn the nurse. Underlying the model of caring is the concept of giving care. The concept of caring is the rubric, or the framework, within which all nursing that is moral and centered on the well-being of humans occurs.

The theories of morality that are analyzed and applied throughout this book are means, guidelines, beacons, and principles that guide the nurse's conduct toward patients, colleagues, families, institutions, and society. Benner and Wrubel aptly illustrate the concept of caring: "I went into the room and he yelled at me, 'Are you listening?' I said 'yes' pretty calmly, and he began crying softly and talking. He knew I was listening." (Mary Culname, RN.)[23] To Benner and Wrubel, caring means that "persons, events, projects, and things matter to people."[24] Caring covers "a range of involvements, from romantic love to parental love to friendship, from caring for one's garden to caring about one's work to caring for and about one's patients."[25] Here are some examples of sentences using the word *care:* (1) Be careful; (2) Take care; (3) Handle with care; (4) That mother and father care for their children; (5) That couple cares for each other; (6) She cares for her roses; (7) He cares for his grandmother; (8) Alan Jones, RN, cares for Steve Moss, his 92-year-old patient; (9) Ms. Bariel, RN, cares for the abused child in Room 403; (10) Some countries provide health care to everyone; and (11) Some poor people received a "care" package. These examples illustrate that to care is to give of oneself to an object or persons.

According to Benner and Wrubel, caring is a response to stress.[26] Stress, in turn, is connected to suffering. Caring is a form of coping or helping those in distress. Nursing is an aid in restoring other people's health care interests.[27] Nurses give care by relieving stress and distress in their patients. Caring is commitment, manifested in persistent assistance to stress. Care is practiced with each patient. This may explain the appeal of the slogan, "Individualize treatment." It may also represent respect for persons as individuals with varying needs, desires, goals, values, and lifestyles.

Care in the Context of the Feminist Framework

The care framework ably presented by Benner and Wrubel has its underpinnings in recent feminist writings, such as the work of Gilligan[28] and Noddings.[29] According to Gilligan, writers such as Rawls, Sandel, and Kohlberg who focus on rights, justice, and fairness, as well as aggression and assertiveness, appeal to a masculine orientation in ethics. In contrast, virtues such as love, caring, nurturing, and sympathy appeal to a feminine orientation. To Gilligan, women develop "an 'ethic of care' whose underlying logic . . . is a psychological logic of relationships, which contrasts with the (generally male) formal logic of fairness that informs the justice approach."[30]

To Noddings, caring is reflected in a mother choosing to save her child over a neighbor's if both are drowning and the mother can only reach one. The ethics of caring, rather than the ethics of equality,[31] universality, or impartiality,[32] guides the mother's ethical decision making. According to Noddings, "caring lies at the very heart of morality and gives it stability."[33] The ethics of caring is part of the virtue ethics, the appeal to qualities of character, such as courage, generosity, commitment, and responsibility.

Three Philosophical Sources of Appeal in the Ethics of Caring

The ethics of caring gains its appeal from several sources. One is the Aristotelian emphasis on the development of natural virtues, such as friendship, prudence, wisdom, temperance, and courage. (See Chapter 4 for a further development of Aristotle's happiness-based ethics.) Benner reported this example of a caring nurse:

> "The patient was a 17-year-old male admitted post c-spine fracture . . . significant lung consolidation developed. The doctors decided to intubate. . . . His respiratory rate increased dramatically . . . his PCO_2 was dropping. The doctors were considering increasing . . . sedation to knock out his respiratory drive so that we could totally control his ventilation with the respirator. . . . I knew the complications which could arise. . . . I just knew we could resolve this problem . . . without using such drastic measures. I began to talk with him . . . assuredly, honestly, professionally, and yet personally. I intervened on his behalf with his multiple physicians; I explained my 'gut feeling', my concerns for his recovery, and negotiated for more time to resolve the problem. . . . It took three-and-a-half hours before he began to relax. . . . He needed to be reassured, and most of all to learn to trust us. . . . He needed to know that we cared about him. . . ."[34]

A question for the supporters of the ethics of caring is not only how well this view helps to resolve questions of ethics, such as charges of subjectivity and relativism, but also how well the ethics of caring helps us resolve major ethical issues in nursing. We will consider this question in subsequent chapters.

Another source of the ethics of caring is found in altruism or love-based ethics, presented by St. Thomas Aquinas, who saw virtues oriented by religion as pivotal to the good life. A third source of the ethics of caring is found in the early Greek hedonists and later in David Hume's utilitarianism, which bases ethics on people's wants and likes and the avoidance of their dislikes and aversions.

THE ROLE OF THE NURSE IN ETHICS

In their innovative proposal ". . . to meet the specialized health care needs of complex patients"[35] through tertiary nurse practioners, Keane and Richmond acknowledge that:

> . . . it is inadequate to prepare the tertiary nurse practioner (TNP) solely for advanced clinical practice. They must also be taught to develop a framework that guides their decisions in the use of technology in order to continue . . . to function as patient advocates. The ANA's *Code for Nurses* serves as the theoretical foundation of ethical

decision-making in patient care. Models of patient advocacy are included in the theory courses. Values clarification and ascending values, beliefs, and preferences serve as the basis of the appropriate application of technology.[36]

Mila Ann Aroskar, a nurse ethicist, writes that during the 1960s and 1970s, "Ethics in nursing began to emphasize advocacy for individual patients, respect for patient autonomy and promotion of patients' rights in health care institutions, a search for more autonomy in nursing practice, and the development of a more holistic approach to patient care."[37] Aroskar discusses the expansion of topics in nursing ethics in the 1980s to include the nurse as moral agent, obstacles to the ethical practice of nursing, ethical issues for nurses in each practice setting and specialty, and evaluation of the feminist and caring theories.[38] The 1980s saw empirical research in the moral development of students and staff nurses using Lawrence Kohlberg's theory of the six stages of moral development. Individual and shared decision making crossing interdisciplinary lines was and continues to be a constant subject of analysis. "Discussion of justice, politics, and health policy as they relate to nursing goals and concerns . . . influenced by changes in political climate, social problems, cost-containment efforts, and discussion of explicit rationing, reappear in the nursing literature."[39]

In 1992, the ANA released its health care reform agenda of universal health care, with an emphasis on primary care and prevention. This followed a 1977 position statement that called for a national health policy providing care for everyone "based on the belief that health care is a basic right of all people."[40] The statement recommends a national health insurance program, national coordination of planning for integrated systems of health care, new approaches to the delivery of health care services with nurses prepared for roles in primary care, accountability of the professions for monitoring member services, health education, home care, and a national policy for the aged, mentally ill, and children.[41]

THE INTERDISCIPLINARY ROLE OF THE NURSE IN ETHICS

Nurses struggle daily with ethical uncertainties and quandaries that arise from involvement with patients, families, and colleagues in the decision-making process. Nursing ethics and health care ethics, according to Toulmin,[42] consist of the triangulation and interplay of cases (real and imaginary), laws and customs, and philosophical theories of morality (Fig. 1–2). To practice nursing ethics or health care ethics is to deal with all three of these aspects.

Increasingly, hospitals are providing expert help, usually via a philosopher, to educate staff, facilitate analysis of problems, alleviate stress, and help in mediating conflicts among conflicting ethical positions. Sometimes the patient's family is included in the process. Multidisciplinary ethics committees are now commonly found in health care institutions. The 1992 Joint Commission on Accreditation of Healthcare Organizations (JCAHO) Supplement of the Accreditation Manual for Hospitals states that an "organization should have in place a mechanism for the consideration of ethical issues arising in the care of patients and to provide

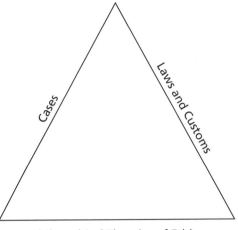

Philosophical Theories of Ethics

Figure 1–2. The triangulation and interplay of cases, laws, and philosophical theories of ethics.

education to caregivers and patients on ethical issues in health care."[43] JCAHO criteria specified that "all health professionals [are] to participate in the discussion and resolution of ethical issues and be given the educational resources needed to evaluate alternatives."[44] The manual called for nursing participation in these committees because nurses are close to patients during hospitalization and need a "defined mechanism" to address the ethical issues that will certainly ensue.[45]

Ethics Rounds is a mechanism by which nurses can review clinical questions in everyday practice in order to raise ethical problems and concerns. The National Commission for the Protection of Human Subjects requires each hospital, medical center, formal caregiving institution, college, and university to form an institutional review board for implementing the Commission's regulations regarding research. Lastly, a combination of formal- and clinically based education will best help nurses to fulfill the role of patient advocate, and to engage in multidisciplinary deliberations concerned with patient care and well-being.

SUMMARY

Throughout the evolution of nursing, health has been regarded as a primary value, with nursing playing a central role in helping individuals, families, groups, and society to achieve maximum health potential. Nurses accord high value to the concept of total well-being. Nursing practice presupposes the value of care as essential to the concept of the good. However nursing is defined, the central question of nursing ethics remains: What are morally justifiable reasons for my nursing actions? This text addresses these and related questions to provide clarification and illumination.

Nursing is a moral activity. Nursing consists of doing good to patients and avoiding harm. A variety of ethical values, some of which conflict with one another, orient nursing and are well-expressed in the *Code for Nurses*. These include beneficence, nonmaleficence, justice, fidelity, veracity, and respect for patient autonomy. A pivotal ethical value perceived by nurses is the concept of caring. This concept has been well-defined in the theory and practice of nursing, even though it presents conceptual difficulties in its application.

Discussion Questions

1. Can one be happy without health? Is Aristotle or Kant right about this? Can one be happy if one is poor? Are people who are rich, good-looking, smart, healthy, and have good parents, good children, and good friends happier than those who are poor, ugly, stupid, sick, and have bad parents, bad children, bad friends, or no friends? Give reasons for your answer. (For part of an answer, consult Chapter 4 on Virtue Ethics or Chapter 6 on Duty-Based Ethics.)
2. In what ways is nursing an ethically good activity?
3. How does technology affect what counts as ethics?
4. How do science and technology help dissolve some moral problems?
5. In your own view, what are some major benefits and drawbacks with the concept of care?
6. What, if anything, makes an answer the "right" one in nursing ethics?

REFERENCES

1. American Nurses Association. *Nursing: A social policy.* Kansas City, Mo: 1980;7.
2. American Nurses Association. *Code for Nurses, with interpretive statements.* Kansas City, Mo: 1976;4.
3. Patridge KB. Nursing values in a changing society. *Nursing Outlook* 1978;26(6):356.
4. ibid.
5. Aristotle. *Nicomachean ethics.* Indianapolis: Bobbs-Merrill. 1962;21.
6. Abbott TK, Fox M (trans). *Fundamental principles of the metaphysics of morals.* Indianapolis: Bobbs-Merrill. 1949;11.
7. Speak up: Health care rationing tops list of pressing ethical issues. *The American Nurse* 1994;26(3):11.
8. ibid.
9. ibid.
10. What nurses are saying. *The American Nurse* 1994;26(3):11.
11. ibid.
12. ibid.
13. Speak up: Health care rationing tops list of pressing ethical issues. *The American Nurse* 1994;26(3):11.
14. ibid.
15. Hoffman PB. Decisions near the end of life: Resource allocation implications for hospitals. *Cambridge Quarterly of Health Care Ethics* 1992;1(3):230.

16. ibid.
17. ibid.
18. American Nurses Association. *Code for Nurses.* Kansas City, Mo. 1985.
19. ibid.
20. Benner P, Wrubel J. *The primacy of caring.* Menlo Park, Calif: Addison-Wesley. 1989;166–167.
21. Herodotus. *Custom is king.* In: Ladd J (ed). *Ethical Relativism.* Belmont, Calif: Wadsworth. 1973;12.
22. Grube GMA *Plato's Republic.* Indianapolis: Hackett Publishing Company. 1974;5–6.
23. Benner P, Wrubel J. *The primacy of caring.* Menlo Park, Calif: Addison-Wesley; 1989;166–167.
24. ibid.
25. ibid.
26. ibid, xiii.
27. ibid.
28. Gilligan C. *In a different voice.* Cambridge, Mass: Harvard University Press. 1982.
29. Noddings N: *Caring.* University of California Press. 1984.
30. Gilligan C. *In a different voice.* Cambridge, Mass: Harvard University Press. 1982;73.
31. Fried C. *An anatomy of values.* Cambridge, Mass: Harvard University Press. 1971;227.
32. Williams B. *Moral luck.* Cambridge, Mass: Cambridge University Press. 1981;21.
33. Noddings N. Doubts about radical proposals on caring. In: Burbules N (ed.) *Philosophy of education.* Normal, Ill.: Illinois State University, Philosophy of Education Society. 1986;83.
34. Benner P. *From novice to expert.* Menlo Park, Calif: Addison-Wesley. 1984;52–53.
35. Keane A, Richmond T. Tertiary nurse practitioners. *Image* 1993;25(4):281–284.
36. ibid.
37. Aroskar MA. Ethics in nursing and health care reform: Back to the future? *Hastings Center Report* 1994;24(3):11–12.
38. ibid.
39. ibid.
40. American Nurses Association. *A national policy for health care: Principles and positions.* Kansas City, Mo; December, 1977.
41. ibid.
42. Toulmin S. The tyranny of principles. *Hastings Center Report* 1981;11:31–39.
43. Joint Commission on Accreditation of Healthcare Organizations. *Accreditation Manual for Hospitals,* 1992 Supplement (Patient Rights, Section RI. 1. 1.6. 1);10.
44. ibid.
45. ibid.

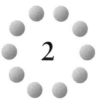

2

Models of Professional Relationships

Study of this chapter enables the learner to:

1. Examine the physician-patient relationship.
2. Evaluate models of physician-patient relationships for their relevance to the care of patients.
3. Analyze models of nurse-patient relationships.
4. Justify the role of nurse as patient advocate.
5. Examine professional codes for their moral and practical implications and applications.
6. Evaluate the functions of professional codes.
7. Explore how the *Code for Nurses* provides moral and professional guidelines for defining, justifying, and limiting nursing activities.

OVERVIEW

Models are idealized patterns, greatly simplified, for looking at complex events in terms of their essential qualities. A model is an abstract representation of a significant portion of reality. Models essentialize the most general aspects of a given phenomenon. They have been called "candidates for reality,"[1] conjectures of what reality is like. A model is an abstract representation of reality, and need not necessarily be pictorial or visual.[2] A model both simplifies and highlights "important features of the subject."[3]

Models oriented by values show different perceptions for understanding the health care process. The use of models supports the conception that health care is value laden and helps to clarify clashes of values as they occur in practice between health professionals.

MODELS OF PHYSICIAN-PATIENT RELATIONSHIPS: EMANUEL AND EMANUEL

Emanuel and Emanuel[4] present four models of the physician-patient relationship to help define the ideal. They describe the physician-patient relationship in decision making as the struggle between autonomy and health, and patient values versus physician values and physician dominance. Each of the models represents different physician goals, obligations, patient values, and patient autonomy. The paternalistic model, also called the parental or priestly model, directs the physician to provide patients with those interventions that best promote their health and well-being.[5] It assumes that patient and physician share similar values and choices. The patient is expected to assent because the physician-guardian places the patient's interest above his or her own. This model is justified in emergencies.

The informative, or the scientific, engineering or consumer, model requires the physician to provide the patient with all relevant information.[6] The information includes the patient's disease state, the possible diagnostic tests and treatments, and the risks and benefits of both the known and the unknowns. This model distinguishes between facts and values with patients exercising control over interventions consistent with their values.[7] In this model, the physician's care for the patient's values, or what the patient should value, is absent because the physician refrains from imposing a recommendation on the patient's known and fixed values. The physician is a technical expert. The authors concede that often persons are uncertain about their actual wants and upon reflection tend to change their preferences.

The interpretive model aims to help the patient identify his or her values and wants and the medical interventions necessary to realize them.[8] The physician provides the necessary relevant medical information and helps the patient articulate values and the medical interventions necessary to their realization by identifying the patient's goals, hopes, commitments, and character. The physician views the patient's life as a narrative whole composed of values and priorities relevant to the medical situations identified in a joint process of understanding with the patient making the decisions.[9]

In the deliberative model, which is considered the ideal, the physician aims to help the patient ". . . choose the best health-related values that can be realized in the clinical situation."[10] The physician provides the information and the values available in the patient's clinical situation, with suggestions regarding the relative worth of the health-related values and what kind the patient could and should pursue.[11] The physician engages in moral deliberation limited to those values that affect or are affected by the patient's illness and treatments, and together they judge these values' worthiness.[12] In this model, ". . . the physician acts as a teacher or friend engaging the patient in dialogue on what course of action would be best . . . The conception of patient autonomy is moral self-development; the patient is empowered not simply to follow unexamined preferences or examined values, but to consider through dialogue, attractive health-related values, their worthiness, and their implications for treatment."[13]

The Emanuels' deliberative model reflects the recommendations of the President's Commission. The model advises physicians to help patients understand the medical situation and possible courses of action in a collaborative process.[14] The Emanuels believe it to be a distortion of autonomy to permit a person to select, without any restrictions, a course of action from a list of options.[15] "Freedom and control over medical decisions alone do not contribute to patient autonomy. Autonomy requires that individuals critically assess their own values and preferences; determine whether they are desirable; affirm upon reflection, these values as ones that should justify their actions; and then be free to initiate action to realize the values. The process of deliberation, integral to the deliberative model, is essential for realizing patient autonomy understood in this way."[16]

The Emanuels believe that the informative model has become the dominant model that reduces the physician's role to that of a technologist.[17] They define the essence of medical practice to be a combination of knowledge, understanding, teaching, and practice by a caring physician, who integrates the patient's values and medical condition into a worthwhile approach.[18]

NURSING MODELS

Sheri Smith draws analogies between models of the physiciant-patient relationship with models of the nurse-patient relationship. In the surrogate mother model (the traditional nursing model), the nurse, like a mother, is primarily committed to and responsible for the patient's (child's) care and safety. The nurse's ethical responsibility to the patient is strong, as is her obligation to act in the patient's best interests at all times similarly to a mother to her sick and dependent child. In this model, the values of the nurse determine the decisions made in the best interests of the patient. The nurse may persuade a patient to accept a particular treatment or decide the appropriate goals for treatment based on the nurse's own values. These are all assertions of the nurse's choice of care on behalf of the patient.

This model is the earliest and most traditional model of nursing care and is no different from the severely criticized model of paternalism that is usually attributed exclusively to male physicians and administrators.[19]

The Nurse as Technician
This model is developed from the view of nursing as a clinical science providing scientific treatment, knowledge, and skills to patients in an objective way that avoids the imposition of values and choices on the patient. The patient's needs are biological. The care and best interests are determined by the patient. As technician, the nurse provides information and skills to the patient and physician and the best correct care as requested, without moral judgments or values attached. The nurse abstains from moral judgments (to the extent that doing so is possible), and the patient is in charge. This model is widely supported by those who take the position of relativism or subjectivism, in which each person, culture, or sub-culture is free to decide.

The Nurse as Contracted Clinician

This model is analogous to the medical model developed by moral philosophers such as Brock, Veatch and Szasz. This model attempts to explain the nurse-patient relationship as "arising from a contracted agreement in which the nurse provides specific care to that patient . . . The patient has the right to control both what happens to his body and the role which the nurse takes with him in providing nursing care."[20] Because the relationship is based on an agreement, the nurse can disagree and thus refuse to participate on the basis of her values and beliefs. The fundamental value, however, is the patient's right to self-determination.

The Nurse as Patient Advocate: Sally Gadow

Gadow proposes a conception of advocacy unlike that of the patients' rights movement, in which anyone can be an advocate, which she calls consumerism. She prefers an existential advocacy for which the nurse alone is uniquely suited. In Gadow's model, the patient and nurse freely decide what their relationship shall be.[21] Gadow regards existential advocacy as the core of nursing because the nurse participates with the patient in determining the special meaning that attaches to his or her personal experiences of health, illness, suffering, or dying. The nurse is in the ideal position to experience the patient as a human being, with unique strengths and complexities, in the process of comprehensive and continuous nursing care. Within this context, Gadow rejects the opportunities for paternalistic acts and attitudes that limit the rights and liberties of the person by providing a good not wanted by the one it supposedly benefits.

The defenders of paternalism view it positively as assistance. Therefore, the professional's responsibility is always to act in the patient's best interests, and to protect the patient's rights to the best possible care as set forth in the previous section. Thus, paternalism becomes confused with advocacy: Paternalism violates self-determination and advocacy by acting for another.[22] What Gadow means by existential advocacy is that individuals can be helped by nurses to exercise their freedom of self-determination "reaching decisions truly theirs . . . that express beliefs and values important about oneself and the world."[23] Sickness threatens prior values so that persons must either recreate their values or their situations to do what they clearly want to do.[24] Gadow regards freedom of self-determination to be the most fundamental human right.[25]

THE ROLE OF THE NURSE AS PATIENT ADVOCATE

The nurse carries out the role of securing the patient's interests by every means at her disposal, sometimes as the patient's eyes and ears or arms and legs. The nurse sometimes singlehandedly embodies the role of caretaker, protector, and advocate, especially in circumstances when no one else is in a position to fight as hard to help the patient to win the final battle of life over death. In these multiple surrogate roles, the nurse also becomes a therapist and source of personal strength during the patient's health crisis. The nurse identifies herself as the human equal of the patient, as a person with fellow feelings, rather than as one who imposes values and preferences paternalistically on the patient. The nurse never loses touch with respect for the patient's autonomy as an individual on an open, democratic, and pluralistic basis.

The nurse who understands the advocacy role promotes, protects, and thereby advocates patients' interests and rights in an effort to make them whole and well again. Where that is not possible, the nurse makes patients as comfortable and free of pain and suffering as possible. In any event, the nurse recognizes that the first duty is to protect and care for the patient's health and safety. In safeguarding the patient, the nurse supports and thereby advocates the patient's interests in the restoration of the patient's health and well-being.

As Minnie Goodnow held at the turn of the century, the role of patient advocate presupposes that "the patient comes first,"[26] that the patient defines what nursing is about, that the patient has rights, and that patients' rights depend on significant others who will protect and care for their rights when they themselves are unable to do so. Thus, the nurse as patient advocate is the touchstone that highlights and guides all other nursing functions.

THE IMPORTANCE OF ADVOCACY

Why is advocacy so important? Because without advocacy and effective protection of rights, there are no rights. Rights depend on backup rights, the rights to be effectively protected in claiming one's rights. We contend that there are no rights without the kinds of backup rights effectively protected by advocates and by a society that recognizes the role of advocates in providing relief and remedies against wrongdoing. The role of advocates is to safeguard clients against abuse and violation of their rights.

Two arguments have been put forth to refute the view that having rights entails advocacy and protection of those rights. One argument, proposed by supporters of "natural law," contends that to have a right is to have a right regardless of particular social circumstances in which such rights may not be honored in practice. Thus, slaves in ancient Greece or slaves in the United States had the right to be free, even though they were unjustly deprived of those rights. Similarly, Jews incarcerated in Nazi concentration camps during World War II never lost their rights to be free and the right to live in the natural-law view; their rights were violated. So too for a woman who is raped; her rights are violated, but not lost.

A second argument against the need for advocacy, proposed by J. S. Mill, is that "the rights and interests of every or any person are only secure from being disregarded when the person interested is himself able and habitually disposed to stand up for them."[27] Consequently, we lose the rights we cannot effectively claim by ourselves. We must be our own best guardians of the rights we hold. If we do not safeguard our own rights, it is our own fault if we lose them.

We maintain that rights are only as strong as the ability, willingness, and resourcefulness of the people of a society that cooperates to protect and care for all the rights of its members. Mill's argument, while true in part (because each individual cares more for his or her rights and interests than anyone else does), is partly false. The rights of anyone or of all depend on the willingness and ability of other relevant persons to bear correlative responsibilities implied by those rights. No one can protect his or her rights alone unaided by others. This is especially true of sick and frightened patients who are unsure of what is happening to them and of their source of help. There are therefore no rights without advocacy of those rights by others. Clearly, the nurse is in a strong position to advocate for patients' rights and interests.

Thus, the reasons there are no rights without advocacy are that individuals may not always be in a position to defend their rights, whereas other persons may be in such a position. Secondly, there are no rights without claims effectively made on behalf of such rights, claims sometimes made by other persons on behalf of rightholders. The right to claim is not necessarily vested in a rightholder alone. Others can and have made claims on behalf of those whose rights have been ignored or violated.

A slave, an infant, or a patient has rights, even if he or she cannot claim them effectively, because even though these persons are helpless to claim such rights, other people as advocates can represent their interests. The problem of claiming rights can be surmounted, because suitable and effective representation can and does in fact occur. If a child or a patient is helpless, a parent or parent surrogate, sponsor, or advocate can step in to protect him or her. Nurses can also—and do quite frequently—protect patients' rights.

THREE MODELS OF PATIENT ADVOCACY

There seem to be three models of patient advocacy. The first, suggested by Abrams, is modeled on "civil disobedience."[28] On this model, a nurse acknowledges patient advocacy that conflicts with established authority involving risk taking and consequences for noncompliance.

The civil-disobedience model puts the nurse on the defensive by having to show a hypothetical or shadowy court of rational authority that his action is the right one. The burden is on the nurse to make good this claim against the practices of established authorities. This can be hazardous to job security.

A second, related model of patient advocacy compares the nurse to a guerrilla fighter, struggling against the health care system.[29] This model of nurse as patient advocate who combats established authority suffers from a similar defect as the model of nurse as civil disobedient. Both models place the enemy, opposition, or problem in the wrong place and upon the wrong set of persons. The problem is not the nurse, rather it is that patients' rights are disregarded by an indifferent system in which no one advocates for the clients' rights to participate actively in their own health care.

Instead of health-professional conflict, there is or ought to be a natural alliance between nurse, patient, and physician against ill health and disease. In this respect, health professionals derive more role guidance and support from the concept of a health team than from either the civil disobedience or guerrilla model of client advocacy. To advocate for the client's need is to be part of the health team, working with others for the health of the patient. However, the nurse requires the mutual respect of other health professionals to be a member of this team, which negates the need to behave as a civil disobedient or guerrilla fighter.

The nurse as a client advocate and health team member is part of a third model. The nurse has professional "standing," a concept borrowed from a legal term that is given to those whose views are granted a serious hearing and consideration before a decision-making board or tribunal, without necessarily being accepted. Before such a team, group, committee, board, or tribunal, the most rational view prevails, one that can be verified as providing the best alternative for patient care. This model gives standing to a nurse as a patient advocate. The appropriate use of moral and cognitive authority is preferable to a model of a nurse as a civil disobedient or urban guerrilla.

ARGUMENTS FOR AND AGAINST THE NURSE AS PATIENT ADVOCATE

Three arguments of varying strength are directed against the concept of nurse as client advocate. The first is that patient advocacy carries no system of institutional supports. The nurse who is willing to advocate a patient's rights when it matters most, in situations of conflict between nurses and physicians, is at risk of losing his job. It is argued that the portrayal of a nurse as client advocate flies in the face of institutional, political, and economic realities.

A second argument is that at least some physicians regard themselves as the basic protectors of their patients' rights and resent intrusion by other health professionals into their contractual prerogatives with their patients.

A third argument, stemming in part from the two foregoing arguments, is that nurses have too many other roles to spend time and resources as client advocates, and that another's wrongdoing is adequately corrected by persons other than nurses (i.e., lawyers).

To rebut the first argument—that patient advocacy lacks institutional supports —the nurse's role of advocacy is to ensure the patient's status as an autonomous human being in a milieu dominated by technology. Patients' rights need to be protected; nurses have a natural alliance with their patients. Moreover, institutions are vulnerable to lawsuits and are sensitive to negative publicity when violations of patients' rights are exposed. Consequently, nurses are natural candidates for advocacy roles in patient care. For example, when Barry Adams, a member of the Massachusetts Nurses Association, stood up for quality patient care and blew the whistle on management, he was fired. The National Labor Relations Board ordered him reinstated and he then helped his state nurses association to pass legislation to protect nurses who speak out against unsafe patient care.[30]

A rebuttal against the second argument is that physicians are not always responsible and accountable. The health care system of "checks and balances" calls for resources, skills, and abilities aimed at protecting patients' rights that are not always guaranteed or implemented by physicians. Moreover, nurses, who increasingly show evidence of higher education, quite naturally provide a form of effective advocacy in the delivery of increasingly complex nursing care. Evidence of high-quality nursing judgments in medical centers point to a natural advocacy role for such nurses.

Finally, in response to the third argument (nurses have too many important technical roles to have the time, skill, and ability to function as advocate): no other group has more continuous and intimate contact with patients and families than do nurses. Therefore, nurses often have the most familiarity with patients' and families' values and ethical choices, and are in good position to protect those interests in serious situations.

MORAL IMPLICATIONS IN CODES OF ETHICS

Essential characteristics of present-day professions are said to be the development of a code of ethics guiding practice, specialized educational programs, a particular service to society, standards of education and practice, an economic and welfare program, and legal practice acts with licensing and self-government as common elements.[31] Because a code of ethics is a standard incorporated in varying degrees in all practice, education, legislation, and licensing, codes for nurses and physicians will be analyzed and evaluated in these respects. Professional codes function as a means of self-regulation. They serve as guidelines for individual and collective responsibility in response to societal needs for trustworthy, competent, and accountable practitioners. Professional codes are regarded as systems of rules and principles by which a profession is expected to regulate its members and demonstrate its responsibility to society.

Since its adoption in 1950, the *Code for Nurses* has undergone revisions in response to the social context and changes within the profession. The core of the *Code*, however, remains a stable entity reflecting the moral values and obligations of the profession.[32] There is a growing awareness of the role of increasing autonomy for both nurses and patients. The *Code* reflects and must continue to support both constancy and change. Nurse advocacy is a constant but the concern for social and economic conditions that undermine health care delivery has become a critical factor. There is a growing recognition in nursing that some changes are not necessarily good. Technology will create nursing roles and new ethical problems that call on the nursing profession to respond in terms of its considered values and obligations.

THE AMERICAN NURSES ASSOCIATION (ANA) *CODE FOR NURSES*

The current *Code for Nurses* functions as the basis for professional status in four ways. First, the *Code* shows society that nurses are expected to understand and accept the trust and responsibility invested in them by the public.[33] Second, it provides guidelines for professional conduct and relationships as the basis for ethical practice.[34] Third, the *Code* defines the nurse's relationship to the client as one of patient advocate, to other health professionals as a colleague, to the nursing profession as a contributor, and to society as a representative of the discipline of nursing. Fourth, it provides the means of self-regulation to the profession.[35]

The *Code for Nurses* is a public statement of belief expressing the moral concerns, values, and goals of nursing. The *Code* aims to justify ethical decisions. It uses both the consequentalist and the absolutist models of morality. The principle of respect for persons is considered the most fundamental value in the *Code*. From the principle of respect comes the principle of autonomy, which places the patient at the center of rational decisions. The principles of beneficence (doing good), nonmaleficence (avoiding harm), veracity (truth-telling), confidentiality (respecting privileged information), fidelity (keeping promises), and justice (treating people fairly)[36] support the value of respect for persons.

Specific Provisions of the *Code for Nurses*

1. The nurse provides services with respect for human dignity and the uniqueness of the client unrestricted by considerations of social or economic status, personal attributes, or the nature of health problems.[37]

The nurse begins to fulfill this provision by accepting the patient or client as a person who is shown interest, respect, and courtesy. Respect for the patient is unaffected by socioeconomic status, personal attributes, or the nature of the health problem. The nurse is committed to the principle of the patient's right to be "fully involved in the planning and implementation"[38] of his or her own care. Each person has the moral right to decide what will be done to him or to her, as well as the right to have the information necessary to make those decisions, to understand the consequences and, on that basis, to accept, terminate, or refuse treatment.

The process of patient or client self-determination may involve the nurse in the roles of resource person and technical expert. The nurse may supply relevant information as well as seek the assistance of other professionals in supplementing the patient's, the family's or significant others', or the nurse's own knowledge. The nurse gives emotional support to enable the patient to explore feelings of fear, dependency, suffering, and hopes for total recovery. The nurse enlists the patient or client and significant others in the process of problem identification, analysis, and resolution of health care needs. The collaboration is directed toward the goal of recovery, optimum function, or dying peacefully and with dignity.

A nurse who opposes the nature of the health care delivered, such as a decision to abort a fetus or to withhold treatment from a deformed and retarded infant, is justified in refusing and withdrawing from the situation as soon as other arrangements are made to provide nursing care to the patient.[39]

The nursing care provided to the dying is expected to enable the patient to live with all possible physical, mental, and social comfort. It is, above all, the nursing care of the dying that "will determine to a great degree how this final human experience is lived and the peace and dignity with which death is approached."[40] The nurse seeks to protect values of respect for human dignity "while working with the patient and relevant and significant others to arrive at the best decisions dictated by the circumstances,"[41] until the last moment of life.

2. The nurse safeguards the client's right to privacy by judiciously protecting information of a confidential nature.[42]

The relationship between nurse and the patient or client is expected to be one of trust and mutuality. The patient may share intimate, previously hidden facts unrelated to current problems on a confidential basis. This confidentiality may extend to a court of law, where the nurse may or may not be able to invoke the principle of privileged communication. Otherwise, the nurse is committed to the client's right of privacy on a moral basis that respects human dignity. However, data relevant to the client's health status need to be shared with other members of a health care team who have common goals of client welfare.

Information about the patient's diagnoses, treatment, and care that must be released for third-party payment, peer review, and quality assurance procedures are expected to be kept confidential according to rigidly enforced written guidelines.[43] The client's consent must be obtained before the record is used for research or other purposes.[44]

3. The nurse acts to safeguard the client and the public when health care and safety are affected by the incompetent, unethical, or illegal practice of any person.[45]

The role of advocate is defined in this provision as one in which "the nurse's primary commitment is to the patient's or client's care and safety."[46] As a corollary, the nurse is expected to be alert to practices by any health professional or the system itself that are unethical, incompetent, illegal, or against the patient's best interests.[47] This requires knowledge of both state practice acts and institutional policies and procedures, as well as a clarification of the term "ethical."

The process of correction begins with the individual who may have caused harm to the patient. If necessary, institutional channels and established procedures are expected to be used for further reporting. Documentation is expected as well.

If the appropriate behavior "is not corrected within the employment setting and continues to jeopardize the client's care and safety . . . the problem should be reported to other appropriate authorities such as the practice committees of the appropriate professional organizations or the legally constituted bodies concerned with licensing.[48] Although a written grievance must be provided to regulatory bodies, every effort is made to protect the confidentiality of the patient advocate.

An effective measure to protect clients and improve practice is the peer review, which is based on published criteria and the procedures for making recommendations. It is intended as a method for improving health care delivery services and the safety, health, and welfare of clients.[49]

4. The nurse assumes responsibility and accountability for individual nursing judgments and actions.[50]

As an acknowledged professional, the nurse is responsible and accountable for the quality, effectiveness, and efficiency of nursing care provided. Moreover, society expects a profession to be self-regulating. However, safeguards for the patient in the form of professional examination and licensure are operative in most states to ensure minimum competencies. Recently, state regulatory bodies have been created for investigating and prosecuting professional misconduct in addition to supporting the profession's responsibility for setting standards of nursing practice.

The nurse is accountable for what is done or not done "to self, to client, to the agency of employment, and to the nursing profession."[51] Accountability includes legal responsibilities. The nurse is responsible for each act or failure to act in a given case. We would add that both the nurse and nursing are accountable to society for decisions at the policy level affecting the future course of a profession, the institution, or health care delivery.

Evaluation occurs at the subjective individual level and is also done by peers. The process of evaluation by self or by others implies that improvement of practice is continuous. Peer evaluation is intended as a means of self-regulation by the profession itself.[52] Through its *Standards of Nursing Practice,* updated nursing practice laws, and accreditation procedures, the ANA demonstrates its accountability to the public.[53]

5. The nurse maintains competence in nursing.[54]

Effective nursing often makes the difference between a client's survival or death, recovery or continued ill health. Therefore, nurses are expected to know what they are doing. Moreover, nurses are expected to maintain competence and remain currently informed of new knowledge.

Present competence measures "include peer review criteria, outcome criteria, and the American Nurses Association program for certification."[55] Continuing education and advanced formal education are means of keeping current with professional, scientific, and technological advances. Scientific advances contribute to the rapidly increasing complexity of nursing service and health care delivery. The process of maintaining competence is self-initiated and self-directed, with the recognition of the need for appropriate consultation with nurse specialists, educators, administrators, or leaders.

6. The nurse exercises informed judgment and uses individual competence and qualifications as criteria in seeking consultation, accepting responsibilities, and delegating nursing activities to others.[56]

The practice of nursing is dynamic and increasingly complex. In primary care and in the specialties of pediatrics, geriatrics, and family health, for example, functions are now performed by nurses that were formerly those of the physician. The nurse performs a physical examination and history as part of the nursing practitioner's assessment and diagnosis. Consequently, nurses are shifting traditionally nursing functions to ancillary personnel. In the process of delegation, the nurse is expected to exercise discretion and judgment in accepting and assigning responsibilities. Consultation is freely used. The primary goal is to ensure safe and effective nursing care.

A second goal is to practice within the limits of the legal practice acts for each profession. In some nursing roles, there is an effort to develop joint policy statements with medicine that will define differences in roles and responsibilities. Existing statements of joint policy represent expert judgment and may have standing in courts of law. A third goal is to influence constructive changes in the law.

The delivery of total health services is now beyond the capacity of any single profession. An interdisciplinary team effort, in which the members share knowledge, skills, and responsibilities for total patient care, nevertheless requires the nurse's recognition of limits of competence. The nurse needs consultation from appropriate sources, including other nurses, physicians, or other health professionals. Distinction in role and functions that are based on education and training are respected without disparagement of individuals having minor roles.

Personal competence, as well as education, training and policy requirements, are assessed before delegating nursing functions to ancillary personnel or accepting medical functions.[57] Any nurse who is unsure of personnel competence has both the responsibility and, in one view, the right to refuse the assignment in question. This protects both the client and the nurse. The same right and responsibility prevail where functions are delegated that are not nursing responsibilities or that keep the nurse from providing nursing care. Similar precautions are expected to be observed in delegating functions to other members of the team who may be unqualified for the assignment.[58]

7. The nurse participates in activities that contribute to the ongoing development of the profession's body of knowledge.[59]

Systematic investigation is necessary for expanding each profession's body of knowledge. Knowledge, implying truth and beliefs based on adequate evidence, serves as the framework and beacon light of the profession's education and practice.

The ANA has developed guidelines for participants in research. Research is expected to be conducted by qualified persons or under appropriate supervision. The purpose, nature, goals, and methodology of the research are evaluated in relation to guidelines for the protection of human subjects. The subject's right of informed consent, privacy, and dignity are thereby ensured. Additionally, the subject has the right to terminate participation at any time. These principles are especially important in research consented to by parents or guardians and performed on children, the aged, and the mentally disabled. The nurse who disagrees with the research because of its problematic aspects has the right to refuse to participate or to withdraw on the basis of its adverse effects on patients.[60]

8. The nurse participates in the profession's efforts to implement and improve standards of nursing.[61]

An assumed public concern of professions is that only qualified persons will be admitted to practice. Nursing competence includes a command of skills, academic success, demonstrated responsibility, and a commitment to improve nursing practice for the benefit of others. The selection of students and evaluation of their abilities is an obligation of educators. Helping people involves more than a generous humanitarian impulse. Therefore, the ANA has developed standards for practice, education, and service that require the participation of each nurse for implementation.[62]

9. The nurse participates in the profession's efforts to establish and maintain conditions of employment conducive to high-quality nursing care.[63]

Nurses are now involved in the process of changing the terms and conditions of employment. This provision of the *Code* emphasizes that economic conditions and general welfare are important factors in recruiting and keeping well-qualified nurses functioning at an optimum level.

The most effective method of defining and controlling the quality of nursing care is collective bargaining. The professional state nurses' associations assist and represent nurses in negotiations with employers. One aim is to ensure professionally approved standards of practice. Equally important is the support for the rights of nurses to "participate in determining the terms and conditions of employment conducive to high-quality nursing practice".[64] The appropriate channel for nurses to improve conditions of employment ethically and with dignity is through the economic and general welfare programs of state and national nurses' associations. Increasingly, work contracts have been achieved in previously unorganized health care facilities. Old contracts are renegotiated and revised to the satisfaction of the majority of employed nurses. Some contracts were secured solely through negotiation. Others were secured only after prolonged, unsuccessful negotiation and a strike threat or an actual strike in which arrangements were made to provide care for seriously ill patients. The dominant theme of revised and renewed contracts is patient safety, to be achieved by nursing participation in determining staffing levels, a step toward nursing control of practice.

10. The nurse participates in the profession's effort to protect the public from misinformation and misrepresentation and to maintain the integrity of nursing.[65]

This section of the *Code* provides for individual advertising of nursing services through listings and biographies in reputable publications. The nurse may use symbols of licensure such as RN, earned academic degrees, and symbols of professional recognition such as Fellow of the American Academy of Nursing (FAAN). No nurse is permitted to endorse, advertise, promote, or sell commercial products, because this may be mistakenly interpreted as an endorsement by the entire profession. In the course of health teaching, several "similar products or services [are expected to] be offered or described so that the client or practitioner can make an informed choice."[66] On the other hand, nurses are expected to advise patients against using products that are dangerous. Violations of these principles by other nurses are expected to be reported to the professional association, as such actions undermine public confidence in nursing.

11. The nurse collaborates with members of the health professions and other citizens in promoting community and national efforts to meet the health needs of the public.[67]

Health care as the right of all citizens is stated in this provision as endorsed by the ANA House of Delegates convened in 1958.[68] Planning for health services to be available and accessible to everyone requires collaboration between consumers and providers of health care at all levels. Nurses have both the right and the responsibility to help achieve quality health care for all by implementing their views through the political process and legislative action. The organization of Nurses for Political Action has been effective in directly communicating the views of nurses on key issues to legislators. The organization has both supported and endorsed political candidates favorably disposed toward nursing interests, health care services, and human welfare.

This provision of the *Code* holds that relationships with other disciplines are expected to be collaborative and supportive. By its very nature, the delivery of complex health care demands an interdisciplinary approach. Likewise, the relationship of nursing and medicine is regarded as interdependent and collaborative "around the need of the client."[69] The changing role of the nurse, particularly primary care or specialty nurse practitioners, requires collegial relationships with physicians combined with discussion of overlapping, similar, and different functions and areas of practice.[70]

The challenge to nurses and nursing organizations is clearly set forth. Nurses serve all of the people. Therefore, nurses have the right to a voice in all deliberations and decisions affecting the quantity, quality, and distribution of health care and nursing services.

Code Revisions

The decision was made by the ANA, through its committees and House of Delegates, to revise the *Code of Ethics for Nurses*. The *Code's* mission statement of nursing emphasizes the nurse's primary commitment to serve the health care needs of individual patients, groups, and communities, both locally and internationally. Ethical obligations are not only to the health care, well-being and safety of the patient, but also to protection of the moral integrity of the nurse involved in practice, education, research, and management.[71] Patient's rights are also underscored, as are working conditions that threaten patient care.

Nurses are expected to advance the profession by assuming leadership and mentorship responsibilities in professional and civic activities committed to nursing and health care policy changes at the state, national, and international levels. The nurse administrator or manager is charged with responsibility for conditions of employment that promote practice within accepted standards with autonomy and self-regulation. Nurse educators are responsible for graduating only those students who possess the essential knowledge, skills, and commitment to safe professional practice.

In the proposed revision, the nurse's advocacy role is acknowledged in the use of medical technologies, such as resuscitation, withholding and withdrawing of life-sustaining therapies, provision of nutrition and hydration, and advance directives. The nurse may intervene to relieve pain and other symptoms even if this act shortens life, provided the goal is not to end life.[72] (This appears to be an application of the principle of Double Effect, discussed in Chapter 4). Collaboration with relevant parties is required in planning and decision making.

The responsibilities and accountabilities of the nursing role extend to administrators, educators, and researchers, who share in participation for the quality of nursing care of those they supervise and instruct.[73] The individual nurse is responsible for delegating nursing care tasks to other health care workers and evaluating the safety and quality of their work. Management and administrative nurses have a responsibility to support and facilitate appropriate delegation.[74] Nurses' concerns regarding the safety, fairness, and morality of the work environment may seek redress through collective action through their state nurses' associations.[75]

A great deal of emphasis is placed on the influence of the environment on nurses fulfilling their moral obligations. Such virtues as honesty, trustworthiness, fairness and caring are seen to be supported and nourished or thwarted and diminished by the practice environment. Such environments include working conditions and policies, group norms, organizational structures, grievance procedures, ethics committees, compensation systems, and disciplinary procedures. Just and fair treatment of employees and support for practice standards promote the values of nursing. The individual nurse, and nursing administrators in particular, are responsible for treating employees fairly and for involving nurses in practice decisions. Acquiescence in unsafe, unfair, or immoral practice is equivalent to condoning that practice.[76] Collective action through the State Nurses' Association, acting as advocate, may be the most effective route to appropriate changes.

The last provision of the proposed revision asserts the values of nursing to its members and to the public. The profession pledges its continued efforts to clarify nursing's accountability to society through its standards of nursing practice and education, the development of nursing knowledge and research, and evaluation practices. The *Code* will be maintained and enforced through critical reflection and self-examination, with change directed toward its ideals. The national and state associations have the professional responsibility to speak for nurses collectively on health care policy and legislation. Healthcare is broadly understood to include related issues as hunger, homelessness, violence, human rights, poverty, and the stigma of illness.[77]

THE INTERNATIONAL COUNCIL FOR NURSES CODE OF ETHICS

In 1948, the International Council of Nurses was officially recognized by the World Health Organization (WHO) as the voice for all nongovernmental nursing. The Council is now the official representative of all nursing at WHO meetings.[78]

As a guideline for conduct for nurses all over the world, the International Council of Nurses' *Code* of ethics recognizes that nursing practice must reflect and respect cultural and religious differences. As a result, nursing may differ in fundamental respects from one area to another. The *Code* contains the seeds of conflict if the nurse carries the laws and customs of the home area to a different one. Respect for the values of a subculture or minority group is a position that raises the dilemma of whether to respect harmful values or to work for change. For example, an African nurse may be forced to choose between psychotropic drugs and the activities of a local healer for control of the hallucinations and thought disorders of a patient with an acute schizophrenic episode.

The *Code* defines the nurse's relation to people as one in which nursing care is provided in an environment that respects individual values, spiritual beliefs, and customs. Information of a personal nature is to be held in confidence unless the nurse judges that it should be shared.[79]

The nurse's responsibility for practice is one of continual learning in order to maintain competence.[80] In specific situations, the nurse sustains the highest possible standards of nursing care and uses judgment in delegating and accepting responsibilities. Personal conduct reflects credit on the profession.[81]

The nurse's relation to society is one of shared responsibility for the initiation and implementation of the health and social needs of the community.[82]

The nurse's relation with co-workers is cooperative. (The physician is not distinguished from other co-workers.) The nurse protects persons receiving care by taking appropriate action when they are endangered.

The nurse's relation to the profession is that of an active role in developing and implementing desirable standards of nursing education and practice, and in contributing to nursing knowledge. Moreover, the nurse is expected to be active in securing fair economic and social working conditions through the professional organization. Female nurses must still struggle for equality and recognition as persons whose professional lives are separate from their personal lives. The *Code* supports the definition of a professional nurse as a person with rights and responsibilities for self, clients, co-workers, community, and profession, and their nursing and health care needs. WHO recognizes the *Code* for supporting nursing education and practice. It is used as a guide to curricula development, licensing, and legislation in countries involved with shaping their health care systems to better serve their people.

THE FUNCTIONS OF A CODE FOR NURSES

According to *The American Heritage Dictionary,* a code is a "systematic collection of regulation, rules of procedure or conduct."[83] A code, in the case of law is a "complete system of positive law officially promulgated. . . ."[84] Ideally, a professional code regulates the professional conduct of its members by instituting sanctions, directly or indirectly, and thus enforcing its provisions.

The word "professional," as used in these discussions of codes, is employed as a persuasive definition. That is, it is used as a value term that urges the reader to agree with the writer or speaker. The use of a persuasive definition is in contrast to a lexical or reportive definition that is true or false, such as that of an island as a body of land surrounded by water. The terms "professional" and "unprofessional" may also be used persuasively. Ms. Jolene Tuma, RN, for example, had her license revoked by the Idaho State Board of Nursing in August 1976 on the grounds that her conduct was "unprofessional" for advocating Laetrile and "disrupting" the patient-physician relationship. Ms. Tuma appealed to the *Code for Nurses* to support her view that she was acting professionally.[85]

The *Code for Nurses* provides moral guidelines to nursing practice in accordance with consumers' health care interests and rights. The *Code* holds nurses accountable for professionally acceptable standards of nursing care. As the *Code* has evolved, this standard of acceptable nursing care has increasingly placed the client at the center of health care. Meanwhile, both the patient and the nurse are increasingly invested with rights and responsibilities.

The use of rights language in codes for nurses reflects not only that patients have rights but also that nurses have a role as patient advocates. To carry out their role as client advocates, nurses have special "earned" rights and privileges, which they may invoke even against physicians if their orders are medically or scientifically contraindicated. The advent of patients' and nurses' rights implies a conceptual redrawing of the physician-patient relationship as well as a higher set of educational and professional role requirements and responsibilities placed on nurses.

Growth of the nurse's advocacy role may also occur as a result of such landmark cases as *Memorial Hospital v. Darling*.[86] Here, the physicians were found negligent along with the nurses in a case involving Dorrence Darling's broken leg, which turned gangrenous and had to be amputated. By holding nurses and physicians responsible for negligence, the nurses' judgment was identified as a causal factor, one that could have made a difference in the outcome. By holding nurses responsible, the Illinois Supreme Court acknowledged the role and importance of nursing judgment, thereby altering the physician's role from the traditional "captain of the ship" to that of a key team member. To hold nurses jointly responsible for negligence against Dorrence Darling, as the state supreme court did, called for nurses to have greater treatment autonomy and the professional right to advocate clients' rights against physicians if necessary. The nurses in the *Darling* case were cited for not reporting the condition of Darling's leg cast, even if doing so meant reporting a physician's negligence. This kind of reporting is now known as "whistle-blowing."

One function of the *Code for Nurses*, then, is to upgrade the nursing profession, thereby benefitting both patients and nurses by investing nurses with rights and responsibilities. Rights enable nurses to care more effectively for clients' health care interests and rights—rights which, some nursing scholars believe, cannot be entrusted to physicians alone. But the rights of nurses are not rights *against* patients, for such rights would defeat the point of nursing and nursing advocacy. Rather, nurses' rights are rights to act *on behalf* of their clients and include nurses' rights against other health professionals, including physicians and other nurses. These rights are invoked if other health professionals fail to promote the rights and interests of patients. Thus, patients' rights come first and justify the earned rights and privileges of other health professionals, on the condition, of course, that professional rights and privileges are consistent with and compatible with patients' rights.

A second function of the *Code* is one consistent with and implied by the first function of upgrading the quality of health care. This function is to set standards to regulate the conduct of nursing practitioners, holding them accountable and morally liable for failure to live up to the standards. The *Code* functions as an oath or promise made by the profession collectively to the public that these standards will be upheld by each individual nurse.

To regulate the conduct of nurse practitioners, the profession, by logical extension through its *Code for Nurses*, attempts to influence licensure, institutional accreditation, and curricular content.[87] The *Code for Nurses* would otherwise be an exclusively ceremonial statement, without influence in the governance of nursing practitioners. Nurses would possibly pay lip service to the *Code*, but it would lack what may be termed "performative" meaning; namely, that the *Code* gets things done.[88] The *Code* would have no teeth if it had no "performative force." To have performative force, the *Code* regulates nursing practitioners by influencing the guidelines for licensure, institutional accreditation, and curricula.

THE AMERICAN MEDICAL ASSOCIATION CODE OF ETHICS

The American Medical Association adopted a new code of ethics in 1990, and updated it in 1994.[89] The physician is characterized as an ally of the patient by serving as an advocate of patients and their rights. These rights are identified as the right to receive information regarding the benefits, risks, and costs of treatment options, and a professional opinion about them as the basis for patient acceptance or refusal. Patients have the right of confidentiality and to obtain copies or summaries of their medical records. Patients have the right to continuity of care, to coordinated activities of the physician with other providers, and to receive adequate notice of discontinuation of treatment. Patients have the right to receive adequate health care and the physician is expected to work toward that goal and for society's provision of adequate resources so that no patient is deprived of care because of cost. Physicians are expected to continue to assume some responsibility for the essential medical care of those who cannot afford it and advocate for patients dealing with third parties.

EVALUATION OF PROFESSIONAL CODES

A criticism of the *Code* and of professional codes in general is that they reflect vested interests. These interests mask deeper conflicts between the interests of the public and the profession around what Paul Goodman used to call "pork-chop" gains in the form of higher salaries and benefits. The evidence is that the *Code for Nurses,* while promoting the interests of the nursing profession, is clearly oriented toward serving patients' interests and rights and placing the interests of nurses second to those of patients. The interests of patients and nurses do not collide, but rather dovetail. There are natural points of alliance between patients and nurses, due in part to being undervalued and underserved and also to the caring core of the profession.

SUMMARY

Nurses, who have a natural kinship with values of life and death and the quality of life and health care, show increasing awareness of value questions; the protection of patients' rights is a natural outcome. Patient advocacy is integral with the expanding relationships nurses have in the care of their patients. Models of nurse-patient-physician relationships show that patient advocacy by nurses is essential to patients' health care rights.

The *Code* provides a moral basis for justifying nursing action through its functions of: (1) upgrading nursing by investing it with rights and responsibilities for caring for patients; (2) setting accountable moral standards for practitioners; (3) influencing licensure standards; (4) influencing educational and curricular standards of performance and conduct; and (5) appealing through its manifesto-like principles for legal incorporation and public acceptance.

Codes may have important symbolic and regulating functions for professional practices, including nursing. A symbolic function is to remind nurses and those in other professions of the status and importance of nursing in health care. The *Code for Nurses* carries out this role by stressing the human rights of patients and nurses to self-determination and well-being. The regulating function of the *Code* is to influence standards and practices of nursing.

Discussion Questions

1. Given mother surrogate, technician and nurse as advocate models, what is your conception of an ethically justifiable model of nursing?
2. What are some major advantages and drawbacks of each of the following models: civil disobedience, urban guerrilla, and legal standing?
3. How does the *Code for Nurses* influence and guide a nurse's conduct in deciding whether to refuse to help a patient?
4. In your view, which of the provisions of the *Code* regarding the right to refuse to treat is ethically justifiable and for what reasons?

REFERENCES

1. Hesse M. Models and analogy in science. In: Edwards P (ed). *The encyclopedia of philosophy.* New York: Macmillan. 1967;5:358.
2. Black M. *Models and metaphors.* Ithaca, NY: Cornell University Press. 1962;236.
3. Scheffler I. *Reason and teaching.* Indianapolis: Bobbs-Merrill. 1975;68.
4. Emanuel, EJ, Emanuel LL. Four models of the physician-patient relationship. *JAMA,* 1992;267(16):2221.
5. ibid.
6. ibid.
7. ibid.
8. ibid.
9. ibid, p. 2222.
10. ibid, p. 2222.
11. ibid, p. 2222.
12. ibid, p. 2222.
13. ibid, p. 2222.
14. ibid, p. 2224.
15. ibid, p. 2225.
16. ibid, p. 2225.
17. ibid.
18. ibid.
19. Smith S. Three models of the nurse-patient relationship. In: Spicker SF, Gadow S (eds.). *Nursing images and ideals.* New York: Springer. 1980;177–179.

20. ibid, p. 181.
21. Gadow S. Existential advocacy. In: Spicker SF, Gadow S (eds). *Nursing images and ideals*. New York: Springer. 1980;81.
22. ibid, p. 83.
23. ibid, p. 85.
24. ibid, p. 85.
25. ibid, p. 84.
26. Goodnow M. The patient's bill of rights and the nurse. *Nursing Clinics of North America* 1974;9:557.
27. Mill JS. *Utilitarianism, liberty, and representative government*. London: Dent. 1948; 208.
28. Abrams N. Moral responsibility in nursing. In: Spicker SF, Gadow S (eds). *Nursing images and ideals*. New York: Springer. 1980;153–159.
29. Kosik SH. Patient advocacy or fighting the system. *Am J Nursing* 1972;72(4):694.
30. Whittaker S. Issues update. *Am J Nursing* 1998;98(8):58.
31. Flanagan L. *One strong voice*. Kansas City, Mo: American Nurses Association. 1976;23.
32. Fowler MD. Ethics relic or resource? The *Code for Nurses*. *Am J Nursing* 1999; 99(3):56.
33. American Nurses Association. *Code for nurses with interpretive statements*. Kansas City, Mo. 1985;2.
34. ibid, p. 1.
35. ibid.
36. ibid.
37. Ibid, p. 4.
38. ibid.
39. ibid.
40. ibid.
41. ibid.
42. ibid.
43. ibid.
44. ibid, p. 7.
45. ibid, p. 8.
46. ibid.
47. ibid.
48. ibid, p. 9.
49. ibid.
50. ibid.
51. ibid, p. 10.
52. ibid.
53. ibid.
54. ibid, p. 11.
55. ibid.
56. ibid, p. 12.
57. ibid, p. 13.
58. ibid.
59. ibid, p. 14.
60. ibid, p. 15.
61. ibid.
62. ibid, p. 16.
63. ibid.

64. ibid.
65. ibid, p. 10.
66. ibid, p. 18.
67. ibid, p. 19.
68. Flanagan L. *One Strong Voice*. Kansas City, Mo: American Nurses Association 1976; 629.
69. ibid, p. 20.
70. ibid.
71. Daly BN. Ethics: Why a new code. *Am J Nursing* 1999;99(6):64–65.
72. American Nurses Association. *Code for Nurses:* Proposed Revision, Draft #8; 1999.
73. ibid.
74. ibid, p. 20.
75. ibid, p. 23.
76. ibid.
77. ibid.
78. Flanagan L. *One Strong Voice*. Kansas City, Mo: American Nurses Association. 1976; 624.
79. International Council of Nurses Code for Nurses. *Ethical concepts applied to nursing.* Geneva, May 1973.
80. ibid.
81. ibid.
82. ibid.
83. *The American Heritage Dictionary of the English Language,* (3rd ed.). Boston: Houghton Mifflin. 1996;366.
84. *Black's law dictionary.* (7th ed.). St. Paul, Minn: West. 1999;250.
85. Tuma J. Professional misconduct. *Nursing Outlook.* 1977;25(9):546.
86. *Dorrence Kenneth Darling v. Charleston Community Memorial Hospital,* 33 111, 326, 211 (NE 2nd 253 1965).
87. Transcript. *The matter of Ms. Jolene Tuma.* Board of Nursing. Idaho. August 24, 1976; 186–188,234–235.
88. Austin JL. Performative utterances. In: Austin JL (ed). *Philosophical papers.* New York: Oxford University Press. 1970;233.
89. American Medical Association. *Principles of medical ethics.* Chicago, 1996.

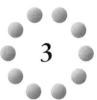

3

Self-Interest Morality

Study of this chapter enables the learner to:

1. Identify self-interest theories of morality used in health care delivery relevant to nursing.
2. Recognize the role of self-interest ethics in the development of the social contract.
3. Identify and distinguish between subjectivism, relativism, objectivism, skepticism, and nihilism in relation to nursing issues.
4. Examine the benefits and drawbacks of subjectivism and relativism (two expressions of self-interest morality).
5. Examine the benefits and drawbacks of objectivism and skepticism.
6. Use the appeal to the self-interest theory of ethics to justify moral decisions.

OVERVIEW

Moral problems arise in nursing whenever a nursing act results in doing good or harm. However, two philosophical questions arise: What is good? And what is harmful in the context of health care ethics? We consider these questions in this and succeeding chapters. To begin with, all health care policies and practices have consequences—some trivial, some serious, and some even life-saving. As significant members of the health care team and as patient advocates, nurses are involved in making decisions that vitally affect the well-being of patients, families, colleagues, and other members of society.

Nursing decisions and policies, such as those expressed in the *Code for Nurses* reflect moral values, issues, and problems in everyday practice.[1] Attempts to solve or resolve these issues are expressed through moral views or beliefs or ways of acting. These moral views, which concern predominant ways of looking at, or examining values, may be seen as ethical theories. A practical model provides an account designed to orient and guide practical activities.[2] A theory of ethics characterizes a perspective for viewing moral relationships (where ethics and morality are used interchangeably). These theories of ethics or morality, which reflect ways of life, overlap and are best understood as existing in a dynamic relationship with one another.

A major theory of morality is self-interest or egoist morality. This theory may take one of several forms. It may be short-term or long-term; it may be subjectivist or relativist, which are closely related although not identical. Self-interest theories play a role in several related theories, such as the social contract, and extend to contemporary elaborations, such as present day existentialism. Self-interest ethics also plays a role in hedonism, which emphasizes individual pleasure and avoidance of individual pain.

In Book Ten of his *Ethics*, Aristotle provides a sympathetic critique of hedonism, which is associated with pleasure. Early Greek hedonism is a forerunner to a later well-developed theory called utilitarianism. Hedonism, however, can be evaluated as not being sufficiently complex to account for the deep and subtle facets of human nature. The desire for pleasure, especially the "here and now" pleasures of the moment, are not one's only desires. These facets of human nature may also include stoicism or the denial of one's pleasures, possibly for the sake of some other goal or process in life that may, however, be identified as a gain for oneself. Thus, it often depends what one means by the self. Is oneself enriched by gratifying or denying the desire for pleasure? In one respect, it seems that one cannot reasonably deny the role of oneself in any morally reflective theory or practice.[3] A saint or a hero or a "selfless" actor gives something of herself or himself to others and hopes or expects to receive something in exchange. Even the golden rule, which says to treat others as one wishes to be treated, reflects an interest in oneself. One may identify the golden rule as the rule of reciprocity. The rule of reciprocity, which is implicitly endorsed by numerous ethical theories, has its "acid test" against a self-interest theory. If it shows anything, the golden rule shows that there is rarely a selfless act. An example of a selfless act, however, is a married nurse with children who donates her own kidney to an unrelated child who was in need.

Ordinarily, the desire for pleasure is part of the self. For some thinkers, pleasure per se is a good, even if not the only good. Moreover, the idea that pleasure is good is easily refuted, as G. E. Moore did when he pointed to bad pleasures.[4] Examples of bad pleasures abound: smoking, unprotected casual sex, substance abuse, and spousal abuse. Finally, one person's temporary pleasure may be another's permanent pain. At any rate, we consider some mild reservations to self-interest ethics with this brief discussion of hedonism, as it originated in ancient Greece, in order to highlight some limits of self-interest ethics. These limits of self-interest ethics may also help one to recognize the strengths of that theory.

PERENNIAL ISSUES IN NURSING ETHICS: SELF-INTEREST ETHICS IN RELATION TO ALTERNATIVE THEORIES

Egoism, Subjectivism, Relativism, Objectivism, Skepticism, and Nihilism

A nurse's effort to do good and avoid doing harm involves her familiarity with several perennial issues, including egoism, subjectivism, relativism, objectivism, skepticism, and nihilism. These "isms" raise questions to which ethical theories help generate proposed answers. Egoism says, "Me first and last." Subjectivism says, "Whatever I say is right." Relativism says, "Each individual or group decides what is right or wrong for herself or himself or itself, even though there is actually no right or wrong." Objectivism says there is a higher good independent of any person's desires. Skepticism casts doubt on all ethical theories, and challenges them to provide adequate justification for claiming to be right. Nihilism denies that any ethical theories can be justified.

Some Further Elaborations

Egoism.   Early Greek sophists (400 BC) championed egoist values as their theory of ethics. They believed that all ethics begins and ends with self-interest. "What is in it for me?" and "Only do something if it pays off for me," they said. They cared about being paid. Teachers' and physicians' fees were basic to their performance of services to others. The function of physicians and health practitioners was to look after themselves and charge as much money as the market would bear.

Thrasymachus, a leading sophist and egoist of his time, and an opponent of Socrates, defines justice "as the interest of the stronger."[5] In effect, he meant that whoever has the power decides what justice is, and to have one's way is to achieve power. An important aim of egoism is to achieve power. Moreover, self-interest morality provides a distinction between the self and the world. The self characterizes consciousness, from which emerges the slogan, for right or wrong (or in part right and in part wrong), that what is good for the individual is good for the country or group. If there were no individual who could be satisfied, there could be no idea of the good. The good does not derive from some abstract plan; it derives from the individual. That is part of the force and appeal of self-interest morality.

As a theory of morality for nursing, nurses who embrace egoism look to patients and institutions solely for the good they can get for themselves. Such nurses look for assignment options that do not include patients with AIDS, tuberculosis, or other infectious diseases. Such nurses negotiate for the highest possible salary, and do so solely for the power that the highest salary achieves for them. For egoist-oriented nurses, their interests come first and the patient's health care interests are the means to such nurses' well-being.

According to egoism, people are and ought to be oriented by self-love. Self-love is a natural trait. As previously stated, justice is defined by Thrasymachus as the interests of those who have power. The sophists initiated conceptual work on the notion of "interests"; they emphasized the value of the self, as in self-interest as a motivation of human acts.

Subjectivism.   The sophists also developed a related philosophical concept called subjectivism, in which there is no truth or goodness in ethics outside of one's own perspective. Individuals and societies decide for themselves what is good or harmful. To some moral philosophers, sophist egoism is difficult, if not impossible, to refute.

Relativism.   A connected sophist value is relativism, in which all values are relative, differing according to the individual or society that holds such values, and that individuals or cultures have immunity against the judgments of others, no matter how distasteful or repugnant their values and practices may seem. For example, the female genital mutilation practiced in some African countries is the moral prerogative of those countries.

Pros and Cons of Subjectivism and Relativism

According to subjectivism, each individual decides what is morally right or true and is the source of justification and authority for making such decisions. In the subjectivist view, "beauty is in the eyes of the beholder," as are truth and goodness. This view is aptly phrased in Shakespeare's *Hamlet*, when the prince remarks that "nothing is either good or bad, but thinking makes it so."[6] On this view, the Nazis thought they did no wrong. However, objective examples of Nazi mistreatment, such as those illustrated in the film *Schindler's List* (1993), refute relativism and subjectivism

Some patients, nurses, and allied healthcare providers subscribe to relativism (there is no universal right or wrong and values are relative to individuals or cultures). For example, in culture A, hemodialysis is not given to those 65 years of age or older. In culture B, dialysis is given to anyone in need, without age or diagnostic restrictions. According to the relativist model, neither culture is right or wrong. In some cultures, AIDS patients are cared for, whereas in others they are not. But on relativist grounds, there is no right or wrong outside of what an individual or group decides. According to relativists, questions of right and wrong, true and false, are left to each group to decide. But Hamlet's question arises: Is such a view of ethics rationally defensible or justifiable, especially in the presence of glaring counterexamples, such as female genital mutilation? Relativism is closely allied to subjectivism and seems to come to the same conclusions.

An advantage of relativism and subjectivism is that these theories do not impose an absolute standard of morality to be obeyed without question. Additionally, relativism and subjectivism foster tolerance of alternative ways of behaving. (Pluralism, which is closely related to relativism, is often an effective antidote to the narrow constraints of an absolute moral standard.)

A rational antidote to absolutism is not relativism or subjectivism, but skepticism, a challenge to justify one's position. A drawback of relativism and subjectivism is that if nothing is right or wrong, then moral education is seriously limited and is reduced to mastery of conventions. One cannot then effectively argue against the lack of health care, the exploitation of nurses, slavery, segregation, racism, sexism, anti-semitism, Naziism, or any other obvious evil. If there is no transcultural justification of any moral practice, then each culture is the supreme moral lawgiver unto itself, and consequently there is then no higher moral court of appeal. The general unacceptability of this moral conclusion for some kinds of cases leads one to consider an alternative to subjectivism and relativism.

Discerning nurses will examine and evaluate the positive, neutral, and negative aspects of sophism. They will acknowledge that self-interest has value, as does the respect and care one gives to oneself. However, it is morally irresponsible for a nurse or physician to fail to care for a patient's health care interest. A serious deductive consequence of egoism, subjectivism, or relativism is that there are no higher moral standards to which one may appeal in order to rationally settle a moral dispute. Nevertheless, one standard used in self-interest theories of ethics is the "social contract," which may be used to express either short- or long-term self-interest.

THREE VIEWS OF THE SOCIAL CONTRACT

The first important form of the social contract comes from Socrates's answer to Glaucon's challenge related in Plato's *The Ring of Gyges*. Glaucon tells the story of Gyges the shepherd, who finds a ring of invisibility. By turning the ring on his finger, Gyges can become invisible at will. Glaucon raises the question, "Why be just if one could become both powerful and invisible and unjust by way of a magic ring that makes one invisible?"[7] Egoists ask and answer this question, "What is in it for me?" by saying, in effect, "Doing X had better be good for me. Otherwise, I won't do X." Socrates, Thrasymachus, and Glaucon have different and sometimes divergent answers.[8] Socrates's answer is that we do not live alone; we need the help of other people.[9] Plato's profound insight and first form of the social contract theory enables any person to have any one of several motives for entering and remaining in society. One of these motives is altruism. Another is enlightened or long-term self-interest. Plato's position may be identified as *rational paternalism* (considered in further detail in Chapter 4). Here, we consider enlightened self-interest.

A form of the social contract is presented by the English social philosopher Thomas Hobbes (1588-1679), to whom the basis of modem egoism is commonly attributed. The main drive in human nature, says Hobbes, is self-preservation. But in a "state of nature," where people are left to themselves, there can be no society at all. In such a state—one in which people act at all times on their basic motivations solely to survive—there would be a continuous "war of all against all." There would be no trade and commerce, no growth of knowledge, no arts. Rather, there would be "continual fear of danger and violent death," and human life would be "solitary, poor, nasty, brutish, and short."[10] Hobbes's ingenious solution is to convert this unbearable state of nature into the nature of a state, to be brought about by a social contract. This contract provides for individuals to agree to give up their liberty to preserve themselves in a state of nature by any means, and to transfer their individual liberty and power to a sovereign whom they agree to obey. The sovereign, in exchange for everyone's obedience, ensures peace and protection. This social contract provides for the exchange of freedom for security. The sovereign keeps individuals obedient by developing a deputized peace force of persons to coerce and control people into continual compliance with civil laws. However, the difficulty lies in that we are never far from our basic interest in ourselves. Our reason for joining society is self-interest.

What Is the Social Contract?
The social contract, which stems from the individual, is an important doctrine with implications for social and and institutional behavior. Therein lies a paradox: Does one comply with agreements that are made without one's consent? Not at all. To

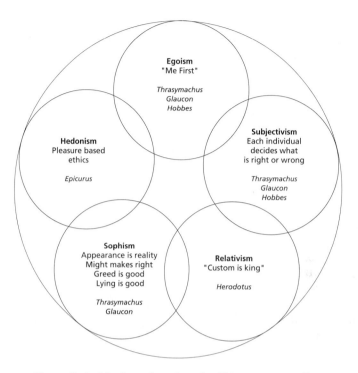

Figure 3–1. Modern theories of self-interest morality.

agree is to give one's consent. However, the social contract was made prior to our birth, so we could not give our consent. Yet we agree to live by the provisions of this agreement, a basic agreement that generates all other agreements.

One answer to this paradox is to consider that the social contract asks us to suppose as a counterfactual, conditional judgment with provisions that everyone would agree to if everyone in a position to do so. One way to make the social contract agreeable to everyone is to make its provisions mutually beneficial (see Chapter 7 for J. Rawls's appeal to the "Veil of Ignorance" for an account of such an agreement).

On an alternative interpretation of the social contract, nurses may find that the conditions of patient care in a given hospital are so deplorable that they have no choice but to go on strike. Nurses have a prior agreement to live by the principles of their professional code. However, the *Code for Nurses* implies that under harmful conditions of patient care, nurses have a right and a duty to protest and perhaps even to strike as a form of remediable action. A principle that orients a social contract in a "free society" is that those who provide services do so based on fully informed consent. Such consent includes conditions under which nurses are obligated to withhold their services.

A question arises: Is morality invented or discovered? If morality is discovered, one looks to an external authority to establish it. If morality is invented by people, then they decide what is right and wrong. The social contract generally implies that one invents morality rather than discovers it. Egoism generates two doctrines: 1) the social contract and the conception that morality is invented by people, and 2) such a contract is designed to serve people's interests. Under altruism, morality is discovered by some external and superior source of authority. Altruism appeals to natural law. Thus, egoism and altruism generate two forms of the social contract: positive law (or human-derived law) and natural law (ostensibly derived from some higher power). The contracts we know are agreements that we accept and act in accordance with. The social contract provides that we agree to abide by previous agreements, including the law, and that we not take agreements, promises, or "the law into our own hands." On this interpretation of the social contract, the very idea of nurses striking violates a fundamental tenet of the social contract. On one interpretation as the source of all contracts, the social contract requires nurses to accept working conditions in hospitals without resorting to public demonstrations of their refusal to work.

A social contract is the agreement to live by agreements, even though those agreements may predate one's own lifetime. When Socrates was convicted and sentenced to death by the citizens of Athens, he took the fatal hemlock rather than accept the help of friends to escape. He thereby showed his acceptance of the social contract he (hypothetically) had with Athens. A question arises in nursing whether it is morally permissible for nurses to abide by a contract that compromises patient safety and well being. A justifying reason for nurses to strike is to correct and remedy unsafe and inadequate patient care, such as poor staffing ratios and poor staff qualifications.

In any event, egoism generates the social contract as an alternative to the war of individuals against one another, living alone without a society. One agrees to abide by laws and regulations peaceably and reasonably out of one's own self-interest. The alternative to accepting the social contract is social chaos and fighting at every turn, which is unthinkably harmful to all concerned and worse than a bad agreement. But the validity of the social contract is up to each individual to decide, at least according to the subjectivist interpretation.

A strength of self-interest morality or egoism is that it speaks to people's motivations. Human beings who are rewarded by money, power, recognition, status, and prestige, are apt to redouble their efforts. A difficulty with egoism is, as Plato pointed out, that people live together and need one another's help. Plato saw that people need to have their behavior controlled in order to help and not harm themselves and others. For people to do whatever they wish (a belief expressed by the bumper sticker, "If it feels right, do it") may be inappropriate. One might, for example, fail to respect traffic lights or fail to answer a patient's call light because one feels that patient is a chronic complainer.

Under the theory of egoism, one claims the freedom to do anything one wants, such as engaging in patient-nurse, spouse, child, or substance abuse. A strength of rational paternalism (discussed in Chapter 4) is that it places rational restraints against harming ourselves and others. Even John Stuart Mill's celebrated essay *On Liberty* (1869) argued that the principle of "Do no harm" sets limits to liberty. This principle, known as nonmaleficence, seems to prevail over other forms of the social contract in nursing ethics.

INDIVIDUALISM IN RELATION TO COLLECTIVISM, EXISTENTIALISM, AND PHENOMENOLOGY

Collectivism

An example of a contemporary moral issue involving conflicting theories is that of individualism versus collectivism. To appreciate the strengths and also limits of individualism, we present its polar opposite, collectivism. Individualism emphasizes individual liberty, individual self-determination, initiative, self-reliance, and self-realization. To an individualist, social institutions are the sum total of individual efforts and actions.

In contrast, collectivism helps one to appreciate and to evaluate the strengths and difficulties of individualism. Collectivism is the belief that capitalism is responsible for human problems, including widespread starvation, lack of drinking water, and lack of health care in many parts of the world.

One form of collectivism originated with Karl Marx (1818-1883). To Marx, individuals are not free, rather only groups of people with power are free in capitalist societies. Those with power are free to exploit others, thereby turning the majority into wage slaves. This form of collectivism calls for total social change rather than piecemeal social change proposed by existentialists and by Bentham (see Chapter 5).

There are strengths and weaknesses in each of these theories. Individualism emphasizes attractive qualities associated with individual liberty, individual initiative, hard work, and rewards for individual merit. However, individuals can amass power and consequently abuse others. Out of such abuse, through exploitation, comes the appeal of collectivism. This doctrine promises to do for individuals what they cannot possibly do alone, namely to organize to form better rules for achieving social and economic justice. Appeal to collectives, sometimes identified as corporate bodies, can also provide for more widespread needs and wants than is possible by appeal to individualism, e.g., the construction, maintenance, and operation of roads, hospitals, museums, libraries, and schools.

Collectives including corporate organizations and institutions, provide security for the basic human wants. They sometimes do so, however, at great cost to individual liberty and to individual self-development. One form of capitalism that affects nursing is "managed care," which emphasizes cost containment in health care delivery systems and in a quite positive sense, requires that health care resources must be paid for to avoid bankruptcies in health care institutions, sometimes to the detriment of emphasizing profits over patients' health care needs and interests.

Existentialism

One form individualism takes is existentialism, which holds individuals responsible for their actions and inactions (or their actions and failures to act) equally. Early 19th century existentialist writers included Soren Kierkergaard (1813-1855), and Friedrich Nietzsche (1844-1900). Kierkergaard discusses and commiserates with the plight of the "solitary individual," and chooses a Christian form of existentialism as the way out of this plight. Nietzsche identifies with a robust form of anti-Christian existentialism, and distinguishes two kinds of morality, one for slaves and slave-minded followers, and one for those who rise to become leaders and decision makers in what he names and prefers as "master morality." For both thinkers, we are responsible for our self-development. For example, if a nurse fails to put the guard rails of a bed up and an 80-year-old patient falls out of bed, breaks his hip, develops pneumonia, and dies, then the nurse is (at least in part) responsible for harming the patient. Her failure to act is equivalent to a harmful act. We are all responsible for our omissions as well as for our commissions. But this question arises: To what extent can a nurse be held responsible? Part of the answer to that question depends on interpreting an important principle of Immanuel Kant's (discussed in Chapter 6), which states that "ought implies can."

An eminent existentialist, Jean-Paul Sartre (1905-1980), holds individuals responsible because "we are all condemned to be free."[11] To live is, as for Hamlet, to have to decide. One can be held responsible for one's acts only if one is free to choose. To Sartre, to decide is to be free, to choose is to be responsible. Freedom implies full responsibility for one's actions and inactions.

Existentialism and Phenomenology

On existentialist and phenomenological grounds, nurses as conscious agents are responsible for their patients as well as for all other persons for whom they can provide nursing help. If a nurse can help people who are in misery but does

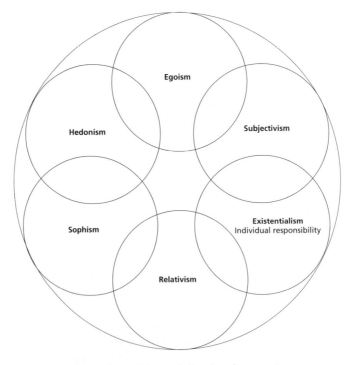

Figure 3–2. Existentialist developments.

nothing to help, then that nurse is morally blameworthy. According to the existentialists, we are all responsible for human suffering everywhere.

Another aspect of existentialism is its focus on "here and now"[12] or particular acts in place of abstract universals. Closely related to existentialist ethics is phenomenologic ethics, which is concerned with people's consciousness and awareness. Both theories converge in the emphasis they give to thinking about human acts and taking responsibility for those acts.[13]

Much is made, therefore, of the existentialist notion of "lived experience," which readily applies to patients' thoughts, experiences, and feelings, and which appeals to the role of the literary arts in bioethics and nursing ethics. Patients' and nurses' search for "the meaning of life" is captured by attention to narratives, parables, stories, and patient-nurse scenarios.

Unlike egoism, existentialism seems to place extraordinary burdens on everyone. Some critics argue that the existentialist theory of responsibility places too heavy a burden on any individual, a violation of Kant's "ought implies can" principle, which holds that individuals are not obligated to do what they cannot do.

However, a strength of the existentialist and phenomenologic theories of responsibility is that it points to a morally inexcusable example to what Thomson refers to as violating "minimally decent Samaritanism."[14] One example of this neglect is that of Kitty Genovese, who was stabbed repeatedly in Queens, New York, in the 1960s while 38 onlookers from neighboring apartments did not even bother to phone the police. Another example is worldwide indifference to Jewish appeals in the 1930s to immigrate to non–Nazi-held countries. A third example is the ignoble Tuskeegee racist experiment involving 385 African American men with syphilis who were not given readily available penicillin, in use everywhere to treat that disease, until exposed in the mid 1970s.

NURSING DILEMMAS IN DECIDING WHAT TO DO

There is a problem brought out in conceptual or definitional ethics defined by philosophers from Socrates (470-399 B.C.) to G. E. Moore (1885-1957). All efforts to identify good with any (natural or supernatural) value (such as health, pleasure, happiness, nobility, honor, or holiness) fail to answer a crucial objection. Others may present alternative ethical theories identifying good with some other, even incompatible, values. They cannot all be good. To illustrate, if Nurse A defines the good as pleasure, and Nurse B defines good as duty or holiness, how do we know which definition of good is correct?[15] If these values are incompatible or in conflict, as they may at times be, then there is no rational way to choose between these definitions of good. Nurse C defines a good patient as a quiet patient. Nurse D defines a good patient as an assertive, self-aware, even talkative patient. This type of example shows why "good" is not definable in a satisfactory way.

Moore pointed out that good cannot be defined simply as pleasure, because there are bad pleasures. One could also point to bad duties, such as the Nazis following Hitler's orders, or following the orders of an evil physician, nurse, or patient. Similarly, as Plato (428-347 BC) reminds us, what is regarded as holy may not be. We have first to answer this Socratic question presented by Plato in the *Euthyphro*[16]: Is what the gods love good because the gods love it, or do the gods love it because it is good? To adapt this example to current life: Is what people desire good because they desire it, or is it desired because it is good? Is tasty food good because we like it or do we like it because it is good for us? Plato argues for the second, whereas utilitarians (discussed in Chapter 5) argue for the first. To apply this question to a current health care setting: Is a policy of large public expenditures for liver transplants good because patients and health providers desire it, or do patients and health care providers desire such a policy because it is good?

SUMMARY

In either of these forms, self-interest provides a movitation for being moral. In the area of moral psychology, self-interest morality wins hands down. But in the area of justification, in the justification of "ought" judgments, self-interest morality encounters a serious conceptual obstacle. This obstacle occurs when individuals, groups, or societies oppose one another. The question then arises: Who wins? Who is right? Is appeal to power the way to resolve conflicts or dilemmas? Not when doing the fair, wise, or benevolent thing or when acting out of love for another is the best way to resolve a health care conflict or dilemma. As might doesn't always make right, as appearance is not always reality, and as desire is not always what is desirable, to do ethics is to consider further alternatives. This is not to disparage self-interest morality, which is the springboard of action, but to supplement it and to enrich it, and to bring together what we cannot do apart from one another.

There is one further sphere where self-interest morality stands out, where it may function to take a last stand. There are moral irreconcilables, where conflicts can and do remain unresolved, or where people live in insularity (such as some nation states) with divergencies. In such cases, there may be no winner or loser, and no right or wrong answer.

Discussion Questions

1. Which of the following options is in the self-interest of the mother and which option is in the self-interest of the daughter? The mother, Mrs. Smith, has one functioning kidney. Her daughter has lost the use of both kidneys and her mother is the best match. If the mother donates her kidney, she will depend on dialysis until or unless she receives a transplant. She is glad to do so, but a second child appears to be developing renal failure from the same cause as her sibling.
2. What are some examples of nurses who act on morally permissible forms of self-interest? What are some examples of morally impermissible forms of self-interest by nurses?
3. What difference, if any, is there between short-term and long-term self-interest?

4. Can one love another person without first experiencing self-love?

5. Can love ever be conceptually separated from desire?

6. What, if anything, is the moral difference between good and bad forms of love?

7. How many other kinds of love are there besides self-gratification; love of one's spouse, children, parents, friends, patients, church, money, power; love of art; and love of ideas?

8. Are love and caring conceptually interchangeable? How are love and caring ever different?

9. How many kinds of caring are there? What difference do these make in patient care?

10. In the example of Kitty Genovese, a young woman who was repeatedly stabbed and witnessed by 38 onlookers who did nothing, what would a minimally good samaritan nurse do?

11. What moral responsibilities does a nurse have toward the hospital in which she is employed if the union calls a strike? What moral responsibilities do nurses have toward their patients, their supervisors, and their colleagues?

12. How does self-interest morality play a role in justifying nursing and health care practices?

13. Is a nurse's self-sacrificing act ever an obligation? What does a nurse justifiably do, for example, in the case of a burning building?

14. When does "if it feels right, do it" not work for a patient?

15. How does Plato's argument that "we all live together" possibly refute some forms of egoism? What answers may an egoist give to such an argument?

REFERENCES

1. American Nurses Association. *Code for nurses, with interpretive statements.* Kansas City, Mo: 1985.

2. Scheffler I. Philosophical models of teaching. In: Scheffler I (ed). *Reason and teaching.* Indianapolis: Bobbs-Merrill. 1975;67.

3. Mackie JL. *Inventing right and wrong.* London, England: Penguin. 1977.

4. Moore GE. *Principia ethica.* Cambridge, England: Cambridge University Press. 1902;1.

5. Plato. *Republic.* In: Jones WT et al (eds). *Approaches to ethics* (3rd ed). New York: McGraw-Hill. 1977;29-46.

6. Shakespeare W. *Hamlet.* Wright LB, Lamarr VA (eds). New York: Washington Square Press. 1975;48.

7. Plato. *Republic.* Comford F (trans). New York: Oxford University Press. 1945;15.

8. ibid, p. 23.

9. Plato. *Republic.* In: Jones WT et al (eds). *Approaches to ethics* (3rd ed). New York: McGraw-Hill. 1977;29-46.

10. Hobbes, T. Leviathon. In: Jones WT et al (eds). *Approaches to ethics* (3rd ed). New York: McGraw Hill. 1972;182.

11. Warnock M. *Existentialist ethics.* London: Macmillan. 1967;39-49.
12. ibid.
13. ibid.
14. Thomson, J. In defense of abortion. In: Munson R (ed). *Intervention and reflection: Basic issues in medical ethics* (6th ed). Belmont, Calif: Wadsworth. 1999;70-79.
15. Plato. *Euthyphro.* In Edman I (ed). *The philosophy of Plato.* New York: Random House. 1928,46-48.
16. ibid.

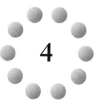

4

Virtue Ethics in Nursing

Study of this chapter enables the learner to:

1. Understand major aspects of virtue ethics, which includes the ethics of Socrates, Plato, Aristotle, St. Augustine, and St. Thomas Aquinas.
2. Clarify the role of virtues in the character development of health care providers.
3. Use virtue ethics to help justify ethical decisions in nursing.

OVERVIEW

Ethics or morality is not always easily defined. An ethical or moral issue arises whenever good or harm results. It follows that almost anything one does in nursing may cause good or harm. Helping a patient recover health and self-confidence is good. A smile, a frown, a grimace, eye contact or aversion, or a hand extended to another can communicate affection, friendliness, disapproval, rejection, or abuse. Doing good or harm or having them done to us occurs frequently, and these interpersonal actions affect us for better or worse. Deciding what to do for a hopelessly defective neonate or an elderly prostatectomy patient whose need for surgery is ignored results in good or harm. The difficult question is how to explain and justify what is said to be good or harmful. For example, is "pulling the plug" on a 10-year-old comatose patient good or harmful?

In Chapter 3 we discussed several self-interest theories of ethics. There are alternative theories of morality that develop out of self-interest morality, that overlap with virtue ethics such as the ethics developed by Friedrich Nietzsche (1844–1900). His theory of morality stresses nobility, courage, stamina, and the role of great leaders in place of equality and democracy. To understand ethics, one cannot take one theory of ethics for granted as providing the true and final answer.[1] The moment one settles on such prized values as democracy and equality, an alternative ethical view emerges, such as Nietzsche's that opposes democracy in favor of elitism. Related views, such as those of René Descartes (1596–1650) and Joseph Fletcher (1905–1991), emphasize consciousness and reasoning. Virtue ethics more or less originated with Socrates's method of argument applied to ethics, which consisted primarily in examining moral ideas that were generally accepted and in refuting irrational conceptions of ethics (i.e., Thrasymachus's claim that "justice is the interest of the stronger"). Socrates's famous student, Plato (427–347 BC), followed up the method of refutation by introducing moral speculations, hypotheses, and ideas that comprise a good life (in Plato's view), which we call "rational paternalism." (discussed shortly). Contrary to Plato, his beloved teacher, Aristotle (384–322 BC) taught that justice was not the basic value of society; rather, it was friendship. Aristotle defended this important moral idea admirably. Other philosophers also expressed their arguments, including St. Thomas Aquinas (1225–1274). Aquinas was influenced by Aristotle, and applied the Greek values of Plato and Aristotle to Christian ethics, giving Christian thought a corpus of intellectually defensible values. This was just the beginning of the story of virtue ethics.

The 14th century saw the rise of art, science, and technology, known as the Renaissance. Unlike the preceding philosophical views of Aquinas, the Renaissance was characterized by secularism (skepticism about religious beliefs), individualism ("I am captain of my soul," "I am an island," "I can do anything"), voluntarism (one's will leads the way), and statism (the big state). These four effects have exerted powerful influences on modern moral thinking and have determined, to some extent, the life, health, and death of individuals.

One ethical-philosophical response to the rise of science and technology is the conceptual adaptation of golden-rule morality to shifting times and circumstances. A second response is the continuing struggle between religion and science. A third ethical-philosophical response is the conceptual development of the social contract, which in turn spawned goal-based or utilitarian ethics, the duty-based ethics of Kant, and rights-based moralities that developed from the 17th century to the present.

FOUR VIEWS OF THE SOCIAL CONTRACT: ALTRUISM, OBJECTIVISM, SKEPTICISM, AND NIHILISM

As we have already discussed self-interest ethics or egoism, we proceed with alternative theories of the social contract on the grounds that self-interest ethics is not the exclusive source for the formation of the social contract. Proponents of virtue ethics also provide a conception of the social contract, beginning with Socrates's account as to why he is morally bound to obey the law.

To reiterate, a social contract is the agreement to live by agreements, even though those agreements may predate one's own time of life. When Socrates (469–399 BC) was condemned to death by the citizens of Athens for impiety and "corrupting the youth," he took the fatal hemlock in preference to escaping from Athens, thereby showing his refusal to disobey the laws and his acceptance of the social contract.

On interpretation of the social contract, nurses may find that the conditions of patient care are so deplorable that they have no choice but to strike. Nurses have a prior agreement to live by the principles of their professional code. The *Code for Nurses* implies that under harmful conditions of patient care, nurses have a right and a duty to protest and perhaps strike. Another principle orienting a social contract is that in a "free society," those who provide services do so based on fully informed consent.

Altruism

Altruism justifies a nursing action by appealing to the golden rule to (treat others as you want to be treated), and not by appealing to an individual's self-interest. The golden rule, in turn, is justified by appealing to a "higher law."

A difficulty with appealing to a higher religious or humanistic law is the lack of proof that such a law exists. A compromise that enables us to retain the strengths of both egoist and altruist social contract traditions is to recognize the need for appealing to rational and impartial third-party principles and bodies to adjudicate disputes.

Objectivism

Limitations to sophistry, subjectivism, and relativism give rise to objectivism. According to this moral point of view, there are allegedly "higher values" of good and evil that can be objectively determined. This view is sometimes associated with the "best interest" standard and is opposed by the "substitute judgment" standard, which seeks to sympathetically project a health care provider into the "shoes" or person of a patient and, to the extent possible, to do what the patient wishes. Conversely, the best interest standard appeals to an allegedly objective and rational basis for deciding what to do for and to a patient. As such a standard does not always live up to its claims, one may reasonably regard this standard as an ideal, rather than a standard that is necessarily operative in each and every case of health care decision making.

A practicing nurse in a modern hospital is well-advised to use the strengths of objectivism. These strengths include the idea that a nurse or physician does not decide what to do in a patient's interests unaided by the "checks and balances" provided by other health professionals. Objectivity is provided for the diagnosis of physicians and nurses by precise instrumental findings, such as blood tests and x-rays, that detect signs and symptoms.

Objectivism, sometimes identified as absolutism, points to the pitfall of nurses or physicians deciding for themselves what the right thing to do is in particular instances. For example, Jolene Tuma, RN, who advocated the use of laetrile, an unproven substance, to a distraught patient who did not want to begin chemotherapy for cancer.

Another example of a lack of objectivism is the case of *Darling v. Charleston Community Memorial Hospital*. The nurse's failure to report the patient's too-tight leg cast and cold blue toes resulted in gangrene, which forced physicians to amputate Darling's leg.[2] Here, nurses and physicians failed to appeal to objectivist values. Objectivism has its problems; it can be too distant to nurse-patient feelings and desires. Objectivism can be misused or abused by those who appeal to a higher authority to disguise their power motives.

Skepticism

A resulting approach to the controversy between subjectivism and objectivism is skepticism. One way to use skepticism is to apply the method of *reductio ad absurdum*, which uses counter-examples to refute a generalization. One counter-example to any ethical theory or principle shows a limitation of that theory in practice. If, for example, a health care instructor says, "Never treat a patient without a physician's orders," one could imagine an emergency situation when no physician is present where a nurse's action makes a crucial difference to the life or death of a patient. Such a situation would invalidate the generalization to never to treat a patient without a physician's orders.

Skepticism brings into moral discussion the dialectical processes of moral or ethical reasoning. Dialectics means a two-way conversation about important issues of good and evil, truth and falsity, meaning and nonsense. The dialogue is conducted according to rational rules and principles of discourse.

Nihilism

Ethical nihilists believe that every effort to solve moral problems of life and death, health and disease, is doomed to futility. In their view, the universe and all of life will come to an end. There is therefore no point in arguing for or against any ethical theory. Nihilists claim that nothing is worthwhile; there is no hope.

To its critics, nihilism does not prevent any basis for moral reasoning. Realistically, the world is largely self-limiting. We all die. The world may come to an end, yet we go on. Viable moral approaches celebrate hope and "here and now" reality, and a finite future of possibilities rather than a surrender to futility. One need not be a nihilist to accept futility at times, as does the stoic, as an appropriate response in the presence of tragedy.

THE USE OF THE SOCRATIC METHOD IN NURSING ETHICS

Socrates was a model of incorruptibility, courage, questioning, and the love of wisdom to succeeding generations of philosophers and teachers. Contemporary existentialists, to whom we later refer, praise him as a great decision maker, a man who was true to his reflective beliefs and unintimidated by authority, as well as a formidable intellectual challenger against any poorly formulated ethical arguments.

Several examples of the Socratic method are found in the early pages of Plato's *Republc.*[3] After Thrasymachus propones justice as the interest of the stronger, Socrates asks, "Now tell me about the physician in the strict sense. Is it his business to earn money or to treat his patients?"[4] Socrates then confirms Thrasymachus's grudgingly given answer, "So the physician as such studies only the patient's interest, not his own. For . . . the business of the physician in the strict sense is not to make money for himself but to exercise his power over the patient's body."[5] To Socrates and Plato, justice consists in functioning appropriately.

The significance of the socratic method for nursing ethics is that, as Socrates put it, "the unexamined life is not worth living." Critical intelligence in nursing consists in reflectively examining arguments for and against ethical theories, with a view toward exposing and confronting counter-examples, moral slogans, and principles that seem good, but which on careful philosophical investigation, are not what they seem.

PLATO'S RESPONSE TO PERENNIAL ISSUES AND TO SELF-INTEREST ETHICS: RATIONAL PATERNALISM

One ethical theory that affects the treatment of patients is that of paternalism versus libertarianism. *Paternalism* holds that the state, as a "father" figure, knows best and that each individual is obligated to comply with the authority figure, be it a patient, a nurse, a physician, or the state. Brian Clark's play *Whose Life is it Anyway?* illustrates an issue between a paternalistic physician and an individual determined to exercise his own will regarding his health. The physician gives the quadruplegic a tranquilizer against his objections. He also believes the patient should be kept alive despite the patient's wish to die. The patient acts on a libertarian ethical theory, which holds that individuals have a right to decide what happens in and to their bodies. One may notice some resemblance between current libertarianism and some of its conceptual origins in subjectivism and even its current doctrine: "Do your own thing."

One can appreciate that Plato is the major philosophical proponent of what might be called *rational paternalism,* which is closely associated with objectivism or absolutism. In his dialogue, the *Gorgias,* Plato shows that the good in a person's own view or what a person desires, such as eating fatty foods, is not necessarily good. Plato cites as an example that a person may desire cream puffs at the bakery and confuse such desires with the good. A contemporary life example is a mother who wishes to "pull the plug" on her comatose son, which may not be the wise thing to do. The sophists (sometimes known as egoists, subjectivists, or relativists) defended the virtues of selfishness, of looking after oneself first and last, and argued that "might makes right."[6]

Plato opposed the sophists and believed that looking after oneself first and last—or doing whatever one wants if one has the power or can get away with it by stealth, pretension, or lies—leads to moral and social destruction. He showed that we live well only by living together according to rational principles of justice—we need one another. Plato proposed a social scheme showing how people may live well together. His form of paternalism is an appeal to knowledge, wisdom, and rationality, rather than to force, tyranny, or ignorance. Plato favored a value scheme for individuals and societies in which reason dominates will, and will dominates appetite. He opposed the reverse, with appetite ruling will and reason.[7] Plato's rational paternalism rules out the practice of some physicians and other health professionals who place their personal wealth above a patient's health. A subjectivist rejoinder, however, is that life without individual freedom is not worthwhile. A Platonic response is that civilized survival is more valuable than individual liberty or freedom. Thus, one issue between rational paternalism and subjectivism in relation to health care and nursing is that of freedom versus rational security and control.

In the *Republic,* Plato relates the account of a challenge, known as *The Ring of Gyges,* which Glaucon (a sophist) makes to Socrates. Gyges the shepherd tells of finding a ring, which on turning one way or the other, enabled him to become reliably invisible or visible at will. With this power, the shepherd contrived to enter the king's palace, where he then murdered the king and raped the queen. Glaucon reminds Socrates that the drive for power undermines all objectivist morality. A nursing ethics corollary would be to ask, "If we could become invisible, would we care to be objectively good?" The challenge to Socrates was to show that justice is intrinsically good and that it is worthwhile for everyone to be good.

Plato responds to Glaucon's challenge with his ethical theory or rational paternalism. Plato recounts Socrates's question (by now Plato's creation in the *Republic*), "How is a society formed? Why do we have a society?" Plato's answer is that we all live together. None of us can live alone. To live together, we have to form agreements, or a social contract, that binds us to recognize and to comply with the requirements for being able to live together. There has to be integrity and trust for a society to exist.

Although some people lack self-control and temperance and try to take unfair advantage of others, society cannot allow the Gyges ring phenomenon or the abuse of power to occur. To allow people to do as they wish undermines all of us living together. To allow the abuse of power to exist means that we no longer trust and value one another nor will we be able to live well with ourselves. We will always be on guard lest someone or some group molest or destroy us.

Plato's teacher, Socrates, then provides an hypothesis as to how a society might be formed. People live better together than alone. In a hypothetical society, one finds four types of vital occupations: farmers, builders, weavers, and shoemakers. To Socrates, all four tradesmen are better off specializing, exchanging, and sharing their services, rather than trying to do all four things alone. Exchanging and sharing is a more efficient way to live than doing everything alone.

In a complex society with many more occupations and professions, a similar social, economic principle operates and is known as the division of labor. There must be those who supervise workers, those oversee the supervisors, and those who ultimately ensure that the principles of social and economic justice effectively govern the entire society. When everyone does the right thing, it is known as functionalism. Persons are what they do, not what they appear or pretend to do. To Plato's rational paternalism, "knowledge is virtue." A health care example is that a pregnant woman ignorant of her HIV positive status is likely to infect her fetus. Plato argued that knowledge is a virtue and ignorance is evil, as this example illustrates. Against the thesis that "Ignorance is bliss" or "What you don't know won't hurt you," Plato's rational paternalism reminds us that "What you don't know will hurt you," and that what hurts us is evil. Therefore, relativism or subjectivism, which neglects or ignores this principle, is morally wrong.

ARISTOTLE'S CONCEPTION OF ETHICS APPLIED TO NURSING: HAPPINESS THROUGH SELF-REALIZATION

Eudaimonism: Happiness-Based Ethics

Aristotle (384–322 B.C.), another great philosopher and a student of Plato, introduced several major ideas at variance to Plato's that apply to bioethics. These include his contribution to method, the practical syllogism, the concepts of experience, self-realization, weakness of will, and the meaning of happiness. To Aristotle, there is no single method of achieving the good life or in understanding truth or beauty. There are as many methods as there are inquiries, activities, processes, and goals. Plurality replaces unity. There are many goods (i.e., health, wealth, victory), not just one.[8]

Using Aristotle's view, the good for nursing is different from the good for medicine. And these may be different from the good of the patient. These are all good as long as they aim at some action, inquiry, or pursuit which, when applied to nursing ethics, benefits the patient, which results in eudaimonism or happiness for the nurse, patient, and family.

Practical Syllogism.   Another major idea of Aristotle is that of the practical syllogism. This contains a major premise, which is evaluative, and a minor factual premise, both of which imply a decision to act. A contemporary health care example of Aristotle's practical syllogism is:

- Major evaluative premise: All women ought to live a full, healthy life.
- Factual minor premise: The early detection and elimination of breast cancer for all women promotes a full and healthy life.
- Practical conclusion: Therefore, all women ought to seek early detection and elimination of breast cancer.

One readily recognizes and appreciates the relation of ends and means in Aristotle's practical syllogism. One may also use this syllogism to promote good health care policies and practices and eliminate bad ones.

Experience.   Aristotle believed that experience is tangible and concrete; we learn by doing. Contrary to Plato, Aristotle argued that humans rightly prize their senses; sensation is part of human nature. Finally, Aristotle comes to intelligence, which enables human beings to "live well." These qualities of experience and intelligence combined with bodily capacities enable human beings to live well or happily. To do so involves individuals seeking self-realization of their capacities.

Self-Realization.   The good for humans is happiness, which can be achieved through individual self-realization. A nurse can make a patient happy by giving the patient hope based on trust. To show how one can achieve self-realization, Aristotle presents *The Doctrine of the Mean*, in which he compares ethical action to aiming at a target. One responds appropriately, neither too strongly nor too weakly. To respond appropriately to a patient's health problem—physical, mental or emotional—is to do what is apt, and to avoid extremes that are excessive or insufficient. To Aristotle, for example, generosity is part way between being extravagant and being miserly. Confidence is a mean between arrogance and shame. Courage is a mean between cowardice and foolhardiness.

Friendship.   An important aspect of Aristotle's ethical theory is the importance of friendship. Friends show their caring for one another through the actions they take. They are moved to act out of virtue, and virtue generates other virtues.[9]

Friendship is more important than justice, according to Aristotle.[10] Between friends there is no need for justice; however, people who are just need the quality of friendship.[11]

There are different kinds of friendships. Some are prompted by utility or pleasure, and some are prompted by mutual caring and regard for one another. Friendship, happiness, and virtue are closely related—one cannot have friendship without virtue, nor happiness without virtue. Happiness, which marks the aim of human life, is basic to self-realization.

Weakness of Will. To Aristotle, the opposite of good is not always evil, but rather the inability to achieve the good due to "weakness of will" (akrasia). Persons who abuse alcohol, smoke, and overeat suffer not from being evil, but from not resolving strongly enough to do what they know is right. They know right from wrong as one knows true propositions, but they cannot live up to what they know. They lack the disposition to act in accordance with what they know to be right. They suffer from "weakness of will."[12]

The Meaning of Happiness. There are several controversial aspects of Aristotle's conception of happiness. First, happiness relies on external factors such as friends, good parents, good children, good health, beauty, and wealth. Platonists internalize happiness and de-emphasize the external factors of happiness.

Second, happiness is acting in accordance with virtue. One cannot be happy without virtue. To Aristotle, happiness does not consist in being amused or in having pleasure. Happiness is a lifelong disposition to act in accordance with virtue. One can be happy only over a full life, not just some part of it, such as a honeymoon or a patient's recovery.

Following are some implications of Aristotle's theory for nursing ethics. Nurses cannot be happy without self-realization. They cannot achieve happiness or self-realization without friendships with co-workers and with their patients. Nurses, like other people, can achieve self-realization, friendship, and happiness through their moral and intellectual virtues. For the happiness of nurses is in accordance with virtue, the virtue of caring, for example.

Epictetus's View of Ethics
Stoicism. Epictetus (c.55–c.135 AD), an eminent stoic philosopher, taught the importance of recognizing the limits of our powers and desires, which may lead to false hopes and illusions. For Epictetus, modesty, apathy, withdrawal, passivity, resignation, and acceptance of one's lot are appropriate virtues.[13] Acceptance of what happens and avoidance of other desires leads to a tranquil life. Epictetus's stoicism influenced Tolstoy's *Death of Ivan Illych,* Dostoevsky's *House of the Dead,* Freud's view that life is a struggle to be endured, and Kubler-Ross's work on the stages of dying, culminating in the resignation or acceptance of death.

The strength of stoicism is that endurance is a virtue, as are modesty and the recognition of individual human powerlessness in the presence of large cosmic events and forces. In nursing, we are ultimately helpless as we face the forces of life and death. Stoicism helps one accept the inevitable when our interventions fail. A difficulty with stoicism is that life, ethics, society, and health care institutions call for doers, thinkers, and pioneers. Persistent, active interventions in health care make a difference to the survival and longevity of individuals, cultures, and societies.

AQUINAS'S VIEW OF ETHICS: LIFE AS A GIFT

Natural Law

St. Thomas Aquinas developed the concept of natural law. To Aquinas, natural law is higher than any human or civil law. One can appeal to natural law to strike down any law or practice that one considers to be repugnant, such as abortion, homosexuality, masturbation, or rape.

Aquinas describes four kinds of laws: eternal, divine, natural, and human. Eternal law is "God's law for ruling the universe in all its aspects. Such laws presumably include the law of gravitation. Divine law commands human beings to act always toward their supernatural goals or ends. Thus, this life is only an initial aspect of one's next life, which is (allegedly) the more important of one's lives. According to Golding, "The most important natural law directs humans to their earthly goals in accordance with eternal and divine law."[14] Human, or civil, law relates eternal, divine, and natural law to human political institutions, which are governed by the (allegedly) rational requirements of consistency, coherence, and fidelity to the "higher laws." These higher laws depend on theological assumptions that not everyone finds to be rationally acceptable. These assumptions of the Christian faith are controversial, and provide a continuing philosophical challenge to both Christian believers and nonbelievers.

According to natural law, the desire for procreation and fruitfulness of the race morally legitimizes sexual activity between duly married individuals of the opposite sex. Premarital or extramarital sex, the use of contraceptives, or rape would be violations of natural law. Homosexuality is considered morally impermissible. Abortion, euthanasia, usury, war, and murder are also violations of natural law. Finally, "human law governs human beings" within communities in accordance with the eternal, divine, and natural law.[15]

A strength of natural law is that it requires legislatures and policymakers to justify laws, policies, and practices. For physicians to require nursing compliance to harmful procedures or medications violates a higher standard. A nurse may appeal to a higher standard in the same way one changes a bad law—by appealing to a higher natural law, as Martin Luther King, Jr., did in his quest for civil rights for African-Americans.

However, there are difficulties with natural law: What truth is there in divine, eternal, and natural law? Can such truths be established, verified, falsified, confirmed, and tested? How does one justifiably decide what constitutes the reliable earmarks of natural law? Rape and usury may be fairly easy to justify as evil, but what about premarital sex, masturbation, or abortion owing to rape? Are these acts all equally in violation of natural law? According to some reasoning skeptics, the case for natural law remains unproved. Other questions also arise: How do we know that natural law is really what its proponents claim? What shall a nurse do about a terminal patient's wish to be helped to die by withholding or terminating gastric feedings? Why isn't abortion morally preferable to giving birth to a person with multiple anomalies?

Christian Altruism

Aquinas is also famous for his development of agapistic, or altruistic, ethics, an important moral point of view that influences and is widely believed to justify moral choices in nursing. Love characterizes enduringly positive interpersonal relations, whether it be sexual love, romantic love, parental love, or love of country, customs, culture, and kinships. Love is the tie that binds humans together. Music, art, and literature have celebrated the force of love in human affairs. People sometimes live for and by one another's love. However, the love people feel for one another is no greater, and knows no greater, than the love of life, which makes all other feelings and love possible. Love is king of the positive emotions, too great and too brilliant to be extinguished or eclipsed even by its rival emotion, hate. Love is the handmaiden of peace, which makes more love possible, but it is opposed by hate, which brings about war and violence. Perhaps it is no surprise, then, that love is the centerpiece of one of the world's most influential religions, Christianity. A contemporary philosopher, William Frankena (1908–1994), characterizes agapism as holding that "there is only one basic ethical imperative [that is] to love."[16] According to Deuteronomy in the Old Testament (and later in Matthew 22:37–40), there are two commandments concerning love (with acknowledgement to Arkadey Gershkovich, a former student, for bringing this important but neglected aspect of Judaism to our attention:

> Thou shalt love the Lord thy God with all thy heart, and with all thy soul, and with all thy mind. This is the first and great commandment, and the second is Thou shalt love thy neighbor as Thyself. On these two commandments depend all the law and the prophets.[17]

St. Francis of Assisi (1182–1226) extends this love of God and of one's neighbor to the love of all God's living creatures. This love, and the test of this love, includes the love of lepers, love of the diseased and dying, love of the poor, love of all living things as God's "creations."[18]

Agapistic or love-based ethics enjoins each person to love others as much as oneself. Such an ethics sometimes calls on people to do extraordinary deeds on behalf of their fellow human beings, which people are not always capable of or interested in doing.

According to Jesus, when someone smites us, we are to turn the other cheek. When there is not enough bread and fish, we are taught to share what there is. On this view, we gain individually by giving of ourselves to others. There are two kingdoms: the earth and a higher, eternal kingdom. We live in the earthly kingdom for a short time, but afterward we live in the eternal kingdom forever.

The ethics of love applied to nursing and health care means that nurses show love, trust, and kindness for their patients. The word "care" is implied by the term "love." Care seems to be a pivotal part of nursing, essential to its calling. An important advantage of love-based ethics is that love is at or very near the core of all positive emotions or, to shift the metaphor slightly, love is the fuel and driving force of all worthwhile human feelings. A positive outgrowth of love and altruism is the development of golden rule morality, which says to treat and care for others as one wants to be treated and cared for.

Several difficulties exist in applying love-based ethics, however. One is that the force of love seems to derive, as does romantic and sexual love, from desire and as such, needs no command or imperative. It is surprising, then, to see love characterized as a commandment in the Scriptures and as an imperative by Frankena. If love flows from the heart, it needs no commandment from any source.

A second, and possibly more insuperable, three-part difficulty is that, as the saying goes, love is blind. It is not always discriminating. One needs a basis for deciding in a pinch to whom to extend love. As the title of one of Bruno Bettelheim's books puts it, *Love is Not Enough* (1950). There is a need for wisdom, reason, and moral priorities. A second, related part of this difficulty is that there are too many beings to love individually, and choices need to be made as to who is worthy of love. Third, (and this may explain the need to issue a commandment to love), while romantic and sexual love may come "naturally," the love of the poor, the diseased, and other beings may not be a love that comes so easily. We are limited not only as to who the recipients of love may be, but also as to whom we are capable of and interested in loving. In either case, to borrow an economic metaphor, the demand for love exceeds the supply. There is just not enough to go around.

Another difficulty in applying love-based ethics lies in the fact that satisfying material conditions of life may be necessary for having feelings of love for anyone. Those who are unloved cannot reasonably be expected to love others. A question arises as to whether the religious account of God, the universe, and the role of human beings in the world, or the humanistic account of the central role of people in human affairs, is a sufficient basis for reducing violence, war, and self-destruction.

Concerning happiness, Aquinas remarks that one cannot be happy in this life at all. One can only be happy in the next life. Whatever interest this view of happiness holds for some religiously devoted people, to reserve the word "happiness" exclusively for the next world, thus making its application to this world unusable, appears to be a linguistically peculiar use of "happiness." There is, moreover an Aristotelian rejoinder to the agapist: One cannot identify happiness or love exclusively with the otherworldly.[19]

SUMMARY

Ethical theories present us with conflicts, dilemmas, problems, tragedies, and stalemates. Philosophical ethics or dialogue between ethical theories also presents reasoned arguments in response to ethical issues in nursing. To the issues of euthanasia, Plato's and Aristotle's ethical theories respond with the idea that a good death is morally preferable to a prolonged, agonizing dying process. To Aquinas, a natural law theorist, taking life even from those who prefer death to life and who suffer from an intractable, unendurable terminal illness, is wrong and a violation of natural law. Who is right? Each theory presents arguments that a rival theory attempts to refute. How does one judge who is right? Ethics is not a science, a finished body of true propositions that yields a certain answer. Nor, however, is ethics purely subjective, for ethics also includes justifying standards that people have for living together to which people of diverse moral views appeal.

To judge between ethical theories, one appeals to *a paradigm case argument*, an example that presents a decisive moral argument and that refutes an opposing argument. In virtue ethics, Socrates presents several such arguments: one against Cephalus's idea of always returning everything, and another against the idea that the primary function of health practitioners is to earn money for their service. The altruistic and natural law doctrines present thoughtful and morally invigorating concerns. These contestable views help us to consider the meaning of good and evil in relation to nursing ideals and practices.

Discussion Questions

1. Do nurses act only out of self-interest? Should they? What is self-interest? Does it overlap with interest in others?
2. Can one love others or oneself exclusively? What is love? How many kinds of love are there? How can nurses and patients show love to one another?
3. What is the difference between a nurse's motivation and justification for caring for an intensive care unit (ICU) patient on a double shift? Can there by any kind of love that does not result in caring? Can caring be paid for, or is caring its own reward?
4. Should nurses receive fees for individual patients, like physicians? Or should physicians receive institutional salaries, like nurses?
5. What is a morally justifiable basis for compensating health professionals on different levels of qualifications in the giving of primary, secondary, and tertiary care?
6. Are there true or false statements in ethics? If so, what is an example of a true or false statement in nursing ethics? If not, are there standards for judging right and wrong in nursing ethics?
7. What is the relation of facts and values in nursing ethics?
8. How do facts or clinical assessments of data contribute to moral decision making in nursing?
9. Benner cites the case of an intubated, quadriplegic patient who could not speak in which the nurse expert says, "I just knew we could resolve this problem . . . so I intervened in his behalf with his multiple physicians."[20] How could this nurse use clinical data and a model of morality to make a difference in this patient's life?

REFERENCES

1. Rachels J. Can ethics provide answers? In: Caplan A, Callahan D (eds). *Ethics for hard times*. New York: Plenum. 1981;1–30.

2. *Dorrence Kenneth Darling v. Charleston Community Memorial Hospital,* Ill., 326, 211 (NE 2nd 253,1965. Certiary denied 383, U.S., 946, 1966).
3. Plato. *Republic.* In: Jones WT et al (eds). *Approaches to ethics* (3rd ed). New York: McGraw-Hill. 1977;29-46.
4. Plato. *Republic.* Comford F (trans). New York: Oxford University Press. 1945;15.
5. ibid, p. 23.
6. Plato. *Republic.* In: Jones WT et al (eds). *Approaches to ethics* (3rd ed). New York: McGraw-Hill. 1977;29–46.
7. ibid.
8. Aristotle. *Nicomachean ethics.* Ostwald M (trans). Indianapolis: Bobbs-Merrill. 1962;21.
9. Thomson JAK. *The ethics of Aristotle.* London: Penguin. 1955;311.
10. ibid, p. 259.
11. ibid, p. 459.
12. ibid, pp. 89, 124, 226–231.
13. Epictetus. *The Encheiridion.* In: Jones WT et al (eds). *Approaches to ethics* (3rd ed). New York: McGraw-Hill. 1977;84.
14. Golding MP. *Philosophy of law.* Englewood Cliffs, NJ: Prentice-Hall. 1981;31.
15. ibid.
16. Frankena W. *Ethics* (2nd ed). Englewood Cliffs, NJ: Prentice-Hall. 1973;56–59.
17. ibid, p. 56.
18. Jones WT et al (eds). *A history of western philosophy* (2nd ed). New York: Harcourt Brace. 1969;11, 149–152.
19. Aristotle. *Nichomachean ethics.* Oswald M (trans). Indianapolis: Bobbs-Merrill. 1962; 21–22.
20. Benner P. *From novice to expert.* Menlo Park, Calif: Addison-Wesley. 1984;52–53.

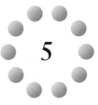

5

Consequentialist
or Utilitarian Ethics

Study of this chapter will enable the learner to:

1. Understand and clarify consequentialist or utilitarian values as the basis of moral priorities.
2. Distinguish between consequentialist and alternative theories of morality.
3. Justify decisions in nursing ethics in relation to the consequentialist theory of ethics.
4. Evaluate the development of consequentialist ethical theory in relation to nursing.

OVERVIEW

Theories of ethics or morality intersect with one another in formal, inductive, intuitive, and dialectic ways, and within institutions, societies, epochs, and cultures in a dynamism and momentum of their own. Changes in conventional ethics occur fairly frequently. Chinese women had their feet bound for centuries. People once smoked in office buildings. Child labor was once accepted. African Americans in southern states endured the humiliation of using segregated bathrooms, schools, and churches. Some of these customs, identified with conventional ethics, have undergone changes. But to trace such changes is to do one part of ethics, conventional ethics, but not to fulfill other vital parts of ethics, namely dialectical ethics, which is to justify conduct in a health care context.

Advances in medical science and technology and the technology of human reproduction have changed the character of moral problems. In this chapter, we consider some major utilitarian ethical theories that affect nursing ethics.

UTILITARIANISM

A modern effort to combine the strengths and to minimize the weaknesses of egoism, altruism, and rational paternalism is found in utilitarianism. Utilitarianism began with David Hume (1711-1776), a great Scottish philosopher. To Hume, ethics depends on what people want and desire. "Reason is and ought to be the slave of the passions."[1] The passions determine what is right and what is wrong. Reason has only two roles in deciding what actions to take. Reason can tell us what is true or false or what the facts are, and reason can tell us what means will achieve our ends. But the ends are up to us and depend on our passions. Hume's ethical theory marks a departure from Plato on the moral priority of reason.

To Hume, we act because of our passions. Our passions drive us to prefer pleasure to pain, and we learn to judge these by noticing the uses and consequences of our actions. Moreover, Hume illuminated the concept of justice. According to Hume, "the cautious jealous virtue of justice would never have a place in the catalogue of virtues" if justice was useless. He then cites four conditions under which justice would be useless. First, if there is complete abundance in the world, there would be no need for justice.[2] Second, justice would be useless if present scarcities continue, but because people are so kind, generous, and loving, they are happy to give scarce items to those in need. On this condition, all people love others more than themselves. Third, Hume considers the opposites of conditions of abundance and altruism, namely extreme scarcity and villainy. (For example, if there are acute shortages of respirators or medications or of nurses that cannot be alleviated, then one again finds the appeal to justice useless). For in times of extreme deprivation, people revert to laws of "necessity and self-preservation," and abandon their ordinarily high regard for justice. Fourth, if scarcities continue, but all people are homicidal monsters, then again there is no use for justice.

Hume's view of justice stands in stark contrast to Plato's, where justice is the main virtue of individuals and societies. Who is right in crunch nursing cases remains an unresolved issue. Hume does not, however, deny the role of justice. Despite Hume's skepticism about the centrality of justice, he makes this further observation: "Human nature cannot by any means exist without the association of individuals; and that association never could have taken place were no regard paid to the laws of equity and justice."[3]

One application of Hume's view of justice for nursing is: Hospitals consist of highly trained people, such as nurses and physicians, who come together in joint efforts to help the sick. These efforts could never occur without recognizing equity and justice.

A second concept that Hume presents is the relation of facts to values. According to Hume, every system of morality starts with propositions using "is" or "is not" and then suddenly concludes with propositions that are invariably connected to "ought" or "ought not." To Hume, this change is imperceptible, but is, however, of the last consequence. For

> as this ought or ought not expresses a new relation . . . it is necessary that it should be observed and explained; and . . . that a reason should be given for what seems altogether inconceivable, how this new relation can be a deduction from others which are entirely different.[4]

An example of the is-ought fallacy would be to argue that nurses in Hospital X have always received wages equaling less than 20% of physicians' wages, and therefore that practice should continue. To say that what is now the case ought to be the case, or what is not the case ought never to be the case, commits the is-ought fallacy that Hume exposes. The is-ought fallacy is a serious error in moral reasoning. Hume states that there cannot be more terms in the conclusion (e.g., ought) than there are in the premises (e.g., factual propositions).

A further example of Hume's is-ought fallacy in nursing is a supervisor telling a nurse that in Hospital Y, "We have always taken orders from physicians without question. Therefore, we ought to continue to do so." As nurses with moral reasoning skills can appreciate, an ought conclusion does not follow from the factual premises alone, because missing in such faulty reasoning is ample reference to justifying reasons for a moral conclusion.

Lastly, one may note the utilitarian stand in Hume's concepts. He views ethics not deductively, but rather inductively, by observing human nature and drawing moral norms, like equity and justice from his study of the facts and passions of people. A question arises, however, about the role of reason, passion, and facts. If the facts determine what is true, how on Hume's grounds does one justifiably conclude with an ought judgment? This question is especially serious if on Humean grounds, reason has only two roles to play—determining the means required for achieving a given end, and determining what the facts are. Hume's answer is that worthwhile passions of what is good, and therefore what ought to be, provide us with moral premises. These premises, along with facts, imply a justifiably moral conclusion. Hume cites this example of a worthwhile moral premise: Why do people choose to exercise? They do so to maintain their health. Why, Hume asks, do they wish to maintain their health? In order to live, says Hume. And that, Hume says, is the end of this series of "why" questions.

CLASSICAL UTILITARIANISM IN NURSING ETHICS

Classical utilitarianism was developed by Jeremy Bentham (1748-1832) and John Stuart Mill (1806-1873). Bentham was the first to develop a "hedonistic calculus." He noted that no matter what moral philosophers and moralists say, we are all governed by two masters: pain and pleasure. The point about ethics is to minimize the first and maximize the second as much as possible. This is now called cost-benefit analysis, which some people refer to as cost-risk-benefit ratio. One may ask about any desire: What does it cost? What is the risk? What is the benefit? To Bentham, the basis for judging any pain or pleasure, (the principle of utility) depends on seven criteria: 1) intensity; 2) duration; 3) certainty or uncertainty; 4) propinquity or remoteness; 5) fecundity . . . or the chance it has of being followed by "similar" sensations; 6) purity, as a pleasure of being followed by more pleasure rather than pain, and 7) extent . . . the number of persons to whom it extends or . . . who are affected by it.[5]

An example of utilitarian ethics applied to everyday nursing is the nurse's decision to give pain medication. This decision depends on the medication's predicted effect of diminishing or eliminating the intensity (Bentham's first criterion) of pain considered in relation to its side effects, such as the slowing of respiration. Similarly, some people drink alcohol to obtain a pleasure of some intensity.

Intensity also figures in the most intimate human experience, namely, sexual intimacy leading to and including sexual intercourse. Richard Wasserstrom, a contemporary philosopher, argues that the high degree of intensity in sexual intercourse is a basis for marital exclusivity in our present culture. According to Wasserstrom,

> It is obvious that one of the more powerful desires is the desire for sexual gratification. . . . Once we experience sexual intercourse ourselves and in particular once we experience orgasm, we discover that it is among the most intensive, short-term pleasures of the body.[6]

Duration, a second criterion of pleasure and pain, is also of concern to everyone. "How long will this pleasure last?" is a common question. Vacationers and honeymooners often dread the end of their bliss in some Paradise Island for return to the drudgery, dreariness, drabness, boredom, and monotony of their everyday lives and work. Conversely, how long a patient has to continue a particularly painful treatment again speaks to the relevance of duration in judging pleasure and pain.

Bentham's third criterion, certainty or uncertainty, is an important consideration in health care. Even the most innocuous, routine treatment, such as an aspirin tablet or a tonsillectomy, contains an element of risk. For certain patients, either of these beneficial therapies could end in death. Considerations of sureness and risk are relevant in evaluating which pleasures and pain to live by.

Propinquity or remoteness, Bentham's fourth criterion, concerns the nearness or distance of an intended pleasure or pain. Patients farthest away from the nursing station are apt to get the least attention. An example of fecundity or fruitfulness, Bentham's fifth criterion, that applies to nursing is continuous patient care, preferably by similar personnel, as basic for a patient's healing process.

Purity, Bentham's sixth criterion, refers to unmixed feelings. An example of mixed feelings, the opposite of pure pleasure is an excess of alcohol followed by headaches. The aim of nursing is purely that of relieving suffering and promoting health. Nursing is impure when mixed with business dealings with the patient. Lastly, extent, to Bentham, concerns the numbers of people affected by a consideration of pain and pleasure. Nurses with six to eight acutely ill patients in their charge will have to distribute their nursing services to a greater extent than if assigned to half that number.

An advantage of Bentham's classical utilitarianism is that it puts us in touch with feelings of pleasure and pain. A strength of the utility principle is that, in questions of resource allocation, it appeals to the principle of *sufferability*, one that includes the capacity of all sentient beings to suffer. The principle of *resource allocation* is based on the utilitarian and also democratic maxim framed by Bentham: "Everybody is to count for one, nobody for more than one."[7] This means that the pleasure-pain calculus considers that "the equal pains or pleasures, satisfactions or dissatisfactions . . . are given the same weight, whether they be Brahmins or Untouchables, Jews or Christians, black or white."[8] The idea that each individual counts for one is basic to the principle of social equality. In nursing, the equality principle means that nurses are to treat all patients with equal consideration.

A difficulty of Bentham's utilitarianism is that it leaves too little room for moral values other than pain and pleasure. Other important values are freedom of the will, duty, love, respect for the individual, truthfulness, or even saving an individual's life if doing so collides with the application of the pleasure-pain calculus.

John Stuart Mill attempts to remedy Bentham's difficulties. According to Mill, an action is right if it conforms to "the greatest happiness principle."[9] Using the utilitarian principle, one appeals to the greatest happiness for the greatest number.[10] This ethics is called "goal-based" because it renounces *a priori* or absolute preconceptions of how best to provide the good that is defined by the greatest-happiness principle. Rather, utilitarian ethics follows inductive methods of trial and error, currently called cost-benefit analysis, with the avowed aim to help the maximum number of persons to flourish. Mill says, "actions are right in proportion as they tend to promote happiness, wrong as they tend to produce the reverse of happiness."[11] To Bentham's criteria, Mill adds the quality of pleasure or pain, a quality appropriate for human beings. He adds this further requirement: "Utilitarianism requires [a person] to be strictly impartial as a disinterested and benevolent spectator. . . . In the Golden Rule of Jesus of Nazareth, we read the complete spirit of the ethics of utility. 'To do as you would be done by' and 'to love your neighbor as yourself' constitutes the ideal perfection of Utilitarian morality."[12]

Mill offers a proof for the principle of utility:

> The only proof capable of being given that an object is visible is that people actually see it. The only proof that a sound is audible is that people hear it. . . . In like manner, I apprehend the sole evidence it is possible to produce that anything is desirable is that people do actually desire it.[13]

In this passage, Mill commits the is-ought fallacy by inferring that what is desired is therefore desirable. That is like saying that, because Hospital X policymakers desire nurses to work a double shift on occasion, such a policy is therefore desirable and ought to be put into practice.

An advantage of Mill's greatest-happiness principle is that it takes the consequences of our actions seriously, a point which no opponent of utilitarianism can ignore. However, despite this and other strengths, there are several difficulties. Although Mill invokes the ethics of Jesus, utilitarianism is concerned with aggregate happiness, doing good for the greatest number, which is not equivalent to caring for and loving everyone. A few examples may show the difference between the ethics of Jesus and Mill's utilitarianism. If a tank with 10 soldiers and an innocent hostage tied visibly to its front is firing at you and 60 friends and neighbors, more lives are to be saved by destroying the tank and all its occupants, including the innocent hostage. Therefore, doing so is not wrong on utilitarian grounds. But such an action is morally wrong, according to the ethics of Jesus. Similarly, in triage health care problems in which some lives can be saved, utilitarian ethics emphasizes help to the greatest number. In the face of limited resources, an application of utilitarianism calls for the subordination of some people, such as the terminally ill, to the care of the majority of persons.

However, to pick an analogous problem, if 85% of the population of a hypothetical society live well at the expense of 15% who live miserably, utilitarianism seems to have no constraint against such a policy. Some would argue that such a practice is morally wrong. A difficulty of utilitarianism is that an appeal to majority happiness overlooks the value of the individual who, although in a minority, may deserve help. For example, the health care needs of mentally ill, retarded, aged, and other vulnerable patients may call for taxes that the majority opposes. Utilitarianism has no answer for these and other difficulties as to what to do about sacrificing some individuals for the good of the majority. One response is that situations occur during wartime or disasters in which there is no way other than to consider the well-being and health of the majority while sacrificing individuals. The use of triage—of sorting out the wounded into those who will survive without help, those who will die anyway, and those who can most benefit from help—is an example of the application of utilitarian principles. A prominent example of concern for the majority's happiness is the military draft, which places a number of persons, usually young men, at risk in defense of the large majority of citizens. Another example of utilitarian ethics is the distribution of scarce resources in response to majority happiness. An example in health care is the risk nurses and physicians take when they are exposed to patients with contagious diseases, such as AIDS, tuberculosis, and hepatitis. An objection to utilitarianism arises, however: Any such policies, which subordinate certain individuals or groups of individuals, can never be just.

CASE 5.1: Competition for Scarce Resources.   Two adult HIV patients, Ben and Herb, both desire the new experimental medication X. In addition to HIV, Herb has serious cardiac and kidney problems. Because Herb has these severe problems and a poorer chance for living longer, the health care professionals decide to give the new experimental medicine to Ben. Herb dies soon afterwards.

The utilitarian principle is to maximize benefit and minimize harm. Giving the only available experimental medicine to Ben satisfies the utilitarian principle in Case 5.1.

RECENT UTILITARIAN FORMULATIONS AND APPLICATIONS

Joseph Fletcher, a contemporary utilitarian ethicist, restates the biological/ biographical distinction used by utilitarian moral philosophers. Whereas biology refers to life, biography refers to one's ability to write down one's thoughts, and therefore to think. Fletcher cites several conditions for being regarded as a person, including a minimum intelligence quotient of 20 to 40, self-awareness, a sense of the past and future time, the ability to have human relationships and to show caring and concern for others; and to exercise some self-control over material and psychological conditions of existence. Fletcher's criteria boil down to the presence of consciousness. How are these criteria relevant to consequentialism in health care ethics? Fletcher characterizes his form of utilitarianism as "situationalism," which by his account, deals with "here and now" health care problems. According to Fletcher's "situationalism," health care is restricted to patients who can benefit from health care resources in relation to quality of life standards, such as enjoying neocortical functioning.[14]

The value placed on having a conscious life stems largely from a 16th century philosopher, René Descartes. Even though he was a nonutilitarian, his formulation of the nature and function of consciousness influenced succeeding thinkers to accept a definition of a person as one who is conscious. This aspect of a person, namely to have a conscious life, provides an invaluable although unstated premise of utilitarian ethics.[15]

A contemporary utilitarian philosopher, Thomas Scanlon, addresses the quality of life question. Scanlon argues that a rational person chooses to "maximize utility" not as a quantity but as a quality that enhances well-being, and this well-being "takes place against a background of utilitarianism."[16] He elaborates on the meaning of these thoughts in a recent book *What We Owe One Another* (Harvard University Press, 2000).

SUMMARY

Philosophical ethics can present conflicts, dilemmas, problems, tragedies, and stalemates. Such ethics or dialogue between philosophical models or morality also presents reasoned arguments in response to ethical issues in nursing.

For example, to controversy surrounding abortion, the agapistic ethics responds that abortion is murder, whereas to a utilitarian, the permissibility of abortion depends on circumstances. Each model presents arguments which the other or others may attempt to refute. How does one judge who is successful? Ethics is not a science, a finished body of true propositions that yields certainty. Nor, however, is ethics purely subjective. For ethics also includes justifying rules that people have for living together. Some ethical theorists express the way people live together through the social contract, which is the basis of all other contracts. The social contract bears a resemblance to Kant's idea of promising. For example, without believing in and honoring promises, we could neither write or cash checks nor trust anyone. The social contract expresses the values of making and keeping promises, which include keeping one's word; it also involves trust and abiding by rules and agreements. The appeal to the social contract, moreover, morally sets aside arbitrary and irrational excesses of people's wills (i.e., racism, sexism, terrorism, antisemitism).

Some forms of the social contract are too ambiguous to bear close scrutiny, e.g., altruism and natural law. A compromise form of the social contract is utilitarianism which, like egoism, has as one of its strengths the power to motivate people, including nurses, to accept its provisions, e.g., the greatest happiness principle. A feature of utilitarian morality that may appeal to nurses is its use of golden rule morality.

Following is a test case that distinguishes utilitarian and Kantian ethics: One can imagine an egoist or utilitarian physician refusing to treat an AIDS patient, leaving treatment to the nurses. One can evaluate nurses and physicians by who treats AIDS patients. Jones, an AIDS patient, will suffer avoidable harm—a violation of a fundamental principle both of ethics and of medicine—if he is not treated.

Discussion Questions

1. Is there a way to evaluate the value of nursing care at a patient's bedside using egoist, altruist, utilitarian, duty-based, and voluntarist ethical theories?
2. How can one justify an ought judgment in nursing?
3. How can Hume's concept of justice be defended in nursing ethics? What arguments are there against Hume's concept of justice in nursing practice?
4. How does a will-based theory of ethics, associated with voluntarism, contribute to the principle of respecting a patient's autonomy, and to a substitute judgment standard in health care?
5. How do rational paternalist, love-based, and duty-based ethical theories contribute to the best-interest standard?
6. What are some major strengths and difficulties of a utilitarian and a Kantian approach to the treatment of an AIDS patient?

REFERENCES

1. Hume D. A treatise of human nature. In: Johnson OA (ed). *Ethics* (4th ed). New York: Holt, Rinehart, and Winston. 1978;212.
2. Hume D. An inquiry concerning the principles of morals. In: Jones WT et al (eds). *Approaches to ethics* (3rd ed). New York: McGraw-Hill. 1977;214–216.
3. Hume D. Inquiries concerning the human understanding and concerning the principles of morals. In: Selby-Brigge L (ed). Oxford: Clarendon Press;206.
4. Hume D. A treatise on human nature. In: Selby-Brigge L (ed). London: Oxford University Press. 1973;469.
5. Bentham J. Morals and legislation. In: Jones WT et al (eds). *Approaches to ethics.* (3rd ed.). New York: McGraw-Hill. 1972;260.
6. Wasserstrom R. Is adultery immoral? In: Arthur J (ed). *Morality and moral controversies* (2nd ed). Englewood Cliffs, NJ: Prentice-Hall. 1986;19.
7. Hart HLA. Between utility and rights. In: Ryan A (ed). *The idea of morality: Essays in honor of Isaiah Berlin.* New York: Oxford University Press. 1979;79.
8. ibid.
9. Mill JS. Utilitarianism. (1861) In: Peist O (ed). *The Library of Liberal Arts.* Indianapolis: Bobbes-Merrill. 1957;10.
10. ibid, p. 10.
11. ibid.
12. ibid, p. 22.
13. ibid, p. 44. Mill JS.
14. Fletcher J. Four indicators of humanhood—the enquiry matures. *Hastings Center Report* 1974;4(6):5.
15. Fromer MJ. *Ethical issues in health care.* St. Louis: Mosby. 1981;12–14.
16. Scanlon T. Value, desire and quality of life. In: Nussbaum MC, Sen A (eds). *The quality of life.* New York: Oxford University Press. 1996;195.

6

Duty-Based Ethics: Universal Moral Principles

Study of this chapter will enable the learner to:

1. Understand Kant's principles of ethics, known as deontological, which distinguishes the hypothetical from the categorical imperative.
2. Clarify the importance of the categorical imperative, which includes truth-telling and promise-keeping, fairness, respect and equality, and exceptionless morality.
3. Evaluate the strengths and difficulties of deontologic reasoning in ethics.

OVERVIEW

Utilitarian ethics is opposed by Kantian ethics, the equal and uncompromising application of fixed principles, regardless of changing circumstances. If one chooses to treat Ben, the HIV patient in Case 5.1, and not treat Herb, one appeals to a utilitarian principle: Maximize benefit, minimize harm. But if such a patient is a person, not saving is immoral on Kant's, duty-based grounds or on Aquinas's love-based grounds.

Opposed to utilitarianism is the idea of principled morality or deontological ethics, whose major proponent was the philosopher Immanuel Kant (1724–1804).

KANT'S PRINCIPLES OF UNIVERSALITY

The first thing to notice about Kant's ethics is that he opens his book on the "Fundamental Principles of the Metaphysics of Morals" by distinguishing what is good with qualification from what is good without any qualification. He argues that the only thing that is good without qualification is a good will.[1] He then eliminates various candidates for being good without qualification, including intelligence, wit, and judgment, because one can always use these qualities for evil ends. Likewise, "courage, resolution, and perseverance" can be used for evil ends. The same argument applies to wealth, power, and honor. "Even health," he says, can lead one to excessive pride. Finally, Kant also argues that even happiness can be used for evil ends, because one person's happiness can lead to a smugness about the misery of other people. Thus, Kant concludes this early part of his ethics with the argument that the only unqualified good is a good will.

Kant then adds a powerful metaphor to aid his emphasis for distinguishing good will from any other good by introducing an imaginary "rational impartial spectator" into a person's moral deliberations. Such a spectator is contemporaneously regarded as a counterfactual conditional judgment, similar to Adam Smith's metaphor of an "invisible hand." Such imaginary conditions do not have to exist in reality to reveal the nature, function, and importance of the metaphor. One may ask what kind of being is good without qualification; for Kant, the answer depends on what would make "an impartial rational spectator pleasure, and therefore, contribute toward being not only happy, but 'worthy of happiness.'"[2] Kant's ethics, then, is an ethics that is about a person's character; and character depends on one's intentions, not upon the results of one's actions.

A second point to bear in mind when reading Kant's answer to consequentialist ethics is that he distinguishes between two kinds of imperatives. First, these are hypothetical imperatives, or "if-then" judgments and second, categorical imperatives. According to Kant, we all make numerous hypothetical imperatives, such as "If you want the patient to recover from pneumonia, then give the patient appropriate antibiotics," or "If you want to be paid, then show up at work on time," or "If you want to become thinner, then eat a reducing diet," and so on. But these imperatives are not moral imperatives, for each person decides what ends or goals he or she desires; however, some or all of a person's desires may, in fact, not be morally rational and worthwhile. Therefore, hypothetical imperatives do not qualify as moral imperatives.

The second kind of imperatives are categorical imperatives, which are the only kind that are moral imperatives. These address a person's character and intentions. Kant's criterion for judging an imperative is that an act is good if everyone ought to act for rational reasons and in similar circumstances, in the same way without exception. The basis for doing this is that it is rational, universal, free, and uncoerced. This is called the categorical imperative or universalizability principle, and it tells us to act always on that principle on which everyone in the same situation ought to act.[3] One is to act from the point of view of a rational impartial spectator, which alone is a worthy moral position. Kant cites five examples of categorical imperatives relevant to nursing ethics: 1) suicide or the taking any life is wrong, because if everyone committed such acts, then the human race would soon be extinct; 2) keeping promises is right, breaking them is wrong. Social institutions depend on people, including nurses, to fulfill their promises, and to do so without exception. One may note the relation of promise-making and promise-keeping to the social contract, the rule to abide by rules; 3) always tell the truth. To be rational and moral requires one to be truthful, regardless of consequences to oneself; 4) always develop your talents to the utmost of your ability. You owe it to the human race to develop to the optimum; 5) always help those in need. Everyone at some time or other needs the help of others.

On the basis of the categorical imperative and these examples of always preserving everyone's life, keeping promises, never lying, developing one's talents, and helping others in distress, Kant formulates a substantive principle, which is to act so that one treats oneself or another person always as an "end" and never as a "means" only.[4]

STRENGTHS OF KANT'S ETHICS

Paul Freund, a contemporary philosopher, cites an example from World War II to show how the "greatest-happiness" criterion, or majority rule, prevailed over uncompromising principles. A choice between allocating scarce supplies of penicillin to wounded soldiers in Africa or to soldiers with gonorrhea had to be made. The principled action would have been to give the penicillin to the wounded. But the decision was to give it to those "wounded in the brothels,"[5] so that they could quickly be returned to the battlefield. Another outrageous example of utilitarian ethics also occurred during World War II when the Moroccans agreed to help the Allies invade Italy on condition that their soldiers be permitted to rape Italian women, the Allies agreed.[6] These decisions expose a moral difficulty of utilitarianism. Appealing to Kantian moral principles shows no doubt as to who should be given the scarce penicillin, namely those who are wounded in battle. And wartime or not, raping a woman is immoral. However, if one appeals to some version of triage or to the greatest benefit for the greatest number, the appeal to some form of utilitarianism seems to provide the morally preferable decision. To ethical relativists, it depends on one's expected moral principles.

However, there is a price one pays in sacrificing moral principles. A war, a sports contest, or a business deal may be won, or a hospital emergency may be solved, all by ignoring a Kantian moral imperative to keep a promise, tell the truth, or to treat each patient as an end and not as a means only. A price to all concerned is that the moral quality of everyone's life will decline.

There is no room in Kant's categorical imperative for special privileges, irrational acts, or coerced acts. The universalizability principle upholds the right act, regardless of inclination, impulse, convenience, or even of the majority welfare. To act morally is to do what is rational, universal, and desirable for the whole human race, independent of anyone's pleasure and without regard for the consequences.

Despite a superficial resemblance, there is an important difference between the categorical imperative and the golden rule. The golden rule directs that we treat others as we would like to be treated, whereas the categorical imperative says to treat oneself and all others as everyone ought to be treated—freely, rationally, and impartially. For example, if one enjoys smoking or drinking excessively, then on golden rule grounds one may justifiably offer cigarettes and alcohol to others. The categorical imperative rules out such conduct.

Kant distinguishes perfect from imperfect duties. One has a perfect duty if the act of not complying with a categorical imperative violates that imperative, such as keeping one's promises, telling the truth, or refusing to commit suicide, no matter how inclined one may be to do so; or helping those in need; or developing oneself. In marked contrast, one has only an imperfect duty to do an act; for example, rescuing a drowning person who is too far away to save is virtually impossible without sacrificing the would-be lifesaver's life. For example, an aging mother with one functioning kidney need not risk a kidney transplant to save even her own child's life. Kant's important principle of "ought implies can" (as it is widely known in ethics) means that one's obligations depend on one's ability; however, one is not rationally excused from carrying out an obligation on the grounds that one experiences contrary inclinations. A patient's "call button" does not rationally excuse a nurse or physician who has a desire to finish a soda before rushing to a patient in need.

SOME DIFFICULTIES OF KANTIAN ETHICS

One difficulty with Kant's principles is that their application is sometimes impractical, in the sense that it is contrary to someone's inclination. Moreover, the unswerving application of rigid principles is a contradiction of what it means to practice ethics, especially in situations in which flexibility and adaptability are required. Although Kant denies that the categorical imperative is connected toward paying any attention to consequences, one cannot practice ethics and ignore the impact of consequences, even to one's most highly regarded principles. Even Kant's principles generally lead to consequences that are, in principle, good rather than evil, which explains why people are likely to carefully consider these principles. Even if one acknowledges the essential rationality of Kant's principles, this does not mean that one should follow all of his examples to their inevitable conclusions. To lie to an evildoer, for example, is not necessarily wrong. To fail to break one of two contradictory promises, if one clearly overrides the other, is not necessarily evil. If, for example, Nurse Jones promised to return a book to the crosstown college library by 11 PM and an acutely ill cardiac patient in the ICU needs continuous care at that time, then Nurse Jones did not commit an evil act by failing to keep her promise to return the book on time.

Kant's ethics also emphasizes the importance of one's will, which he identifies with one's character. However, the will he endorses is a rational will, which he equates with autonomy rather than self-determination, one's non-rational will, and which John Ladd, a contemporary moral philosopher, distinguishes in a recent lecture. Self-determination is doing what one wishes, such as smoking, disregarding one's diabetes regimen, or engaging in drug abuse, whereas rational autonomy consists in using one's will to carry out a categorical imperative.

VOLUNTARISM: INDIVIDUAL AND SOCIAL

There have been two major moral-philosophical developments influenced by Kantian voluntarism, which emphasizes the role of the will rather than the use of reason in human affairs and in social change. The emphasis in philosophy, up to and including the work of Kant, had been on the use of reason. One form of voluntarism is individualism (discussed in Chapter 3); another form is collectivism, expressed in this century as Marxism.

In response to Kant's moral conceptions (according to a lecture presented by the late Sir Iasiah Berlin), 19th century moral philosophers subordinated questions of truth and falsity to questions of the power of states, groups, and individuals in order to make social changes. Hegel pointed to the power of the modern state. To Hegel, religion provides a thesis in human evolution. This is followed by its antithesis, science. The synthesis of these cultural forces is the modern state, which accounts for change in human events. Hegel, Karl Marx, and Engels stress the power of states and collective groups, including voluntary associations, corporations, labor unions, and professional associations (i.e., American Medical Association, American Nurses Association) to make social change. Marx's epigram captured the new ethical theory: "Philosophers have sought to understand the world, but the point is to change it."[7]

The power of an individual's will, which Friederich Nietzsche terms the "will to power," gave rise to voluntarism as a moral and political theory. The relevance of voluntarism to health care ethics is expressed as "the will to live." To voluntarists, all virtues stem from the will. Schopenhauer (1788–1860) even defined good as whatever satisfies the will, and evil as whatever frustrates the will.[8] These forms of voluntarism, collectivism, and individualism have influenced contemporary ethical theories. Whereas collectivism is expressed as Marxism, individualism is expressed as existentialism and phenomenology (e.g., Kierkegaard's concern with "the solitary individual," and M. Buber with the I-Thou relation).

In modern society, voluntarism celebrates ambition, initiative, courage, nobility, assertiveness, and feminism. Voluntarism deplores submissiveness, obedience, and the "herd mentality" (to use Nietzsche's phrase). In nursing, Florence Nightingale, Virginia Henderson, Hildegard Peplau, Dorothy Orem, and other nursing heroes exemplify the importance of the virtues of voluntarism, courage, initiative, nobility, and assertiveness.

However, challenging questions arise for voluntarism: If there is a conflict of wills, whose will should prevail? Who decides? Is there a rational basis for deciding? A related challenge is this: How can one ignore the immense evils that have occurred under the ethical theory of voluntarism, such as Naziism? In nursing and health care ethics, tragedies unfold because a person's will (whether that of a nurse, physician, patient, or dominant family member) fails to consider the dim voice of reason. The excesses of the will, individually or collectively, remind one of Plato's adage that will is always subordinate to reason. The excesses of the will are expressed as Marxism, individualism is expressed as existentialism and phenomenology.

● W. D. ROSS'S ATTEMPTED SOLUTION: PRIMA FACIE VALUES

An important addition to the Kantian duty-based ethics is provided by W. D. Ross, who regards duties as prima facie (at first sight). These prima facie duties are taken seriously, such as duties of gratitude, of reparation, of reciprocity, and of fidelity. But these duties may be "overridden" in selected moral conflicts by appeal to higher moral duties. Although a nurse may have a duty to care for a hysterectomy patient's wound, a code blue involving at attempt to save another patient's life may override the nurse's initial duty.[9]

A FURTHER ATTEMPTED SOLUTION: KOHLBERG'S STAGES OF MORALITY

Another contemporary response to Kant's work, with an important ethical, psychological, and educational impact on nursing ethics, is the work of Lawrence Kohlberg (1927–1987). He proposes to refute relativism and subjectivism by identifying three levels and six stages of moral growth and development. Level 1 is preconventional, within which Stage 1 is oriented by fear of punishment and obedience to authority, and Stage 2 is instrumental and relativistic ("You scratch my back and I'll scratch yours"). Level 2 is conventional, within which Stage 3 is characterized by "nice guy, nice-girl" behavior, approved by the peer group, and Stage 4 is characterized by conforming to "law and order." Level 3 is postconventional, autonomous, principled behavior. Herein, Stage 5 is a "social contract, constitutional-legal orientation," and Stage 6 is a "universal ethical, principled" orientation.[10] Kohlberg's emphasis is not on conscience, because consciences differ. Rather he appeals to universal principles, such as saving life, preventing harm, and truth-telling. Human beings grow morally in these ways and through these six stages, according to Kohlberg.

There are merits in Kohlberg's stages of moral development. First, Kohlberg provides a good argument against subjectivism and relativism. Second, Kohlberg's analysis suggests parallels between intellectual and moral development. The higher one's intelligence, the more likely one is to be moral. In other words, cognition precedes morality.

There are, however, several flaws in Kohlberg's analysis. First, an account of how one develops morally, even if true, does not imply or justify how one ought to behave or develop. The is-ought fallacy that one cannot use facts alone is to imply values committed here. Second, one may arrive at the right moral decision of preventing harm by a conventional or even preconventional, egoist move. Even Kohlberg's example of a poor man stealing a cancer-curing drug for his wife appeals to self-preservation, a Hobbesian value, at the preconventional or egoist stage. Egoism is not always morally wrong. The egoist action might in some cases be the right thing to do. Should the poor man not steal the drug and thus let his wife die? On the other hand, if we respect property, then is stealing wrong no matter what the consequences? Perhaps a utilitarian theory would alleviate part of this problem by limiting the price of drugs.

Third, there are no proofs that the moral hierarchical method, in which one arrives at universal moral principles, is the valid and sound view in all cases. Fourth, if one's moral development could not be altered by a moral agent, then one could not be said to have a free will with which to make moral decisions. But if one could do nothing to alter one's moral behavior, there would be no point in telling anyone what optimal, desirable, moral development would be. Kohlberg's stages of moral development would be like describing the growth of a tadpole into a frog.

However, if Kohlberg intended his six stages as a proposal as to how individuals ought to develop morally, in which free will is assumed, then people would have a choice. When people make choices, good as well as bad may result. If there is a choice as to how to develop morally, then we would have no sure way of knowing how moral development necessarily ought to proceed. Followers of Nietzsche, Thrasymachus, existentialists, and others who give their moral reasons for denying the moral desirability of the sixth stage have not been shown that their position is morally wrong in all cases. One may prefer truth-telling and doing away with the use of placebos. Yet, in some instances, there are reasons involving the prevention of harm that could justify lying and giving placebos. To reiterate, Kohlberg has not been able to show that stages of hierarchical moral development from the lowest (egoism and obedience), to the highest stage of acting on universal principles is the way to become increasingly moral. Kohlberg has not successfully shown that the questions of ethics have true or justified answers.

SUMMARY

Philosophical ethics is an attempt to find methods of rationally resolving moral disagreements, and responding to stalemates and tragedies. Kant's ethics presents an attempt to provide a rational criterion for deciding what is morally justifiable. Kant's criterion is the categorical imperative.

Moral issues in nursing include the moral permissibility or impermissibility of abortion, euthanasia, and managed care. As previously noted, utilitarian ethics regards the moral permissibility of abortion as dependent on circumstances. In Kantian ethics, since murder is categorically wrong, if abortion is murder, then it, too, is wrong. In Kantian ethics there is a clear answer to what is right or wrong. Utilitarian ethics emphasizes right and wrong as a matter of degree.

Each theory of ethics presents arguments which other theories may deny or refute. How does one judge which theory is successful? Ethics is not a science, a finished body of true propositions that yields certainty or even probability. Ethics is a branch of normative discourse that is concerned with making justifiable value judgments, such as one finds in the arts, religion, philosophy, and politics. Normative discourse consequently does not result in making true or false propositions alone. Nor, however, is ethics purely subjective. For ethics is also concerned with arriving at justifying rules that people have for living as well as possible with one another.

Kant's idea of the social contract is expressed in his emphasis on the morality of promise-making implying promise-keeping. For Kant it is contradictory to make a promise and will to break it. The making and keeping of promises is a vital condition for the survival and continuity of any society.

The writing of checks presupposes that those who accept checks trust those who write them. Those who write checks are morally obligated to make good on their checks, that is, to have sufficient funds; and thus, to keep their promises.

As Plato wisely reminded us, to live as humans is to live together. Kant additionally reminds us that to live together is to make and keep promises. Making and keeping promises involves recognition of a form of the social contract. The appeal to the social contract moreover rules out irrational attitudes, such as those expressed through racism, sexism, terrorism and anti-Semitism. For these isms undermine the promissory aspect of the social contract, which is to abide by rational agreements.

Some expressions of the social contract are either too vague or too rigid and prohibitive. Kant's form of the social contract belongs to the latter. Kant's emphasis on the categorical imperative places excessive demands on the aspirations and even frailties of human nature. For Kant to rule out the desire for good health as a good, on the basis of its leading to pride, is an example of his rigidity.

An example of Kant's principles of promise-keeping and truth telling is evident in the unobserved behavior of the nurse who inadvertently contaminates a sterile package in the operating room but who, despite the disapproval and impatience of the surgeon, admits the fault and secures a replacement. Such examples of admission of error or other unseen errors involving the wrong dose of medication, show how a principled nurse benefits the patient's health and well being.

A feature of utilitarian morality that may appeal to nurses is its use of golden rule morality, which says, "Do unto others as you would have them do unto you." But even this highly venerated rule has its problems (as noted earlier in this chapter), which distinguish it from the Kantian categorical imperative. Whatever the drawbacks of the Kantian duty-based ethics, such as the inflexibility of the categorical imperative, the Kantian use of the social contract is clear and unequivocal (i.e., a promise is a promise), whereas altruism, with its call to express universal love, is too vague; and natural law, in some of its interpretations, is both vague and excessively restrictive to appeal to large-scale human interests and desires. For example, if an infant with multiple deformities and anomalies is kept alive at the risk of depriving three normal but critically ill infants of needed nursing intervention, then there may be ample justification for morally preferring to care for the normal infants.

A test case that distinguishes utilitarian and kantian ethics is this. One can imagine an egoist or utilitarian physician (under the older physician's code) refusing to treat an uninsured patient, leaving it to nurses to treat the patient. One can evaluate nurses and physicians by who treats uninsured patients. Jones, an uninsured patient, will suffer avoidable harm, a violation of a fundamental principle both of ethics and of medicine if not treated. A morally important aspect of both the *Code for Nurses*[11] and the American Medical Association[12] is that both codes point to the health care professional's responsibility to care for patients' needs and interest. This emphasis on responsibility in place of an individual's greed is consistent with Kant's categorical imperative to care for those whose well being morally requires being looked after.

Kantian duty-based ethics remind us of the role of truth-telling, promise-keeping and keeping one's word, and being a person of "good" character. This fidelity to one's principles was exemplified by Martin Luther King, Jr., especially in his "I have a dream" speech, and in his courageous stand against racism. Moreover, Kantian duty-based ethics stresses such human values as equal treatment of all people, respect for every person, freedom and dignity, and regard for human decency. Two closely associated social movements currently express this Kantian concern. Environmental ethics, for example, is concerned with global warming, pollution, and the ill-effects of strip mining. A second, closely related movement is known as communitarianism. Both of these movements emphasize not only virtue ethics (discussed in Chapter 4), but refer more particularly to people's characters, with special attention to the concept of responsibility as it applies both to individuals and to individuals as members of communities. A recent book illustrates this emphasis.[13]

A difficulty of Kantian duty-based ethics is that it is excessively rigid and fails to recognize the need for flexibility. Kantian rigidity may influence a nurse as a moral agent to therefore prefer consequentialist ethics for at least some difficult moral problems, or an appeal to Ross's prima facie view of principled ethics. But there are consequences to a society that is willing to forego principles, such as respect for truth-telling and promise-keeping. (In Chapter 7, we turn to a further effort in the form of rights-based morality, which attempts to resolve some of the difficulties presented by these four theories of ethics.)

Kant is often favorably remembered in philosophical circles for his two substantive principles of morality: 1) to treat any person, whether oneself or any other persons, never as a means only, but also as an end; and 2) to will the end is also to will the means. Regarding the first of these, treating people as ends and never as means only has inspired anti-racism, anti-sexism, and anti-exploitation of all kinds, such as women being paid lower wages than men for equal work. As for the second of these memorable principles, one may paraphrase another Kantian principle, namely that the ends of life, including principles and promises without practical applications and means, are empty.

Discussion Questions

1. What are the major differences between an ethics that emphasizes results and an ethics that emphasizes intentions?
2. Is there a way to evaluate the value of nursing care at a patient's bedside using egoist, altruist, utilitarian, duty-based, and voluntarist ethical theories?
3. Appealing to a duty-based ethics, how can a nurse justify a moral judgment about telling a patient the truth?
4. How can Kant's concept of promising be defended in nursing ethics? What arguments are there, if any, against Kant's concept of promising in nursing practice?
5. How does a will-based theory of ethics, associated with voluntarism, contribute to the principle of respecting a patient's autonomy, and to a substitute judgment standard in health care?
6. How do rational paternalist, love-based, and duty-based ethical theories contribute to the best-interest standard?
7. What are some major strengths and difficulties of a utilitarian and a Kantian approach to the treatment of an uninsured patient?

REFERENCES

1. Kant I. *Fundamental principles of the metaphysics of morals.* New York: Liberal Arts. 1949;38.
2. ibid, p. 46.
3. ibid. (See also Oldenquist A (ed). *Readings in moral philosophy.* Boston: Houghton-Mifflin. 1965;201–253.)
4. ibid.
5. Ramsey P. *The patient as person.* New Haven: Yale University Press. 1971;257–258.
6. Walzer M. *Just and unjust wars.* New York: Basic Books. 1997;133–134.
7. Marx K. Thesis on Feuerbach. In: Engels F (ed). *Ludwig Feuerbach.* New York: International Publishers. 1941;84.
8. Schopenhauer A. The world as will and idea. In: Jones WT et al (eds). *Approaches to ethics* (3rd ed). New York: McGraw-Hill. 1977;275–277.
9. Ross WD. Ethics. In: Munson R (ed). *Intervention and reflection: Basic issues in medical ethics* (6th ed). Belmont, Calif: Wadsworth. 1999;17–21.
10. Kohlberg L. From is to ought: How to commit the naturalistic fallacy and get away with it in the study of moral development. In Mischel T (ed). *Cognitive development and epistemology.* New York: Academic Press. 1971;164–165.
11. Code for Nurses. In: Beauchamp TL, Childress JF. *Principles of biomedical ethics* (5th ed). Belmont, Calif: Wadsworth. 1999;42–44.
12. American Medical Association. *Fundamental elements of the patient-physician relationship.* Chicago: 1996.
13. Baier A. *Moral prejudices.* Cambridge, Mass: Harvard University Press, 1995.

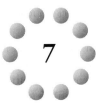

7

Rights-Based Ethics

Study of this chapter enables the learner to:

1. Understand the role, importance, and limits of rights-based ethics.
2. Identify rights as moral priorities in selected health care contexts.
3. Distinguish between alternative theories of morality.
4. Philosophically examine the strengths and difficulties of rights-based ethics.
5. Attempt to justify decisions in nursing ethics in relation to theories of ethics, such as self-interest morality, virtue ethics, consequentialist (utilitarian) ethics, duty-based ethics, and rights-based ethics.

OVERVIEW

Ethical theories and practices intertwine with one another in the four approaches previously noted. These are formal, inductive, intuitive and dialectical. These four approaches have a role within institutions, such as hospitals, societies, epochs, and cultures, often with a dynamism and vitality of their own. As for inductive or conventional ethics, dueling, once regarded as the way men had of settling affairs of honor, is practically extinct. Women in Western countries were once forbidden to wear trousers, to vote, or to smoke. Patients were segregated by race. However, times have changed. Smoking, once permitted in public places, is increasingly banned in public buildings. To avoid committing the is-ought fallacy, one is well advised to recall that the above examples are under the rubric of conventional ethics, rather than dialectical ethics.

The technological aspects of human reproduction have changed the character of moral problems. According to ethical relativists, values change with major changes in society, but is this view of values compatible with rights-based ethics? Do patient's rights, for example, change with time and circumstances? And is the ethical relativist view of values defensible? Were slavery, segregation, sexism, and antisemitism morally defensible at one time and place, even if times have now changed? Or were these views *never* morally defensible? This question, among others, will be considered in this chapter. A further question is whether there is one rights-based theory or several. We argue that there are at least two theories of rights that bear on nursing ethics. In this chapter, we will also consider rights-based ethics in relation to alternative ethical theories that affect nursing ethics.

ETHICS BASED ON JUSTICE: RAWLS

To offset the difficulties of utilitarianism, relativism, individualism, collectivism, and libertarianism, one turns to rights based on justice. John Rawls (1921–) attempted to provide an effective synthesis between utilitarian and absolute ethics. To Rawls, the idea of justice as fairness occupies a central place in ethics. Justice is uncompromising and is ". . . the first virtue of social institutions as truth is of systems of thought. A theory, however elegant and economical, must be rejected or revised if it is untrue; likewise, laws and institutions, no matter how efficient and well-arranged, must be reformed or abolished if they are unjust."[1]

Rawls argues that "rights are secured by justice."[2] As St. Augustine held, rights flow from justice.[3] To Rawls, rights are not merely declared by those who seek power over others or those who benefit from interests that require "the violation of justice."[4] Rights based on principles of justice "are not subject to political bargaining or to the (utilitarian) calculus of social interests."[5]

Rawls arrives at the idea of justice as fairness as a central principle through a powerful thought experiment, called "the veil of ignorance."[6] We are all to imagine not knowing our biological, social, economic role, place, or identity in the world. Imagine that we will not know whether we will be born smart or dull; healthy or disabled; white, yellow, red, or black; rich or poor; male or female; beautiful or ugly.

Rawls's veil of ignorance is a democratic challenge. Anyone is welcome to reflect on what principles a person would accept as a binding form of a social contract. Under this veil of ignorance, what rational rules would we agree to live by? Rawls suggests that we would rationally choose to live by two principles. The first is that we would want all people to have equal political liberties, such as the equal right to vote. This comes from Jeremy Bentham's older principle of "one [person] one vote."

The second principle is in two parts. First, social and economic inequalities arc justified only if they are of "the greatest benefit" to "the least advantaged," consistent with "the just savings principle." (This principle implies saving a fair share of resources for future generations, accruing to the benefit of all.) Second, offices and positions are "open to all under conditions of fair equality of opportunity."[7]

The principle of "the fair equality of opportunity" for filling offices and positions overrides the principle of caring first for "the least advantaged." Fair equality of opportunity generally favors the advantaged. Rawls's second principle consequently undermines the first principle, serving "the least advantaged."

Despite its problems, the Rawlsian conceptual scheme has an important role in health care and nursing in particular, such as fairness and compensation for nurses. Rawls tries to bring together two important values in distributive justice, satisfying large-scale health care needs and recognizing and rewarding individual merit in providing health care. Rawls's scheme attempts to give appropriate consideration for the advantage of all, including those who are least served, and to recognize merit by rewarding persons on the basis of equality of opportunity.

In health care, appeal to justice as fairness rules out certain profitable practices, such as the exploitation of nurses through unpaid overtime and overcharging the government for patient services not given. In short, Rawls's theory of justice exposes gross health care injury. Rawls aims to equalize access to the "primary goods" of life, such as power, money, education, and good health care. His work brings home to health care ethicists, including nurses, that there can be no ethics without justice, and that justice is to ethics what equal access to health care and nursing are to a good life for everyone.

RESPONSES TO RAWLS'S SOCIAL CONTRACT VIEW: LIBERTARIANISM AND EQUALITY

Libertarianism

There have been several notable responses to Rawls's ethical theory. Libertarianism (the view that the most important value is individual liberty) is a morally viable alternative to relativism and to Rawls's social contract. Its progenitor was John Stuart Mill, whose classic essay *On Liberty* provided the basis for valuing personal freedom as high as life itself. Robert Nozick, a major proponent of libertarianism, contends that the best state is a minimal state that protects individuals against force and fraud, or the "nightwatchman" state.

According to Nozick, a society that provides for the "advantage of all" imposes an intolerable burden of taxation in the form of "forced labor,"[8] and such a deprivation of a person's liberty can never be just. Nozick's basic tenet is that a state is morally legitimate only if it leaves people alone, unless they harm or deceive others. An individual has a right to keep what he or she earns. The person who climbs the coconut tree and gets the coconut gets to keep it.[9] Nursing or hospital administrators, physicians, or surgeons are entitled to charge whatever the traffic will bear, and no state is entitled to deprive them of their earnings. For a state to provide more than minimal services of protection against "force and fraud," and then to impose taxes to pay for public services, such as libraries, museums, schools, hospitals, and welfare,[10] is to coerce people into "forced labor."[11] By Nozick's account, forced labor is a violation of one's right to the free use of one's labor and thus is immoral. According to Nozick, if one sees a little boy drowning in a puddle of water, one has no moral obligation to try to save the child. It would be nice if one did, but an individual is not morally at fault if he or she ignores the plight of a drowning child. Such a position seems counterintuitive. A nursing example is that a nurse is not obligated to give mouth-to-mouth resuscitation to a stranger on the sidewalk in a large city. Nozick reminds us that there are limits to one's obligations, and this nursing example reinforces his point.[12]

Robert Sade, MD, a libertarian physician, argues that medical care is not a right, but a "purchasable commodity"[13] on the open market. Sade argues that a physician has a right to make a living just like other professionals.

A strength of libertarianism is that it stresses the moral value of freedom. Taxation that interferes with people's freedom to keep what they earn is considered to be forced labor and a loss of liberty.

A difficulty with libertarianism is that it assumes that the state has nothing to do with helping people achieve economic, social, and political goals beyond the services rendered by a nightwatchman state. This concept ignores the point that helping those in need may benefit the majority. Failure to tax a person's earnings for the common good, such as public education, public health measures for disease control, and public hospitals, results in an ignorant, crime-ridden, unhealthy society. Private earnings are justifiably taxed to provide for the disadvantaged. A person cannot be free if she or he is illiterate, diseased, or hungry. People cannot live free under conditions of ignorance, poverty, and disease. This requirement that we are all to contribute a fair share to help "the least advantaged" is termed by Thomson as "minimally decent Samaritanism."[14]

Equality

Ronald Dworkin presents a different response to Rawls's theories. He argues that the function of states is to protect individual rights equally. To Dworkin, such rights are "political trumps held by individuals"[15] that no state may take away. However, the emphasis in the concept of rights that Dworkin defends identifies rights with the idea of equality rather than liberty.[16] Because individual rights are held equally, people do not have a right to equal shares or equal treatment in the distribution of health care resources, but a right to equal consideration and to treatment as equals. One can recognize that the rights both to liberty and to equality are important to patients and nurses alike.

VALUES IN CONFLICT

To complicate matters even further, some moral values in health care are irreconcilable. For example, people want the prevention of harm,[17] but they also want minimum suffering as well as freedom of choice, as illustrated by the refusal of Jehovah's Witnesses to accept blood transfusions. In everyday life, people want both to eat excessively and to lose weight. People want meaningful democratic participation, fair and equal treatment, and speedy and impartial application of justice. They also want their own way, and some people think justice is on their side. They want virtues displayed regularly. They want the good life. It is virtually impossible to have all of these values.

These alternative moral models show that ethics is not a science with verifiable answers. For some issues, there is no rational way to resolve divergencies and conflicts. Nor can one beat down someone else's position by some definition of what is "ethical" or "unethical," such as may be found in a professional code such as the *Code for Nurses*. Contrary to the idea that there is objectivity in ethics, there are divergencies in moral views, as well as tragedy and stalemate. As the late I. Berlin pointed out, if there is only one kidney dialysis machine to serve two patients, then the excluded patient faces death. For every organ transplant there are numerous applicants with just claims that cannot be met and who are destined to die. What type of ethics should be used in such situations?

An answer to our dilemma of which ethics to choose—justice-based, virtue-based, self-interest-based, consequentialist, or duty-based—is to try to combine them all. People need both justice and care, as well as desires, duties, and regard for consequences. But how are we to bring these together?

POST-RAWLSIAN RIGHTS-BASED ETHICS

Paradigm Case Arguments in Health Care

There is a compromise between the unacceptable alternatives of objectivity and subjectivity in ethics. A promising lead consists of refuting paradigms or standard examples.[18] Paradigms or standard examples are partway between subjectivity and objectivity. A metaphysical philosopher, F. H. Bradley, once argued that "Time does not exist," yet another philosopher, G. E. Moore, refuted this statement by stating, "I had breakfast before lunch." A paradigm in ethics is found in Moore's classic examples of bad desires that refuted Mill's view that whatever is desired is therefore desirable.

An Argument for Rights in Health Care Ethics

An example of how the paradigm case argument may work in nursing ethics is the view held not so long ago that patients and nurses have no rights. To refute this, appeal is made to standard examples of rights in health care; these examples show how rights function. For rights provide the symbol and basis to justifiably override denials or abuses of decent treatment in health care settings.

Tuskeegee Experiment. The ignoble Tuskeegee experiment showed as decisively as any refuting argument can that if there are any morally justified values at all, they include human rights of patients, research subjects, and health professionals to informed consent. From 1932 to 1972, an experiment was performed to study the difference between those syphilis patients who were treated with penicillin and those who were not.[19] A public health nurse helped persuade over 300 African American men with syphilis to forgo the penicillin treatment, even though it had been tested and was available.[20]

According to Elizabeth Carnegie, RN, "experiments performed on human subjects by professionals . . . violate" the rights of subjects if done without informed consent.[21] As this experiment was exposed to public scrutiny, its immorality became obvious. The Tuskeegee experiment was a horrendous evil, a moral outrage, a gross violation of justice.[22] It is also a paradigm or standard example against the thesis that the nurse does not need to know anything, that a nurse just takes orders and keeps quiet. The exposure of the Tuskeegee experiment shows that there is no place for ignorant nursing. Nursing based on ignorance is a contradiction. Ignorance includes the moral ignorance of those who unthinkingly cooperate with an evil experiment. To be effective a nurse is required to have a high degree of knowledge, including the knowledge needed to help make justifiable moral decisions, which is possible in clear-cut cases of this nature. As a paradigm case argument or standard example, the exposure of the Tuskeegee experiment refutes the contention that patients and subjects have no rights, such as the right to informed consent.

Nazi Experiments. A second argument favoring the right of informed consent of patients and subjects is founded on the infamous Nazi medical experiments conducted during World War II. These dehumanizing experiments involved "sterilization techniques, cold water survival, decompression, and heteroplastic transplantation."[23] In addition, the Nazi genocide program entitled "euthanasia," which consisted of "techniques of efficient killing," eliminated "thousands of patients with chronic disease or mental illness."[24] According to Redlich, a group of Nazi physicians, called "doctors of infamy," who practiced under Hitler's chief physician Karl Brandt, carried out the selection and killing of patients "deemed physically or mentally unfit, with injections of barbiturates, phenol, and in most cases through carbon monoxide gas, the lethal component of exhaust gases from motor vehicles."[25] As a result of Nazi medical atrocities, the Nuremberg Code (1946), an international guideline for bioethics, emerged following the trial of 23 Nazi physicians for crimes against humanity. Among its principal points, the Nuremburg Code states that "informed consent must be obtained from all subjects."[26] Both of these paradigms or standard examples count as refuting arguments against the view that there are no rights for participants in health care, such as patients, subjects, and nurses. The infamous abuses of human rights contributed to what some people call Nuremberg morality; this is made explicit and incorporated in the 1975 Declaration of Helsinki.

The Women's Rights Movement. A third argument in favor of the right to informed consent is the women's rights movement and, in particular, Thomson's important article, "In Defense of Abortion."[27] Thomson's argument on abortion, her view of moral rights as a form of self-defense against abuse, contributed strongly to antisexist morality. She emphasized a vital principle in the ethics of health care and in social life that applies to nurses in particular. Thomson's foremost principle is that to have rights at all is to have rights in and to one's body.

Nurses' Rights. In nursing, Claire Fagin and her teacher Hildegard Peplau refuted the idea that patients and nurses have no rights by arguing that nurses have a right to refuse to administer electroconvulsive therapy (ECT).[28] Another refutation in nursing is the argument against the "master-of-the-ship" doctrine that the physician knows best, illustrated by the *Darling vs. Charleston Community Memorial Hospital* case in which physicians were held responsible for neglecting a patient.[29] One nurse was also charged with neglecting to report her observations, which could have saved 18-year-old Darling's leg, which after 14 days in a poorly prepared cast, had turned gangrenous and had to be amputated. The *Darling* case showed that responsibility is not confined to a physician or the hospital alone; it is also attributed to nurses. With responsibility, training, and ability come decision-making rights or privileges to decide within rules, such as those enjoyed by automobile drivers or professional practitioners. One writer calls these "discretionary rights."

Rights as a Form of Moral Standing Against Arbitrary Abuses

Although one may not think too well of some recent abuses or excesses of rights assertions, the paradigm examples cited show the role and justification of human rights. Rights as rallying symbols, cries, and slogans are generated by detecting and exposing violations of justice. To have rights is to have a form of moral standing. When you have rights, such as your right to an earned paycheck, you know where you stand and where others stand. Your right to your paycheck means that you have earned it and your employers, if they have not paid you, owe it to you. The attempt to take your paycheck away from you is a gross violation of justice.[30] A right is a justified option or permission to do, to have, or to claim that which one regards as one's due.

The Meaning and Importance of Rights

There are five conditions that help define rights. First, to have a right is to be free to exercise it or not as one chooses, without being blamed or punished for exercising or not exercising that right. Thus, the right to vote means one may vote, one has permission to vote, and one may rightfully demand or claim that right; but one is not required to vote, and no penalty or harm should be incurred if one chooses not to vote. Similarly, the right to treatment means a patient may demand or claim the right to treatment but is not required to undergo treatment if he or she chooses otherwise.

A second condition of any significant right is that others have a duty to facilitate one's exercise of rights in appropriate ways. The poll watchers and police have a duty to protect a citizen's right to vote if he or she exercises that right. Similarly, a patient's right to treatment means appropriate health professionals have corresponding duties to assure and protect that right.

A third condition of any right is that the right must be in accord with rationally defensible principles of justice. Generally, such principles coincide with equality, impartiality, and fairness. They also reconcile conflicting claims of need and merit in a fair proportion. Rights based on justice rule against legal and institutional rights that are not so based. For example, if Dr. Barney Clark, the first artificial-heart recipient (1982), had been the wealthiest person in need of this operation, then giving him the first artificial heart on that basis would have been unjust.

Another important aspect of this third condition of a positive right includes the right to be cared for or the right to assistance in living. If there is a conflict between a liberty right and the right to be cared for, one tilts in favor of the right to be cared for. People who smoke or patients who are HIV positive cannot be left alone to decide to act on their liberty right to pollute the environment or to have unprotected sex. The right to be cared for overrides one's liberty rights where harm to oneself or others results.

A fourth condition is that a right of importance is enforceable. Other relevant persons must recognize and effectively protect a person in the exercise of his or her rights. According to Becker, a philosopher, enforceability means that "if I have a right to your help . . . and you refuse, some sort of arm twisting is in order."[31] Enforceable rights are specific and special. In nursing, the enforceability provision means that in a hospital which honors a bill of rights, provision is made for "whistle-blowing" for reporting violations of patients' rights. Patient-care and ethics committees may also provide for implementation of human rights in the health care setting.

A fifth and related condition is that if a right is violated, set aside, or overridden in favor of some other right or value, then the person whose right was violated or set aside is given compensation. The concept of rights violations implies that something is owed to the victim.[32] Rights thus imply freedom, duties, and justice. These conditions, in turn, imply enforceability and compensations for violations or infringements. These conditions show how seriously a society takes rights and therefore how important such rights are.

Hare distinguishes three senses of rights.[33] First, to have a right in a minimal sense means that one is not wrong to do X. Second, to have a right means that others are wrong to interfere. Third, to have a right means that others have a positive obligation to assist rightholders to exercise their rights. Hare's distinction helps nurses to assess the strength of patients' and nurses' rights. A patient may have a right in the first sense without having a right in the second or third sense. For example, Jones has a right to play cards in his hospital bed, but not to to disturb others by keeping the lights on after hours. A nurse has a right to advocate higher pay, but she may not have a right in the second or third sense. Hare's distinction between these three senses of patients' and nurses' rights helps nurses decide what kinds of rights they and their patients have.

The Moral Importance of Human Rights in Health Care Ethics

Resulting human rights are moral rights of a very important kind, shared equally by all. These human rights are the union of two kinds of rights: self-determination or liberty rights, and rights to be cared for or well-being rights. To have a full-fledged set of human rights, however, is to have both liberty rights and rights to be cared for. One can critically evaluate legal and institutional rights by reference to human rights. The importance of rights is the conceptual link they provide between being a rightholder and being a person. To deny patients and nurses their status as rightholders, with all the conditions implied, in effect denies their status as persons.

The Appropriate Attribution of Rights

To have moral standing means that persons are entitled to be recognized and heard, and to have their views considered fairly and equally. Rights to protected freedom and care serve as a basis for claims and actions. According to Singer, to have moral standing is to be respected.[34] It is also to act responsibly by respecting the rights of others, and thus work within the rules for achieving and maintaining everyone's moral standing. A right as a form of standing is a social achievement, not a self-evident characteristic found in human nature; nor is a form of standing an inalienable birthright. There are no rights against wildlife or against events in nature, such as snow, rain, typhoons, or lightning. Rights are for people and are accorded by people, and the duties that rights imply are imposed upon and accepted by people as well.

The Justification of Rights

The justification of rights consists in showing, through standard examples, why a world with rights is morally preferable to one without rights. Rights enable people to do things, such as vote, pray, go to school, go to a hospital, receive Social Security payments, and do activities they enjoy. Rights are like red and green traffic lights, showing where people stand. A view of rights that regards rights as a form of moral standing, as entrenched and seriously held social values, places rights partway between moral objectivity and subjectivity; they are in some respects objective and in other respects subjective. Rights, after all, result from interests and desires. Yet rights are also a composite of other values, such as freedom, love, restraints, duties, and justice. Beyond that, rights break down in the recognition that tragedy and stalemate, too, are aspects of the ethical life of human beings that no formalization or objectivity can overcome.

THE ROLE OF RIGHTS AND VIRTUE IN NURSING ETHICS

Critics of rights in health care point to the high cost of malpractice suits and to the loss of trust and confidence that once pervaded health care delivery systems. These critics call for a moratorium on the language of rights and rules and a revival of concern with traditional virtues that contribute to character and community. Notable among these critics are A. MacIntyre, S. Toulmin, C. Gilligan, and N. Nodding, and in nursing, P. Benner and J. Wrubel. MacIntyre emphasizes the cultivation of virtues, such as courage, wisdom, prudence, temperance, caring, honesty, and responsibility,[35] that are developed in families and communities, which are the roots of ethics. Ethics is about character formation, from which laws and rules emerge. But without concrete applications in particular moral concerns, ethics becomes abstract, largely irrelevant, and insignificant to the lives of people in communities.

In the same vein, Toulmin distinguishes the ethics of intimates from the ethics of strangers.[36] Toulmin draws on Tolstoy's symbols of face-to-face interactions. Family members, friends, and neighbors with whom one frequently interacts are intimates. Most of one's day-to-day relationships are with these people. The boundaries of ethics are about these interactions. Then there are the distant relations we have with strangers, people with whom we have no deep personal relationships beyond politeness. The ethics of strangers appeals to formalized principles of justice, rights, and rules. Such rights and rules develop adversarial relations that include malpractice suits. We thereby give up the trust we once had in health professionals.

Gilligan takes virtue ethics a step further, arguing that the justice, rights, and rules orientation is designed by and for male domination. An alternative to this view is a feminist ethical orientation concerned with care and nurturing.[37]

Noddings focuses on the ethics of care, arguing that if, for example, a mother has to decide between saving her drowning child and a neighbor's child, then her first concern is and ought to be her own child.[38]

Lastly, Benner and Wrubel apply the ethics of caring (discussed in Chapter 1) to nursing situations. Caring means patients matter as meaningful persons. "Caring . . . fuses thought, feeling, and action."[39] Caring sets up options for dealing with a patient's stressful situations.[40] A strength of the ethics of caring is that it emphasizes features that are neglected by the rights-based ethics. A system of rights based on justice is not everything; people can lead a good life only if they also receive and give care.

A difficulty with the ethics of caring is that it avoids certain questions: Whom shall one care for? How much shall one care for intimates? How much care do I have to give? One cannot decide these matters without considering questions of the just distribution of health care resources. To avoid questions of justice invites ethical relativism and subjectivism, where people arbitrarily decide who receives what. The result will be a rationalization of whoever one wishes to care for, leaving others uncared for without ample justification.

RIGHTS AND VIRTUES

Can ethics help us to rationally resolve disputes? Are the ethics of rights and virtues compatible? We think so. Rights that are worth having are a composite of certain virtues, such as respect, dignity, freedom, fairness, and care. But rights based on justice are not the whole of ethics either. There are acts of extra devotion, courage, wisdom, prudence, temperance, generosity, friendship, and trust that are fundamental to moral rights. A community or an individual who does not have these virtues has no moral rights either. There is no necessary opposition between rights and virtues, provided that their structure and functions have been carefully thought through.

To offset relativism in judging nursing acts, there are moral principles, guidelines, and composites of the ethics of rights and virtues. These partially overlapping principles include consistency; coherence; truth; respect for rights and for life, liberty, and the pursuit of happiness; autonomy; promise-keeping; loyalty; care; generosity; sympathy; fidelity; freedom; equality; fairness; courage; beneficence; and nonmaleficence. These principles provide parameters and defining characteristics of ethics.

We can apply these principles into reasoned arguments, which appeal to rights and virtues. One might defend the principle that feminism is good as follows:

> Ideas, individuals, and institutions that promote the decent and caring treatment of people are good.
> Feminism promotes treating women decently and with care.
> Therefore, feminism is good.

One may refer to those moral ideas that merit special attention and recognition as rights.

Respect for feminism merits attention and recognition as a right.

Therefore, all feminist principles, like caring, may be identified as rights to be cared for.

SUMMARY

A society with rights based on justice, despite the drawbacks that rights present, is morally preferable to a society without rights, or to a society with rights reserved only for owners of nearly unregulated power over goods and over people. A society that recognizes rights based on justice for all persons, including patients and health care providers, elevates moral standing of all. Truths and rights are to the development of ideas and to social institutions as virtues are to the moral and intellectual development of individuals. Ideas, institutions, and individuals without truths, rights, and virtues are morally unguided. The denial of seriously held truths and rights by ethical relativists and subjectivists undermines their argument. Slavery, racism, sexism, and antiseminitism have always been morally wrong. But the ethical relativist or subjectivist could easily counter that any rights, including patients' rights, are up to the people of any society to uphold or deny.

Discussion Questions

1. Which principles of justice contribute to a just and equitable workload and salary scale for nurses?
2. Why is Gilligan's identification of feminine and masculine virtues, such as caring and justice, appropriate or inappropriate?
3. Is subjectivism refutable? How?
4. Which major ethical theory benefits AIDS patients the most? The least? For what reasons?
5. How would you show that rights-based ethics and virtue-based ethics are compatible or incompatible with one another?
6. Based on the theories of morality, what justification, if any, is there to the American Medical Association creating subprofessional groups, such as physician assistants or registered care technologists (RCTs), to supplement nurses?

REFERENCES

1. Rawls J. *A theory of justice* (2nd ed). Cambridge, Mass: Harvard University Press. 1999;3–4.
2. ibid, p. 4.
3. St. Augustine. *The City of God* (1647). Hammondsworth, England: Pelican. 1972;882.
4. Rawls J. *A theory of justice*. (2nd ed). Cambridge, Mass: Harvard University Press. 1999;3–4.
5. ibid, p. 3.
6. ibid, p. 136–142.
7. ibid, p. 302.
8. Nozick R. *Anarchy, state and utopia*. New York: Basic Books. 1974;169–172.
9. ibid.
10. ibid.

11. ibid
12. ibid.
13. Sade R. Medical care is a right. *N Engl J Med* 1971;285:1288.
14. Thomson J. In defense of abortion. *Philosophy and Public Affairs* 1971;1(1)47–66.
15. Dworkin R. *Taking rights seriously.* Cambridge, Mass: Harvard University Press. 1978;xi.
16. ibid, p. 267.
17. Hutt P. Five moral imperatives of government regulation. *Hastings Center Report* 1980;10(1):29–31.
18. Macklin R. Return to the best interests of the child. In: Gaylin W, Macklin R (eds). *Who speaks for the child?* New York: Plenum. 1982;294–295.
19. Marshal CL, Marshal CP. Poverty and health: The United States. In: Reich W (ed). *Encyclopedia of bioethics* (vol. 3). New York: Macmillan. 1978;320.
20. Carnegie E. The patient's bill of rights and the nurse. In: Nicholls M, Wessels V (eds). *Nursing standards and nursing process.* Wakefield, Mass: Contemporary Publishing. 1977;69.
21. ibid.
22. Cranston M. *What are human rights?* New York: Taplinger. 1973;68.
23. Vastyan E. Medicine and war. In: Reich W (ed). *Encyclopedia of bioethics* (vol. 3). New York: Macmillan. 1978;1696.
24. Gruman GJ. Death and dying: Euthanasia and sustaining life: Historical perspectives. In: *Encyclopedia of bioethics.* (vol. 1). New York: Macmillan, 1978;267.
25. Redlich FC. Medical ethics under national socialism. In: *Encyclopedia of bioethics* (vol. 3). New York: Macmillan, 1978;1016.
26. ibid, p. 1018.
27. Thomson J. In defense of abortion. In: Feinberg J (ed). *The problem of abortion.* Belmont, Calif: Wadsworth. 1973;128.
28. Fagin C. Nurses' rights. *Am J Nursing* 1975;75(1):82.
29. *Darling vs. Charleston Community Memorial Hospital.* 33 IL.326, 211 (NE 2nd 253, 1965).
30. Cranston M. *What are human rights?* New York: Taplinger. 1973;68.
31. Becker L. Individual rights. In: Regan T, Van DeVeer D (eds). *And justice for all.* Totowa, NJ: Roman and Littlefield. 1982;203.
32. ibid.
33. Hare RM. *Moral thinking.* Oxford, England: Clarendon Press. 1981;151–152.
34. Singer P. The concept of moral standing. In: Caplan A, Callahan D (eds). *Ethics for hard times.* New York: Plenum. 1981;31 36, 40–41.
35. McIntyre A. *After virtue* (2nd ed). Notre Dame, Ind: University of Notre Dame Press, 1984.
36. Toulmin S. The tyranny of rules. *Hastings Center Report* 1981;11:31–39.
37. Gilligan C. *In a different voice.* Cambridge, Mass: Harvard University Press. 1982;1–3, 20, 171–174.
38. Noddings N. *Caring: A feminine approach to ethics and moral education.* Berkeley: University of California Press, 1984.
39. Benner P, Wrubel J. *The primacy of caring.* Menlo Park, Calif: Addison-Wesley. 1989;1.
40. ibid, p. 1.

8

Ethical Decision Making in Nursing

Study of this chapter enables the learner to:

1. Use reasonable principles of shared decision making.
2. Apply the principles of self-determination, well-being, and equity as an integral part of shared decision making.
3. Assess the patient's capacity, willingness, and access to essential information as the basis for effective participation in shared decision making.
4. Use nursing guidelines and strategies in supporting the client's full participation in shared decisions.
5. Identify common fallacies of reasoning used in reaching unsound conclusions.

OVERVIEW

The rapid advancement of science and technology in health care has brought about better health, increased quality and length of life, and "new sources of hope for the ill."[1] The "technological revolution"[2] has widened the range of treatment choices within health care. The choice has moved from that of acceptance or rejection of a single intervention to the more complex question of which treatment to choose. Because each of these options carries different estimates of success, side effects, and degrees of intrusiveness, the implications for the patient's way of life are profound.

The mass media provide graphic, intimate details of artificial heart and organ transplants, in vitro fertilization, and fetal surgery to a curious public. The means, ends, and limits of health care are widely debated on television and in the press. Consequently, consumer expectations have changed. Generally, patients expect to maintain control and to be responsible for decisions involving their health consistent with their values, goals, and lifestyles.

The role of the health care professional is being redefined as well. The paternalistic attitude of health care providers is now much less accepted. Patients and families expect that professionals will share their knowledge with them as the basis for informed consent. Thus, the ideal is rational decision making based on fully shared knowledge, explicit ethical principles, and freely given consent. This chapter examines the values related to and supportive of this model. The patient's capacity and competence will be analyzed as necessary conditions for participation as an autonomous person. A guideline that incorporates these concepts is also offered as an approach to decision making. The term "approach" is selected, because ethics is not an exact science. Ethical decisions cannot be reached "simply by following handy formulas. No matter how carefully one issue has been resolved, the solution cannot be applied in cookbook fashion to another problem. Rather each issue . . . must be examined in the context of its particular circumstances."[3] Lastly, because fallacies of argument impede ethical decision making, such fallacies are also discussed.

According to Thompson, "The old-time hospital—the 'doctor's workshop' where physicians ruled without challenge—is fading from the scene."[4] Nurses, administrators, unions, families, patients' rights representatives, and lawyers claim a voice in making health care decisions and in asserting their authority. There is both an increase in numbers and diversity of the people involved in making ethical decisions. There is a problem in attempting to balance these various claims, but Thompson says that "there is no reason to assume that physicians or any other group have a monopoly on moral wisdom in these matters. But neither is there any reason to assume that the only solution is to give equal weight to each group or individual who thinks they have something to contribute."[5]

VALUES SUPPORTIVE OF SHARED HEALTH CARE DECISIONS

The application of the values and principles of autonomy, well-being, and equity are an integral part of the justifications for decisions reached and for the nurse's role in achieving them.

Values Expressed in Nurse-Patient Relationships

The role of the nurse in shared decision making rests on important premises. The first premise is that every competent adult has the right to decide what will be done with his or her person, that is, to accept, terminate, or refuse treatment. The second premise is that the patient's care, safety, and well-being are the nurse's primary commitment. This view places the patient in the center of professional scrutiny and activity with full patient involvement, understanding, and agreement. The third major premise is that the increasing complexity of health care requires an interdisciplinary approach to patient care situations. An important function of the nurse is to promote collaboration on behalf of the patient among professionals involved in that patient's care.

Values and Principles Underlying a Reasonable Decision-Making Process

The Principle of Self-Determination.   Patient self-determination is widely accepted as an important value to be respected and enhanced by nurses and other participants in health care decisions. The American Nurses Association's *Code for*

Nurses supports the self-determination of clients as a moral right.[6] Although the doctrine of informed consent has distinct legal implications, "it is essentially an ethical imperative . . . rooted in the fundamental recognition . . . that adults are entitled to accept or reject health care interventions on the basis of their own personal values and in furtherance of their own personal goals."[7] In addition,

> The right to control one's body and one's treatment and the emphasis given to self-determination, privacy, freedom, autonomy, and emphasis on not being deceived, and being given complete and truthful information, all point to an important aspect of a rights-based view, namely the role of an individual patient's will in individual decision making.[8]

This statement takes the position that respect for persons necessarily supports "self-determination as a shield . . . valued for the freedom from outside control it is intended to provide," and manifests "the wish to be an instrument of one's own and "not of other men's acts of will". . . . As a sword, self-determination manifests the value that Western culture places on each person to be a creator—"a subject, not an object."[9] This position recognizes that people define their values and assume responsibility for their particular lifestyle and health practices. An illustration of reasonable decision making is the Patient Self-Determination Act.

THE PATIENT SELF-DETERMINATION ACT

The federal Patient Self-Determination Act (1990) requires that every individual receiving health care be informed in writing of his or her right under state law to make decisions about that care, including the right to refuse it and to initiate written advance directives. This information must be available to the patient at the time of admission to hospitals and nursing homes, to health maintenance organizations (HMOs) at the time of enrollment, to hospices when care is received, and to home care agencies before care is given.[10]

The Act requires the institutions to provide policies, procedures, and personnel responsible for staff and community education regarding advance directives. The intent of the Act is to encourage adults to provide advance written directives in some form such as a living will or a health care proxy.

Nurses are frequently responsible for implementation of the Act in hospitals, nursing homes and home care agencies. Therefore, nurses need to ensure that patients, proxies, or surrogates (1) have access to the knowledge on which to base

---

Advance Directives

Living will: Document in which a person specifies his or her preference to consent to or to forego treatment in the event of future incompetence or terminal illness.

Durable power of attorney: A document appointing a proxy decision maker in the event of future incompetence.[11]

a treatment decision, (2) have clearly expressed their decisions and desires, and (3) receive treatment in accord with their expressed preferences.[12] Because of their close, frequent and intimate contact with patients and their families, nurses find patients who want to talk about advance directives or patients whose health care status suggests the need to do so. These can be positions of unclear and uncertain authority.

As employees, nurses need to know both formal and informal policies regarding advance directives. Hospitals and nursing homes need clear and explicit procedures for implementing the Patient Self-Determination Act, including lines of responsibility for informing and helping patients to complete an advance directive including the authority to witness.[13] The responsible person may be a social worker or patient representative, but on weekends, evenings, nights or in situations of compelling need, nurses are usually the appropriate sources of information.[14]

The Act holds institutions legally responsible for informing patients of their rights to advance directives. The Act "mandates that institutions educate staff and provide a forum for discussion of issues that become apparent as a result of its implementation."[15] Mezey views nurses as having responsibilities for the institution's compliance met through case reviews, ethics rounds, and quality assurance measures.[16]

Circumstances of admission or lack of understanding of the provisions of the Act may contribute to a patient's uncertainty about the treatment preferences. Nurses may be unsure about how to respond and exactly who is finally responsible. To respond to "morally troublesome cases,"[17] the role of such hospital resources as patient representatives, ethics committees, and risk managers are helpful if it is clearly drawn. Unit-based or interdisciplinary ethics rounds or meetings are also helpful.

Despite a patient's advance directives refusing treatment, he or she still needs continuous comfort care, control of pain, communication, and therapeutic interaction. Physicians may quietly withdraw from terminal patients and their families without acknowledgement of the major role played by nursing care in the well-being of these patients. Lines of communiction between and among the patient, family members, and care providers need to be clarified to help avoid situations in which there is conflict between the family's and the patient's wishes or the patient is simply ignored. Nurses can be pivotal in supporting a patient's decision-making capacity, especially in elderly, depressed, disabled, or non-English-speaking persons. In instances of erroneous assessment of patient capacity or a family member's imposition of his or her decision on the patient, nurses need to consult with an ethics committee or designate. A structure needs to be in place with which a nurse can feel comfortable and safe from reprisal despite calling into question another professional's assessment of the patient's decision. Whether expressed verbally or in writing, a patient's wishes take precedence over any other decision. "The PSDA (Patient Self-Determination Act) provides institutional support for mechanisms that address nurses' concerns about conflicts between patient, and family members and/or health care providers about decisions."[18] However, collaboration, among health care professionals provides the best assurance that the Act will achieve its intended aim of protecting patients' autonomy.

The Principle of Well-Being

Serving the patient's well-being through improving health is another justification for nursing and all other health care.[19] "The nursing profession exists to give assistance to those persons needing nursing care."[20] The obligation to promote patients' well-being is assumed to be the operational principle of the health care system by both consumers and care providers. Well-being is further supported by the principle of beneficence, which says that one ought to prevent harm and promote the good.[21] The nurse sees the nursing role as that of friend in the Aristotelian sense, rather than as servant or master to the patient.

In practical affairs, conditions such as breast cancer and hernias, for example, may be treated in several ways. Most health consumers accept the decision of the professional on the expectation that the patient's well-being is served by the recommendation of the nurse or physician. However, issues such as amniocentesis or termination of aggressive cancer treatment in patients with refractory metastases are value choices rather than purely technical or clinical questions.[22] The patient makes this choice based on furthering his or her well-being. Yet another way of serving well-being is achieved by supporting the patient's preference for one intervention over another that is recommended. For example, a patient with a slipped disc can be treated medically, orthopedically, or surgically. Previous episodes of prolonged bed rest for this specific patient were so depressing that the patient prefers the greater risk of surgery.[23] A professional baseball pitcher may prefer continuous cortisone for his inflamed elbow, rather than move to the outfield.[24]

Evaluating the patient's choices in terms of well-being emphasizes nursing and provider commitment to principles of promoting the good and avoiding harm by limiting the alternatives. Patients cannot demand whatever they wish. The choice is "among medically accepted and available options, all of which . . . have some possibility of promoting the patient's welfare, including always the option of no further medical interventions, even when that would not be viewed as preferable by the health care providers."[25]

Clearly, the definition of well-being is a broader concept than self-determination alone. The concept of well-being takes the patient's best interests into account in relation to the patient's self-determined goals and values. This process requires dialogue between practitioners and patients in which the patients' views, goals, and values are related to the available treatment options. Thus, the principle of self-determination expands to include the contribution of relevant practitioners concerned with the patient's well-being in the process of shared decision making. Self-determination and well-being may therefore be regarded as compatible values. The compatibility of self-determination and well-being takes the form of shared decision making. Shared decision making recognizes the professional's expertise along with the patient's evaluations of the options, the consequences of each option, and the relevance to the patient's well-being. Shared decision making also permits consideration of the well-being, goals, and values of family members. Constraints arise against permitting a patient to exhaust family resources when little or no patient benefit is likely.

The Principle of Equity

The ideal that people be treated "fairly and equally with all concerned"[26] has implications for both consumers and providers of health care. A traditional approach "is the Aristotelian principle of formal justice that like cases be treated alike."[27] This principle is applicable in the practice of government support of all dialysis treatments for everyone with end-stage renal disease. Arbitrariness is, in principle, eliminated. The principle of treating like cases alike also implies that differences are treated differently. To treat patients fairly may be to treat them differently, because their needs differ. There are, however, practical difficulties in applying both parts of this principle. Nursing resources are especially difficult to distribute fairly. Even patients with identical surgery and expected outcomes in the intensive care unit have different physical responses, emotional reactions, and interactional needs. Rarely is the nursing service adequate to meet all the patient care needs defined by responsible nurses. Nevertheless, a major value of nurses is to promote the well-being of their patients. Nurses do this by respecting their patients' rights and treatment options. In this way, patients are treated fairly as equal participants in making shared health care decisions.

ASSESSMENT OF PATIENT CAPACITY AND COMPETENCE

Fulfilling the principles of self-determination, well-being, and equity calls for familiarity with obstacles to reasoning. The nursing goal is to facilitate the patient's participation in decision making, which requires an accurate assessment of capacity.

Errors in reasoning may be committed by persons with the capacity to be rational. But some individuals lack both the capacity for rational thinking and for the correction of their errors in thinking. These differences need to be clearly differentiated because the goal of the decision-making process is to "advance the ability of patients to maintain control of, and be responsible for, decisions regarding their lives and their health."[28] To be an effective participant in the decision process, three factors are essential.[29] First, the patient possesses the capacity to participate. Second, the decision is voluntary. Third, the patient acquires access to essential information relevant to the health problem and to related life goals, plans, and values. (Note the role of chapters 3, 4, and 5 as guides to nurses' moral decision making.)

Patient Capacity to Make Rational Decisions

The capacity to participate effectively depends on the "mental, emotional, and legal" ability to do so.[30] The "decision-making capacity is specific to a particular decision and depends . . . on the person's actual functioning in situations in which a decision about health care is to be made."[31] Obviously, infants, young children, comatose persons, and severely mentally disabled persons are incapacitated, and they require separate consideration. In borderline cases, careful assessment of the patient's comprehension and reasoning by nurses in contact with the patient in various situations and times of day and night is a major contribution to the evaluation process, as in the "sundown syndrome," the case of a patient alert in the morning but confused in the evening. Thus, nurses are in the best position to evaluate the effects of psychotropic drugs on the patient. Through observation, nurses can identify gaps in a patient's information and supply the missing knowledge. Eventually, the patient's capacity or incapacity to make a decision regarding treatment must be established and resolution secured.

Determination of the patient's capacity to make a decision relates to the individual's abilities, the demands of the decision task, and the probable consequences of the choice. The President's Commission[32] views the capacity to make decisions as requiring:

1. Possession of a set of values and goals;
2. The ability to communicate and to understand information; and
3. The ability to reason and to deliberate about one's choice.

A framework of goals and values is necessary for the patient to decide what is good or bad for him or her. The ability to seek, receive, and give information with understanding requires language and conceptual skills sufficient to grasp the task at hand. Life experience is useful for appreciating the significance of alternative medical interventions and lifestyles.[33] The capacity to reason and to deliberate enables the patient to evaluate the effect of alternative decisions on his or her goals and plans.[34] This capacity includes the ability to weigh probabilities and possibilities in terms of present and future consequences to the self.

The President's Commission suggests criteria for assessment of the patient's capacity to make a particular decision regarding treatment.[35] These criteria are:

1. The ability to understand relevant facts and values;
2. The ability to weigh a decision within a framework of values and goals;
3. The ability to reason and deliberate about this information; and
4. The ability to give reasons for the decision, in light of the facts, the alternatives, and the impact of the decision on the patient's own goals and values.

In everyday practice, it is generally only those patients who disagree with a health professional's recommendation who are scrutinized regarding their decision-making capacity. If the patient agrees with the recommendation, and the family does too, then the patient's capacity usually remains unquestioned. When refusal of treatment is considered detrimental to well-being, then there may be grounds for questioning the patient's decision-making capacity. The patient's refusal, however, is the beginning rather than the end of dialogue with the patient about the situation. If the patient both fully understands the situation and demonstrates sound reasoning ability, then the patient's decision to refuse treatment is final and must be respected.[36]

Patient Incapacity to Make Rational Decisions

The terms *incompetence* and *incapacity* are roughly synonymous, although *competence* is a legal concept determined by a court. Decision-making capacity is an important requirement for exercising self-determination rights. Infants, small children, comatose patients, severely retarded patients, and seriously disturbed persons are identified as clearly lacking decision-making capacities. One problem, however, is to determine appropriate criteria for deciding difficult cases that border on incapacity. Examples are patients with mild retardation, young children and adolescents, and those with advancing senility. Especially difficult are patients who refuse treatment that will aid them to achieve autonomy. Macklin supports overriding a psychiatric patient's right to refuse treatment in such cases.[37] Macklin's compelling reason for the apparent arbitrariness is that a patient's rational powers and autonomy are increased by treatment when the patient's consenting organ itself, the mind, is affected.

The reason for having a clear boundary is that a competent patient may forego, refuse, or terminate treatment, whereas incompetent persons' "wishes may be overridden in order to protect their lives and well-being."[38] When persons are considered incompetent, other interested persons exercise decision-making capacities on their behalf. For example, a father, knowing that his 10-year-old son has cancer in his leg, may consent to surgical amputation of the leg while actively seeking the child's understanding and assent to the procedure on the grounds that it is life-saving.

A person who is judged competent (and this is a legal and minimal indicator of capacity) is one who is put in a position to exercise and enjoy self-determination rights.

Best Interest Versus Substitute Judgment

There are two standards to deal with those who lack a decision-making capacity: "substitute judgment" and "best interests." The standard of substitute judgment "requires that the surrogate (the person who stands in for the incapacitated person) attempt to replicate faithfully the decision that the incapacitated person would make if he or she were able to make a choice."[39] There are constraints imposed on the surrogate, namely "the same limitations that society legitimately imposes on patients who are capable of deciding for themselves."[40] There are, additionally, "reasonableness" requirements concerning certain risky procedures, for example; a substitute decision maker may not make these decisions on behalf of an incapacitated person.[41] On the other hand, "decision making guided by the best interest standard requires a surrogate to do what, from an objective standpoint, appears to promote a patient's good without reference to the patient's actual or supposed preferences."[42]

The substitute-judgment standard is intended to be faithful to the tradition that honors individual self-determination. The best-interest standard, on the other hand, is intended to carry out the patient's rational interests, those the patient would choose if he or she were rational. For example, an incapacitated Jehovah's Witness patient who would refuse blood transfusions would be treated differently by each standard. If the standard of substitute judgment is used, a Jehovah's Witness patient may die from lack of blood. With the best-interest standard, such a patient may be given a transfusion and saved. The nurse's role as advocate and watchdog is to protect the patient's best interests and impose rational restraints against legally and morally impermissible health care interventions. But determining which of these standards to use is sometimes an intractable dilemma. If priority is given to a patient's well-being over self-determination, then the best-interest standard is invoked. In emergency situations, the best-interest standard is usually applied. The further away the health care team members are from a patient's circumstances, the more apt these members are to invoke the best-interest standard. A difficulty with the best-interest standard is that appeal to this standard may mask an ambiguity—the patient's best interest or the best interests of other people in society. These two standards do not always coincide. Nevertheless, the best-interest standard may frequently present a rational form of the golden rule. This cannot always be said of the substitute-judgment standard.

The substitute-judgment and best-interest standards may be regarded as bipolarities. Justifiable health care decision making takes appropriate account of both. One guideline for ethical decision making is to respect and develop the grounds for self-determination wherever possible. This value is at the core of personhood, and one's best interests are at the periphery. Well-being depends on self-determination and the fulfillment of one's best interests. When these conflict, as they do for Jehovah's Witnesses, the best-interest standard prevails by the appointment of a guardian to consent to transfusion for a child. However, a conscious, competent adult may refuse blood even at the cost of life.

One may imagine or write down two concentric circles designed to portray the relation between self-determination and one's best interests, with rational self-determination at the core of a person's being. This value is sometimes called *rational independence* or *autonomy.* When independence fails or is inoperative, as it is in infancy and in a comatose state, the best-interest standard comes into play.

Patient Voluntariness

Another necessary condition for informed consent is that the patient's final choice is voluntary, free from coercion and manipulation. The principle of voluntariness is both a legal and a moral imperative that respects patient self-determination.

Serious illness is coercive of both the patient and health professional, because there are often no options or only unsatisfactory options available. The limits are real and beyond human control. Thus, voluntariness is often partial in specific cases. Limited voluntariness in patients who are acutely or seriously ill and dependent on professional expertise for guidance is clearly evident. These patients are particularly susceptible to subtle, or even overt, manipulations of their wills and, consequently, compromise of their voluntariness. A great deal of routine nursing and health care falls into the category of forced treatment, because it is given without the informed consent of patients. For example, patients are expected to turn, cough, breathe deeply, get out of bed, and urinate on the nurse's command. Routine laboratory and diagnostic tests are usually ordered and performed without the patient's consent on the assumption that the patient's admission to a hospital is in itself a consenting act.

Forced treatments include interventions given without patients' consent or even against their objections. Mandatory vaccination, chlorinating public drinking water, and sedating violent mental patients are good examples of forced treatment performed to serve the public good, which is not necessarily wrong, as these examples show.

A coerced decision results when a patient is threatened with undesirable consequences unless he or she agrees to the intervention. Psychiatric patients may be threatened with discharge unless they agree to ECT as the "only hope for lifting depression after drugs fail." Patients who refuse treatment such as getting out of bed when the nurse is ready to administer therapy may receive threats of the nurse's being too busy or unavailable later on. The greater the disparity in power and status between the patient, the nurse, and the physician, the greater the potential for the abuse or neglect of voluntariness among "captive" patient populations, such as those in nursing homes, group homes, and mental institutions. Sometimes the family coerces a patient to accept an unwanted intervention with little hope of benefit. Conversely, the family may either directly or subtly manipulate a patient into refusing expensive treatment with potential benefit.

Manipulation of the patient to secure agreement to an intervention is easily accomplished with clients who completely trust and depend on their physicians and nurses for decisions. Such patients regard themselves as ignorant. They grant health professionals expertise and adherence to the moral principle of serving the patient's well-being. Therefore, it is easy "to package and present the facts in a way that leaves the patient no real choice. Such conduct, capitalizing on disparities in knowledge, position, and influence, is manipulative in character and impairs the voluntariness of the patient's choice."[43]

There are many forms of manipulation. Information can be withheld or distorted. The patient is not informed of alternatives. Risks or possible complications of the recommended treatment are overlooked or minimized. The manner of presenting information strongly influences the patient's perception and response to it. The facial expression, the tone of voice, the relative physical position of the informant and the informed (the informer standing and looking down at the patient), and other aspects of a presentation selectively slant the message toward a particular direction. Information can be presented in so general and positive a way that risks or alternatives are minimized "without altering the content. And it can be framed in a way that affects the listener—for example, 'this procedure succeeds most of the time' versus 'this procedure has a 40 percent failure rate.'"[44]

Patient Access to Essential Information

A third aspect of patient participation in health care decisions is open, continuous communication between health care professionals and the patient related to "the facts, values, doubts, and alternatives on which decisions must ultimately be based."[45] The objective is to establish a dialogue so as to enhance the self-determination and well-being of the patient.[46] A recitation of facts and risks couched in technical jargon, followed by the signing of a standardized consent form, may satisfy legal requirements but hardly fulfills the ethical imperative of respecting a person's self-determination. The President's Commission views the core substantive issues to be discussed by patient and professional as:

1. The patient's current medical status, including its likely course if no improvement is pursued;

    2. The intervention(s) that might improve the prognosis, including a description of the procedures involved, a characterization of the likelihood and effect of associated risks and benefits, and the likely course with and without therapy; and

    3. A professional opinion, usually, as to the best alternative.[47]

The patient's current medical status is recognized as the physician's responsibility in the American Hospital Association's statement of *A Patient's Bill of Rights* (1973). The statement affirms the patient's right to know his or her diagnosis, treatment, and prognosis.

The privilege of a medical diagnosis is reserved by law for licensed physicians. Some states, of which New York is one, use the word "diagnosing" in the nurse practice act. A nursing diagnosis is distinguished from a medical diagnosis as "that identification of and discrimination between physical and psychosocial signs and symptoms essential to effective execution and management of the nursing regimen."[48] Thus, the nurse's role consists of supporting the patient's right to know his or her medical status, and clearly identifying and sharing the patient's psychosocial response to that knowledge so that nursing care restorative of well-being can be provided.

Those medical and nursing interventions that a nurse performs are appropriately discussed with a patient as part of health teaching and health counseling. These functions are explicitly stated in the New York State Nurse Practice Act (one example of laws in states that use this concept), which defines professional nursing as "diagnosing and treating human responses to actual or potential health problems, through such services as case finding, health teaching, health counseling, and provision of care supportive to or restorative of life and well-being. . . ."[49] In the opinion of Jane Greenlaw, RN, JD.

> As long as you make it clear that you're giving your opinion as a nurse, and speaking only from your own experience and knowledge, you can feel free to answer questions about the patient's course of treatment. You can relate your experience in caring for other patients undergoing the same treatment and answer questions about alternative treatments.[50]

On this view, the nurse can discuss medications, temperatures, blood pressures, wound care, and any other nursing or medical interventions that the nurse performs "supportive to or restorative of life and well-being."[51] The nurse can facilitate the patient's discussion of values and goals in relation to the nursing care plan and goals.

Holder and Lewis, a lawyer and a philosopher respectively, view "the negotiations necessary to obtain the patient's informed consent as the responsibility of the person who will perform the procedure. . . . The physician may delegate the discussion to another but retains the legal responsibility to make sure the patient understands."[52] The nurse's legal responsibility for a preoperative consent form consists of witnessing the patient's signature as the act of that person. The nurse's moral responsibility is to support the patient's right to understand the purposes and significance of the proposed intervention. If the patient's knowledge is seriously deficient, the nurse's duty is to inform the responsible person so that the proposed surgery or diagnostic procedure is performed based on a fully informed consent in relation to the patient's own values and goals.

Ironically, minor surgery, for which written consent is routinely secured, may be far less risky than many drugs that nurses give without question to themselves or to patients. In interventions of this kind, nurses have an unusual opportunity to teach the patient regarding drugs and their effects. Drugs are both lifesaving and life-threatening, as when unexpected reactions and interactions occur. This is health teaching directed toward the patient's understanding of the specific intervention used, the benefits, the side effects, and the risks. This function supports the patient's self-determination and well-being.

A third substantive issue is the professional's opinion of the best choice. In cases of surgery or a serious diagnosis, the professional is usually, but not always, the physician. The only justification for any intervention is the benefit to the patient. "The decision . . . has two components: whether to treat and how to treat."[53] The decision belongs to the patient. Studies conducted by the President's Commission found that little or no discussion of treatment options occurred between physicians and patients in hospital settings; physicians generally made the decisions and proceeded to treat without patient participation.[54]

Most treatment refusals studied were related to lack of information regarding the purpose, nature, and risks of the diagnostic and therapeutic measures ordered. "Conflicting information given to patients by different health care professionals"[55] was another source of treatment refusal. This is a predictable occurrence in hospitals where patient care is provided by many different people and communication among these people is not direct. The result is that patients are insecure about who is in charge, who has the qualifications, and who is to be trusted. In situations where the authority structure is clear, where professional roles of nurses and physicians are clarified, and where the lines of communication are open and direct, the nurse and physician can relate to the patient as colleagues who are equally concerned with the patient's participation in shared decisions. Professional collaboration is essential for enhancing patient participation in decisions and for coordinating activities toward this goal. However, the element of uncertainty can never be completely eliminated. Instead, it is given its due in relation to the probabilities of success based on empirical data.

Patients who are acutely ill, distressed, and in pain are constrained in their ability to understand, accept, and use the information communicated to them. The physicians and nurses are usually strangers. The language used may be too technical. The hospital setting may be frightening. If all of the health professionals involved with each patient are clear about what is to be communicated regarding the physician's diagnostic and treatment recommendation, then the discussion can proceed and enlarge as the patient's state of readiness and receptivity improve. Thus, time is required to esure this occurs.

Written and audiovisual materials discussing specific interventions are useful in nonemergency situations. Some physicians require patients to write their own consent forms for elective surgery as a test of their understanding and as the basis for further patient participation in the decision-making process. The inclusion of families can be significant in the patient's understanding of the physician's or nurse's treatment recommendation.

GUIDELINES FOR SHARED DECISION MAKING

Strategies to Maximize Participation

The aim of the nursing strategies used in this context is to facilitate relationships between patients, nurses, physicians, professionals, and families "characterized by mutual participation and respect and by shared decision making."[56]

An important nursing function is to coordinate the medical, technical, and nursing activities on behalf of the patient's well-being into a meaningful process that the patient and family can use in the shared decision process. This function is stated in nursing laws and codes as patient education, health teaching, and health counseling.[57] The process of communicating essential information to the patient may be carried out independently as part of the nursing care. The patient's response is shared with other health professionals and the family as discussion and deliberation around the patient's well-being ebbs and flows with changing needs and concerns. In everyday practice situations, nurses "typically have a central role in the process of providing patients with information."[58] Nurses are increasingly viewed by the public and by themselves as patient advocates. In this role, nurses help patients gain better health and more control of their participation in health care.

Nurses also facilitate patients' informed participation by functioning as interdisciplinary team members working with others to solve patient problems. The client benefits from the improved communication and easier access among professionals whose focus as a team is on the whole patient, rather than on a limited aspect. A team that functions effectively can better manage interdependent problems and integrate services.[59]

Questions of what person or persons or discipline will serve as primary communicator arises when people from many disciplines work with each patient. A related question is how to communicate consistent messages to the patient and the family. A further question relates to the communication of the team concept to the patient and the family.[60] One measure of effective communication is the consistency of messages from health professionals to client, and the accuracy of the client's information.[61] This is in contrast to settings where there is little communication among professionals, resulting in the patient's receiving separate, different, and sometimes conflicting messages from individual professionals.

Whether a decision-making process is used by an individual nurse or a group of practitioners, the same considerations need to be addressed. The sequence may vary because the apparent ethical problem or dilemma may change as more data are collected. An apparently straight-forward issue, such as turning off the life support machine for a brain-dead patient, may become complicated by questions of organ donation, authority conflicts among family members, and differences of opinion among the staff. Data collection, therefore, needs to be extensive. The database includes the identification and definition of the ethical problem and the nature of the ethical conflict, followed by identification of the actors involved and their source of authority; the proposed actions, alternatives, and their consequences; and the justification for the decision in relation to moral theories and the common morality discussed in this work.

Formal interdisciplinary team meetings are the ideal: Meetings or rounds held regularly with a focus on client problems and management issues. Problems are usually aired and settled by the group, which uses negotiation and conflict resolution processes. Meetings enable nurses to communicate patient concerns in a systematic fashion to an interdisciplinary group in which the problem can be analyzed and the nurse's perceptions, inferences, hypotheses, and recommendations are confirmed or disconfirmed by a group whose focus is the patient's well-being. The nurse is recognized as a colleague in a vital professional role. The principle of feedback is used in all interactions. The nurse's contribution to patient care is formalized, recognized, and placed in the context of total care to the patient and family.

PITFALLS OF REASONING: FALLACIES

Despite the best intentions of participants, road blocks to effective decision making occur through errors in reasoning known as fallacies. Exposing and confronting fallacies in reasoning helps to minimize them. The recognition and correction of fallacies facilitates effective and justifiable decision making in nursing.

Fallacies can be committed innocently stemming from ignorance of methods of reasoning or they can be deliberately used to falsify the case or to mislead the listener. Fallacies may be used by anyone. Their use is prominent in advertising, in political rhetoric, and in selling a product or an idea. The health care delivery system and practitioners of all kinds are not immune to the use of fallacies. Among the many formal, inductive, and informal fallacies cited in the literature, the following are the most notable types that interfere with making morally justifiable and effective nursing decisions.

The Is-Ought Fallacy

The *is-ought* fallacy is committed when someone argues that X is the case; therefore, X ought to be the case. (The letter X stands for some practice, policy, procedure, decision or custom). A common fallacy is: This is the way we do it; this is the way we've always done it. What follows is the implication that therefore, this is the way it *ought* to be done.

> This patient is alive because of cardiopulmonary resuscitation (CPR); therefore, all patients *ought* to be resuscitated in cases of cardiac arrest.

One can substitute "dialysis," "life-support systems," or "artificial feeding" for CPR. Another example of this fallacy is:

> Nursing is the bedside care of sick individuals; therefore, nurses *ought* to be trained at the bedside of sick individuals.

An obvious implication here is that formal college education for nurses is unnecessary or that all nurses should give bedside care to patients. Another example of this fallacy is:

> A nurse is required to work a double shift whenever necessary in this hospital; therefore, double shifts *ought* to be required of all nurses during this period of acute shortage.

Still other examples of the is-ought fallacy include:

> A nurse is a low-paid health care provider; therefore, nurses *ought* not to expect high salaries.

> A nurse is subordinate to a physician in rank and education; therefore, a nurse *ought* to obey a physician without question.

Many more examples from nursing are available. The point is that the is-ought fallacy consists of moving from a given present case, practice, policy, decision, or custom (the *is*) to a statement of obligation. The fault in reasoning is that if X is the case, it does not follow that X *ought* to be the case. Not everyone *ought* to be resuscitated, or kept on life-support systems, or undergo dialysis, or receive an organ transplant or an artificial heart. It is fallacious to proceed from the is to the ought, because ought does not necessarily follow.

Appeal to Force

This fallacy consists in making another accept the conclusion of an argument on the basis of force alone. For example, surgeon presents this argument to a patient regarding elective surgery: "If you don't get that fibroid tumor removed, you'll die." Or a physician orders an overdose of morphine that the nurse refuses to give, to which the physician responds "I'll have you fired." Or a nurse who must pick up her two young children from child care and cannot work a double shift is told by her supervisor, "Either you work the next shift, or you'll be fired." These are appeals to the sole use of force and lack of rational support. However, the nurse in the intensive care unit who tells the patient, "I have to give you this injection (or treatment) to relieve your pain (or ease your breathing, or slow your heartbeat, or clear your passageways)," is appealing to force on a rational basis with supporting evidence for her conclusion.

Abuse of the Person

Another fallacy in argument consists in abuse of the person instead of providing rational, relevant reasons for a decision. In the fallacy of *personal abuse*, a nurse may criticize a physician for the repeated resuscitation of a terminally ill patient on the grounds that the physician "cannot accept defeat" or "is afraid of death."

In *circumstantial abuse*, one person blames another for concluding X on the grounds of membership or inclusion in a group that habitually does something blameworthy (X). For example, Nurse A chides Nurse B for refusing to care for an abortion patient on the grounds that Nurse B is Catholic. It may be true that Nurse B is Catholic, but in fact Nurse B's opposition to abortion may stem from her longing for a child of her own and rejection of women who terminate their

pregnancies. Or the fact that Nurse A and Nurse B graduated from the same bac-
calaureate program in nursing and A praises the practice of B does not entitle
Nurse C to accuse, "Oh, but you both graduated from Hunter." Nurse C's argument is irrelevant to whether Nurse B is or is not an expert practitioner.

Another version of abuse is known as *tu quoque,* "You're another." Nurse A goes
off duty early for class and Nurse B also goes off duty early to go shopping, and the
unit is left dangerously understaffed. The charge by either A or B of "You're another
irresponsible nurse" is fallacious because two wrongs don't make a right.

In the genetic fallacy, people are abused on the grounds of their origins,
rather than refuting or accepting evidence on relevant grounds. For example,
"The reason you have AIDS is that you come from the slums." Obviously, AIDS is
contagious and without social economic consciousness.

Appeal to Populace

The fallacy in the argument, "Everybody does it," is that because "everybody does
it" it must be good. For example, Nurse A says that "Everybody is working three
twelve-hour shifts a week; therefore, to do so must be good." Nurse A's argument
does not prove that this schedule is good. Nurses may spend days recuperating
from this schedule. Popularity does not prove worth.

Appeal to Inappropriate Authority

As might be expected, the appeal to inappropriate authority is a frequent pitfall of
reasoning in the health care system. The fallacy consists of persons with authority
presenting themselves as authorities outside or beyond their field or area of expertise. At minimum, to have appropriate authority is to have the required creden-
tials. For example, a physician may decide to resuscitate a young patient with a severe, debilitating form of leukemia who specifically refuses resuscitation. The
physician argues that she knows the value of life far better than the young patient
who does not realize how rewarding it is to be alive. In this case, the physician is
going beyond her appropriate authority.

The Slippery-Slope Fallacy

The slippery-slope fallacy assumes that if one exception to a rule or principle is allowed, then an uncontrollable set of events with unwanted consequences will follow. Thus, if active, voluntary euthanasia is permitted, even under strict controls,
then the killing of elderly persons with Alzheimer's disease or other forms of dementia or senility will follow. Similarly, if abortion is permitted, then infanticide of
the severely handicapped will follow. Likewise, hospital administrators who oppose collective bargaining argue that if nurses are permitted to make salary demands, then the cost of hospital care will be unaffordable to the public.

A counterargument against the slippery slope fallacy can point out that one
can stop anywhere along the line and not have to go all the way. For example, active voluntary euthanasia is practiced in such countries as Holland without any decrease in either the quality of care given to the demented and senile elderly or in
the commitment to their survival. Abortion is legally practiced and morally supported as a means of population control in China. The result is a tremendous

outpouring of love for the permitted child by the parents and a great deal of effort in areas of child care, health, and education. Universal respect for the elderly Chinese as a source of wisdom and authority continues as it has for centuries.

Slothful Induction

This fallacy refuses to allow any evidence that contradicts the conclusion of one's argument in order to protect one's conclusions against criticism. For example, a nurse who supports abortion argues for the primacy of the woman's right to her own body, while a nurse who opposes abortion argues for the primacy or equal rights of the fetus. Neither nurse looks at the evidence of the tragic national need for better sex education and family planning that might decrease the incidence of unwanted or unplanned pregnancies.

The dogmatic beliefs of a group regarding the supremacy or inferiority of members of a race, tribe, class, or culture without regard for contradictory evidence is a futher example of slothful induction. Historically, such groups have raged against the theory of evolution, immunization, and the equality of races and sexes. The antidote to the fallacy of slothful induction is to open all arguments to inquiry and contradictory evidence. A nurse or physician who refuses to question any ethical argument or conclusion because it was put forth by an authority is committing the fallacy of slothful induction.

The Fallacy of Accident

This fallacy consists of the indiscriminate application of an ethical principle to every situation without regard for "accidental" differences or circumstances. For example, the Kantian imperative of always telling the truth, if applied indiscriminately, can have tragic results. Some individuals are terrified by the thought of cancer and consider it an immediate death sentence that, in some cases, they prefer to carry out themselves by suicide or by rejecting all treatment. Most people need support, sympathy, and encouragement during the process of accepting painful truth.

Complex Question

This fallacy consists of asking a question whose answer depends on the affirmative answer to a previous question. The question, "Do you want cardiopulmonary resuscitation?" presupposes that you may experience cardiac arrest. The question to patients, "Will you accept this surgery (treatment, medication) and live, or refuse it and die?" is an example of the fallacy of bifurcation or exclusive alternation or either-or thinking. Boldly presenting two alternatives does not mean that there are not more alternatives or even that one of the two is not a real alternative.

SUMMARY

Choice is an important value for every person. Nursing strategies for facilitating patients' choices enhance the values of personhood, especially at critical times in a person's life, such as when he or she is ill, incapacitated, dying, or vulnerable due to age, mental disability, or socioeconomic status. A nurse often knows what to do and how to do it, and who can best do what is needed for maximizing the patient's well-being. At times, the nurses' priority on behalf of the patient's best interests may conflict with the patient's choices. This may present an ethical problem without a true or final answer. In ethics, one cannot ask for absolutes. As Aristotle long ago pointed out, one cannot expect the same precision in ethics as in mathematics or science. Nevertheless, one may improve ethical decision making in nursing by becoming aware of and avoiding fallacies.

Discussion Questions

1. How do science and technology promote effective decision making in nursing? Cite an example from this chapter.
2. How do science and technology promote morally justifiable decision making in nursing?
3. How have science and technology affected the role of the best-interest standard in relation to the substitute judgment standard?
4. How does one decide whether to use the best-interest standard or the substitute judgment standard?
5. In answering Question 4, refer to the example of the father who decides on surgical amputation of his son's leg.
6. How do fallacies interfere with competent and morally justifiable decision making by nurses?

REFERENCES

1. President's Commission for the Study of Ethical Problems in Medicine and Biomedical and Behavioral Research. *Making health care decisions.* Washington, DC: US Government Printing Office. 1982;33. PB83236703.
2. ibid.
3. President's Commission for the Study of Ethical Problems in Medicine and Biomedical and Behavioral Research. *Summing up.* Washington, DC: US Government Printing Office. 1983;72. PB83236703. PB83236810.
4. Thompson DF. Hospital ethics. *Cambridge Quart Health Care Ethics* 1992;1(1):206.
5. ibid.
6. American Nurses Association. *Code for Nurses with interpretive statements.* Kansas City, Mo: American Nurses Association, 1985;4.
7. ibid.
8. President's Commission. *Making health care decisions.* p. 2.
9. Bandman B, Bandman E. The nurse's role in an interest-based view of patients' rights. In: Spicker SF, Gadow S (eds). *Nursing images and ideals.* New York: Springer-Verlag, 1980;129.
10. Mezey et al. The Patient Self-Determination Act: Sources of concern for nurses. *Nursing Outlook* 1994;42(1):30–37.
11. ibid.

12. *ANA Position Statement on Nursing and the Patient's Self-Determination Act.* Washington, DC: American Nurses Association; 1992.
13. Mezey M et al. The Patient-Self Determination Act: Sources of concern for nurses. *Nursing Outlook* 1994;42(1):30–37.
14. ibid.
15. ibid.
16. ibid.
17. ibid.
18. ibid.
19. President's Commission. *Making health care decisions,* p. 45–46.
20. American Nurses Association. *Code for Nurses with interpretative statements.* Kansas City, Mo: American Nurses Association, 1985;4.
21. Frankena WK. *Ethics* (2nd ed). Englewood Cliffs, NJ: Prentice-Hall. 1973;47.
22. President's Commission. *Making health care decisions,* p. 42.
23. ibid, p. 43.
24. ibid.
25. ibid, p. 44.
26. ibid.
27. President's Commission. *Summing up,* p. 70.
28. President's Commission. *Making health care decisions,* p. 16.
29. ibid, p. 55.
30. ibid.
31. ibid.
32. ibid, p. 57.
33. ibid, p. 58.
34. ibid, p. 59.
35. ibid, p. 60.
36. ibid, p. 62.
37. Macklin R. *Man, mind, and morality: The ethics of behavior control.* Englewood Cliffs, NJ: Prentice-Hall. 1982;90,91–95.
38. ibid.
39. President's Commission for the Study of Ethical Problems in Medicine and Biomedical and Behavioral Research. *Deciding to forego life-sustaining treatment.* Washington, DC: US Government Printing Office. 1983;124. PB83236836.
40. President's Commission. *Making health care decisions,* p. 178.
41. ibid.
42. ibid.
43. ibid, p. 179.
44. ibid, p. 66.
45. ibid.
46. ibid, p. 69.
47. ibid.
48. ibid, p. 74.
49. Nurse Practice Act, Title VIII, Article 139. New York State Education Law, 1972.
50. Greenlaw JL. When patients' questions put you on the spot. *RN* 1983;46(3):79.
51. Nurse Practice Act. Title VIII, Article 139. New York State Education Law, 1972.
52. Holder AR, Lewis JW. Informed consent and the nurse. *Nursing Law Ethics* 1981;2(2):1.
53. President's Commission. *Making health care decisions,* p. 76.
54. ibid.

55. ibid.
56. ibid, p. 36.
57. Nurse Practice Act. Title VIII, Article 139. New York State Education Law, 1972.
58. President's Commission. *Making health care decisions,* p. 147–148.
59. Bradley JC, Edinberg MA. *Communication in the nursing context.* New York: Appleton-Century-Crofts. 1982;278.
60. ibid, p. 278–279.
61. ibid, p. 279.

PART TWO
Nursing Ethics Through the Life Span

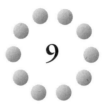

9

Nursing Ethics in the Procreative Family

Study of this chapter enables the learner to:

1. Understand the functions, values, and dynamics of traditional and nontraditional families.
2. Distinguish between ownership, partnership, and club membership models of family relations.
3. Facilitate the family's participation in shared decision making in the clinical and ethical aspects of reproductive technology.
4. Develop the role of the nurse in genetic counseling based on facilitating the family's evaluation of its goals, values, and rational life plans, knowledge of the disease, and the options faced if carrying a defective gene.

OVERVIEW

A new family that brings out the best in each member is usually and desirably motivated by love, including sexual love. The morally idealized union of a young man and a young woman coming together out of love, care, and respect for each other has been dramatized through the visual, literary, and musical arts in love stories such as *Romeo and Juliet*, in operas such as *La Bohème*, and films such as *The Sound of Music*. Love as a form of family interaction may also be depicted in

117

sculpture, as in *The Family of Humanity*, in which a man and a woman with a child between them embrace with expressions of love. For love is the essential ingredient that binds new families together. The love of two people for each other is ordinarily and desirably transmitted to their offspring.

The family is commonly regarded as the source, development, and justification of almost all values. To a newborn, the family is the substance and boundary of its universe. The family gives stability and sustenance to a child's first experiences, once aptly termed by William James as "a booming, buzzing confusion." The family thus converts the child's initial confusion into an orderly ongoing system. The family is the young child's universe. The child's value relations depend on the love and quality of care given by its parents and significant others who share in the parenting.

The first role of the nurse is to strengthen the positive love and to affirm and sustain moral, creative family-life values. The nurse's second task is to help the troubled family achieve the strength and stability of a family that supports each member's worth in the process of growth and development. The nurse's third task is to facilitate the family's participation in shared decision making on the basis of information regarding reproductive technology, genetics, and the associated ethical issues.

FAMILY FUNCTIONS, DYNAMICS, AND VALUES

The values, leadership, size, membership, roles, and functions of the American family are changing. Despite change, it remains the basic social unit, the source of human capacities for relatedness and caring for another. Today's family systems are experiencing value conflicts as new lifestyles are considered and tested. New configurations emerge as single parents, stepparents, parent and live-in friend, surrogate parents, and homosexual parents form a family in conjunction with one or more children.

Burgess' widely quoted definition of the family reflects its changing character. He defines the family as

> ". . . a group united by marriage, blood, or adoption, residing in a single household, communicating with each other in their respective roles, and maintaining a common culture. . . . The family is in transition from a traditional family system controlled by mores, public opinion, and law to a companionship family system based on mutual affection, intimate communication, and mutual acceptance of division of labor and procedures of decision-making."[1]

Mutuality of interests, values, and goals is seen as the basis for becoming partners in a relationship. Increasingly, the goal of individuals starting families is that of happiness and self-actualization through affectionate ties with others. The pursuit of individual goals within a family can sometimes conflict with family utilitarian goals of the greatest good for the greatest number, which may sacrifice the interest of the minority to those of the majority. Kant's ethics of duty can be a powerful force in parental behavior and decision making through the use of a principle that calls for right action without exception. Love is also a powerful factor in doing the right thing.

Some of the functions of the family flow out of its definition. Burgess and colleagues see the family as most valued because it provides emotional support through reciprocal expressions of love and caring acts. Our culture places a high value on the factor of love and choice of mate. Burgess sees the family's second function to be its commitment to the provision of an environment in which its members share experiences, activities, and companionship. The third function Burgess defines as the care and rearing of children. Lastly, the family is one of society's primary agencies for transmitting the culture from one generation to the next.[2] As the primary unit of society, the family is the center of authority and decisions regarding the procreation of children, the provision of comprehensive care regarding their health and education, and all of the necessary supports to life and well-being.

THREE MODELS OF FAMILY AND MARRIAGE

Ownership Model

One model of marriage and family, regarded by some as the traditional model, is the model of ownership. Here, one member, usually but not always the male spouse, has the unshakable conviction that he is the boss, the one who owns every member of the family in a master-slave, dominance-submission relationship. The conviction of ownership may be malevolently expressed in spousal or child abuse, or expressed benevolently in acts of measured and controlled beneficence. The model of owning something finds natural appeal within human nature in the belief learned early in life that if one owns anything, it is one's own body.[3] Moreover, in the early, formative years of an infant's life, parents may act wisely by following the ownership model, which implies close responsibility and care. One speaks, after all, of "Mrs. Jones's children" in a way that clearly communicates a possessive relationship. To own something is to protect and cherish it. For that reason, the association of ownership with one's body and one's life provides a naturally persuasive case for a woman's rights regarding abortion.

In a family oriented by the ownership model, we find a "morally strong role differentiation," to adapt a concept from a work by A. Goldman, who writes that such moral role differentiation entitles one person to have special powers, privileges, and exceptions from the moral rules that apply to other family members.[4] The family sovereign may, for example, be given the best food at the table, the best chair in the home, and the most attention, and may never be expected to help with the dishes, the lawn mower, or the vacuum cleaner. The ownership model invests authority and the source of all family duties in a single individual and requires unquestioning obedience to the will of the master.

One may distinguish three kinds of ownership. In the benign ownership view, the master rules, with most decisions being beneficial to the master as well as to other family members who obey. This view coincides with Plato's rational paternalism. The family sovereign makes reasonably good decisions most of the time and is efficient, consistent, and accountable for the general well-being of all family members. But such a sovereign nevertheless exercises sole decision making with unquestioned authority. If that sovereign is unexpectedly incapacitated, absent, or dead, such a sudden change may throw the family from order into chaos, because in this kind of family pattern, other family members are unprepared to step in and make everyday family decisions.

A second version of the ownership model is a self-seeking, uncaring ruler whose only manifest concern is self-aggrandizement. A third version of the owner-ship model is a malignant sovereign who shows no responsibility for the good of other members of the family. Such a person is likely to squander family resources at frequent and expensive outings and to act impulsively and without regard to obligations to other family members. This person is a tyrant and may systemati-cally abuse the spouse and children and even kill them in a fit of rage or jealousy.

In their article, Robbins and Schacht discuss the role of the nurse in family hi-erarchies: "[Although] we cannot observe hierarchies directly, we can infer them from our observations of the sequence and direction of behavior. For instance, who talks first? Last? Longest? Who talks to whom? When? Where? About what? If one family member consistently approaches the staff about the patient's health care, may we hypothesize that he or she holds an upper position in the family and has the task of being an 'expert' on the patient's status?"[5]

Although Robbins and Schacht are concerned that a "nurse's attempt to com-municate with family members may meet with resistance if the communication in-advertently violates the family communication hierarchy,"[6] our concern is with the nurse's value role in relation to the values of the family. We think that a value-oriented nurse may, for example, question the practices of any fixed hierarchical pattern, one implied by the ownership model, in order to support the patient's right to participate in the treatment plan.

The ownership model may also provide a perspective for perceiving nurse-patient-family relationships. The nurse or other health care team members may view patients as subordinate within the health care hierarchy. Nurses and physi-cians may regard themselves as sovereign beings who "own" their patients, which means that their patients in effect have no right to question them.

Club Membership Model

A response to the difficulties of the ownership model is the club membership model. Here the relation of family members is like that of members in a club, who can come and go as they please, use the facilities and locker rooms, play the sports they like, take a shower, and leave when they wish. The members have only to abide by rules involving relations to other members, the use of the facilities, prompt pay-ment of dues, and respect for the property and propriety of fellow members.

In this model, where each person does "his or her own thing," there is weak moral role differentiation among the members, with scope for relativism and moral anarchy. The club membership model endorses liberty or self-determination rights but few subsistence rights to be cared for. Special privileges and powers conferred by the club override moral considerations to outsiders. The club mem-bership model of a family is one of loose affiliation of its members. Alliances between members may be formed, but without deep and abiding alliances to the club. Moreover, the club membership model tolerates indifference to the lives and quality of lives of its members as well as to persons outside the family.

The club membership model is like professional association, a social institution, or a miniature society. Citizenship is in a society, although small, but a society nonetheless. Here, personal bonds are loose, with scope for individual self-development and a minimum of paternalism. The club membership model is also like some family communes, in which the affiliation is loose, roles are diffuse, boundaries are highly permeable, and the membership is continually changing. In this respect, club membership lies at the other end of the spectrum of the behavior controls exerted by the ownership model. The club membership model also has advantages and drawbacks. One advantage is that it emphasizes individual liberties and noninterference. However, there are too few rules to guide its members to care for one another and as a result, family members show indifference to the welfare of spouse, children, patients, and nurses.

Partnership Model

The difficulties of both the ownership and club membership models call for a third model. This model, one more compatible with rights talk and its principles of justice and fairness in a family, is a partnership model. According to this model, everyone in the family feels that he or she has an investment in achieving wise, benevolent, just, fair, and compassionate decision making. The slogan "all for one and one for all" prompts the members of this family model to cohere. They each stand to gain by committing themselves to the good of the family. All are beneficiaries, and all share the burdens as nearly equally as possible. In a family oriented to a partnership model, there is a weak or even no moral role differentiation between family members, owing their different social roles. On this view, the husband in the ownership model who never wipes the dishes, does laundry and cleaning, or cares for the children, may well be expected to do so based on the fair and equitable distribution of family chores.

A partnership model entails a rights-based view, with a full complement of rights to make decisions and rights to be cared for. These are rights accorded to each family member or held in trust.[7] In a partnership-oriented family, the rights of family members are approximately equal.

Two types of partnership models may be distinguished. In one kind of partnership, there is a senior partner and a junior partner or several junior partners. George Orwell's *Animal Farm* (1945) sardonically points out that "some animals are more equal than others." Likewise, in some families in which partnership is the practice, there nevertheless is a recognition that one member, usually a parent or surrogate, is the senior partner. Perhaps this seniority is owing to age, experience with life problems, an edge in wisdom, financial or physical power within a family, charm, or charisma. But the consequence of such a "senior partnership" may be slippage back to the ownership model.

In this seniority version of the partnership model, a problem arises that is similar to the use of the "team" analogy in health care. On a sports team, there is generally a captain and even a coach, who give the orders which other team members follow. In a sense, a political democracy is a partnership. However, anyone versed in *realpolitik* is aware that despite James Madison's noble sentiments to the effect that the people in a democracy are the governors and rulers, in practice, only one person or a small number of persons make all the important decisions. Thus, the seniority version of the partnership model dominates families and nurse-client-physician-family relations.

A second version of the partnership model is that of virtual equality of all family members in decision making. This may be more of an ideal type, with fewer examples than the seniority version. If rights are taken seriously in nurse-family relationships, then the principle "each member counts equally" is respected. The value placed on partnership in the family may be extended to perceiving the nurse as a partner in the therapeutic process. Benoliel writes that

> . . . a nurse-family relationship that promotes partnership as the central means for seeking solutions and resolutions is an essential component of delivery of nursing care in such a manner that the integrity of each person is preserved.[8]

An advantage of the partnership model is that shared decision making, whenever feasible, distributes burdens and benefits, liberties and duties on a roughly equal basis. This agrees with Rawls's justice-based model. A partnership model provides for open and self-correcting decision-making procedures in a family. This is in contrast to a single decision maker in the ownership model. John Stuart Mill's eloquent reason for freedom of expression readily applies to the partnership model of family life. Mill gives the reason for providing the freedom to dissent as an opportunity to substitute truth for error.[9] To paraphrase Mill, a single decision maker under an ownership model is robbed of the chance to correct mistakes that come with the alternative decision makers found in the partnership model. Benoliel puts the case for nurse-family partnership well: "Partnerships with families require an openness to the possibility that there are many different ways of sharing power within groups."[10] A partnership model also develops strong bonds and existentially felt commitments to the good of the family.

A drawback of this model, however, is that a partnership model–oriented family, sensing few or no bonds or commitments beyond the family, may develop insularity and aloofness toward non-family members. The slogan "One for all and all for one" may exclude others and also result in pitting a family against society. The close-knit family is akin to a close-knit profession whose members may show indifference and callousness to those outside the profession. Likewise, the close-knit family may regard others with suspicion, alienation, and hostility, and erect "high fences" or barriers to keep the family in and strangers out. A result of such family insulation is the development of a dubious notion that the ethics of intimates in the family is all there is and that there is no ethics that applies to strangers.[11] A related difficulty is that a family with strong partnership involvements may suffocate individuals and prevent them from developing separately. Partnerships have their price, the most costly of which may be the chains all of the members unwittingly wear.

Some further issues arise for nursing in the relationship with families. Can the nurse be regarded as a full partner and not as an intruder if the nurse voices views that are unpopular to a family? If the nurse's religious, political, and philo-sophic views affect his or her beliefs on abortion, sterilization, mental illness, eu-thanasia, and experimentation, and these are in collision with the views held by a family, what significance is to be placed on the nurse's values and what on the family's values?

Relations Among These Models

Only in the partnership model are family members likely to develop autonomous relationships of mutual respect and self-respect. For these reasons, although all three models provide points to consider, the one that is maximally rights-based and therefore seems morally preferable to the others is the partnership model. This model provides a full complement of decision-making rights and rights to be cared for. What counts most in this model is the members' caring for themselves and one another. However, the defects that such a model provide, such as neglect of outsiders and suffocating relations within the partnership, call for appropriate consideration of each of the other models as well.

FAMILY DYNAMICS AND VALUES

Whatever its composition, the family is an interacting, interdependent unit that operates by rules and expectations, values, and relations of intimacy. Relations are permeated by feelings of affiliation, loyalty, caring, and pride or conflicting feelings of hate, shame, and rejection. Family experiences are the source of ado-lescent and adult values, which are usually modified or extended but are some-times rejected in adult life. The most basic values, such as respect for human worth, honesty, and truth-telling, have their roots in family experiences. Stephen Toulmin, a philosopher, distinguishes the ethics of intimates from the ethics of strangers.[12] He argues that the ethics of strangers does not take adequate ac-count of individual circumstances and needs. To strike a balance, Toulmin sug-gests that we look to Leo Tolstoy, the 19th-century Russian author of *War and Peace, The Death of Ivan Ilych,* and *Anna Karenina.* Tolstoy held that morality was possible only among intimate relations, as in families, between parents and children, lovers, and neighbors. As Tolstoy saw it, ethics is for those people within a person's walking distance. The moral universe stops when one takes a train, for the people one sees there are casual and commercial contacts, not close relations. Moral relations become less significant as one relates to acquaintances and strangers; and more significant as one relates to intimates. Tolstoy's ethics of intimates is a crucial example of virtue ethics. Nurses deal with strangers as new patients most of the time and are challenged to develop moral relationships within a brief period and to practice virtue ethics.

Although Tolstoy's ethics is regarded as an example of virtue ethics and, in part, provides a model of how one conducts one's life with one's intimates, it pre-sents serious problems for nursing ethics. Patients are not intimates, nor, however, are they strangers, to be neglected and not cared for. A nursing ethics of caring for patients (which also qualifies as a virtue ethics) repudiates Tolstoy's moral position toward strangers. Patients are neither strangers nor intimates. Yet they are to be cared for not as intimates, but as persons worthy of professional nursing care and concern. Tolstoy's ethics, moreover, commits a bifurcation or either-or fallacy, for patients are neither intimates nor strangers.

Family Caregiving

Family caregiving is the process of providing services between family members. The number of dependent persons is increasing as are survivors of leukemia, cystic fibrosis, diabetes, sickle-cell anemia, and end-stage renal disease.[13] Parents who care for chronically ill children must add the physical, emotional, and social demands of siblings to their own response to the illness in addition to the economic burdens of care. The stress can be overwhelming.

The number and proportion of elderly people are increasing in America, with millions of unpaid caregivers assisting noninstitutionalized, disabled elderly persons with one or more limitations in their activities of daily living. As a moral imperative, this too may be a crushing burden to families.

Harding questions the prevailing ethic of patient autonomy as one which ignores or subordinates family interest to the interests of the patients.[14] Saving the life of a newborn with serious defects will affect the rest of the family, as would caring for a family member with Alzheimer's disease, AIDS, or cancer. Depression, separations, divorce, and dysfunction within the family may be but some of the consequences of these unflagging burdens. Harding argues that decisions should be made based on what is best for all concerned, not just the patient's interests. This does not eliminate special consideration for the ill members and necessary sacrifices; rather, it denies exclusive or overriding consideration.[15] There are limits to the sacrifice of all other goods to the care of the ill. Harding points out that the medical setting is so powerful as to subordinate the nonmedical interests of the famuily to the medical interests of the patient. Consequently, the family may need an advocate in the attempt to reach a decision that is fair to all. The nurse as advocate can enable the family to become informed and involved in treatment decisions critical to the family member's well-being and survival.

Abuse

Although love and consideration among family members is desirable, other feelings, such as indifference, hostility, impatience, and verbal and physical abuse, do occur. Awareness of abuse may help expose, confront, and minimize abuse and contribute to its replacement by positive love-generating feelings. Family members reflect social, psychological, and economic realities, which may reveal conflicts between spouses early in marriage. Some couples are known to feel disenchantment soon in their relationship and begin to see faults in the other person that grow to intolerable proportions. Such disenchantment may well lead to abuse and even a habitual pattern of abuse between husband and wife, lovers, partners, or companions. Such couples live together but they cannot stand each other. At worst, they abuse each other. Abuse may become the basic pattern of interaction between partners.

Battered women account for one quarter to one third of women seeking care in the emergency department, nearly one third of those injured, and one quarter of those who attempt suicide.[16] Signs of abuse are to delay in securing treatment, inconsistent explanations of injury, history of trauma, chronic pain with no cause, depression, psychological distress, an overly protective partner, or a partner who won't leave. The woman is probably in danger if there has been an increase in frequency or severity of threats to herself or to the children, or the availability of a gun. These are indications to the nurse to call police.

Abuse is a serious harm or offense. Identifying abuse and knowing what constitutes abuse is important in deciding what to do about it as distinct from some lesser wrong. The occurrence of abuse justifies interference with the abuser's right to freedom. Abuse may be direct or indirect, active or passive, intentional or unintentional. Abuse involves violation of another's rights.

The nurse's role is to support a victim of violence by letting her know what social, legal, and nursing services and remedies are available. By keeping careful records, nursing agencies can join other social agencies in advocating the victim's interests and preventing recurrence of physical abuse. The nurse's role in developing awareness, recognition, exposure, and confrontation of abuse is designed to minimize and eliminate it. Abuse is a serious violation of a person's human rights and is the antithesis of decent human behavior. Nurses as nurturers have both a right and a duty to safeguard people, especially the powerless, against abuse.

The concept of abuse also provides a paradigm case argument against the notion that everything is either subjective or relative. To say, for example, that in some families, communities, or countries, it is acceptable to beat wives and children, is to deny that it may be justifiably judged as abuse by others who are more enlightened. Abuse is morally wrong. A civil society does not condone the "banality of evil" (in political philosopher Hannah Arendt's phrase) This occurs when moral and legal instruments fail to recognize and prevent abuse.

Divorce

Although divorce is a legal event, the process of separation is fraught with moral problems for both spouses and children. Their lives, once intimate and cohesive, become separated, disorganized, and rearranged in new and unfamiliar patterns. Divorce is an increasingly frequent occurrence in American life, involving at least one child in most cases.

Divorce does not end the feelings and ties of parents with children. It simply puts distance between them and enables them to use the children as pawns to continue the conflict if they so choose. Divorce is the end of a marriage, which by its nature places every family member at risk. The process of family rearrangement is slow, involving the ethical, emotional, psychological, physical, social, and economic dimensions of family life over a period of years. The impact of divorce is heavy on each member, but perhaps heaviest on young children whose foundation of security is in the feelings of "omnipotence" and "omniscience" of their parents.[17] The predictability of their world is shattered, and each child carries a load of self-blame and guilt. Children worry about what they did wrong and what they can do to reunite their parents. The child is deeply attached to both parents, and when one parent ostensibly abandons the child, the fear of abandonment by the other parent is usually strong. The family system, however disrupted by marital discord, represents survival to the children affected. Older school age children and adolescents may be more verbal in expressing their rage and frustration at what they perceive as parental failure, but often even they regress, fail in schoolwork, and engage in antisocial activities in the effort to re-unite their parents around their problems.

Levels of vulnerability differ among children, yet all can benefit by adherence to ethical principles governing relations. The process of separation and divorce need not be made any more traumatic than necessary by respecting the rights of every family member to a truthful explanation of reasons for the divorce. Children are powerless, and their rights particularly need to be respected. Children are en-titled to know the truth in terms they can understand. The difference between truth-telling and deception is vital to the development of the child's autonomy, in-tegral to Kant's ethics. If the parents are divorcing because of one partner's alco-holism, crime, mental illness, or desertion, the children need to know this so that they will not fill in the vacuum with self-destructive mythology. If the parents are separating because one prefers another or because of incompatibility, this too needs to be said without blame. In this way, the child is not forced to choose be-tween the "good parent" and the "bad parent."

The parents must exert themselves to the utmost to avoid adversarial, visita-tion, and custodial battles involving children. This causes considerable conflict and ambivalence, with possibly permanent damaging effects. Each parent's right to continue relationships with a child needs to be respected and facilitated by the other parent. Parents need to consider the ethical principles of rights and fairness in their relations to each other so that one parent, usually the mother, does not carry an undue share of the physical, psychological, and financial burden of child care. If both parents adhere to Kantian ethical principles of placing their parental duty to their children above considerations of individual comfort and convenience, it is quite possible for parents to unite around such issues as truth telling and promise-keeping with their children. If the ethical principle of love as concern for the welfare of each family member is paramount, even though parents are di-vorced, it is possible to change the effects of divorce from crisis proportions to an event with "potential for growth and enhanced maturity"[18] for all concerned. The nurse can facilitate that process through exercise of her role as moral agent rein-forcing ethical principles of duty, rights, and fairness.

THE NURSE'S ROLE IN FAMILY ETHICAL ISSUES

What can the nurse do to help a troubled family or parent to decide what ought to be done, in the light of their own value preferences and life situation, about a health problem? The nurse can use a problem-solving method, beginning with an assessment of the facts and a clear definition of the problem by the nurse and par-ents together. A next step may be for the parents to identify their ethical principles and value choice in relation to the problem and the alternatives. The nurse can facilitate the process by raising questions to clarify understanding of all the options.

Family decisions are of several kinds. Decisions can be made unilaterally by one parent who assumes the authority for the whole family, as in the ownership model. The authoritarian family values the duty and responsibility of one or both parents as the main factor in decisions. In some families there is an absence of deliberation and decision-making processes so that external events and forces shape the decision, as in the club membership model. Or decisions can be made by majority vote or by consensus, in which discussion continues until there is commitment to the decision, as in the partnership model. The family seeking consensus of its members values sharing responsibility and commitment to group decisions.

The nurse can serve as a catalyst to the family, identifying the need for decision in the problematic situation in ways that each family considers right for them. The nurse can encourage open discussion of the problem with respect for the rights of all concerned.

ETHICAL ISSUES IN REPRODUCTIVE TECHNOLOGY

Family Planning and Contraception

For some couples, the number of children conceived and brought to term presents no problems. Such parents regard "life as a gift" to be respected and preserved and consider the use of contraceptives unnatural. For them, abortion is both tragic and unthinkable. To other couples, the omission of contraceptives, with consequences of an unintended pregnancy, is tragic and unthinkable. Other couples decide that for personal and social reasons of over-population, they will not have any children, and choose to be sterilized.

Those who morally oppose contraception must contend with the inescapable fact of individual, family, and group obligations to meet the nurturance, nutritional, health, housing, clothing, and educational needs of its members. The tragic consequences of failure to meet those needs are evident in the faces and bodies of millions of starving and diseased people, as well as many of the mentally ill and criminal population.

CASE 9.1: AIDS. A teenaged married couple on welfare have a seriously ill 2-year-old son. This child requires a great deal of nursing care and frequent hospitalizations for treatment of HIV. The parents, Joe and Mary, have been informed of their son's poor prognosis. The 19-year-old father is a high school dropout, unemployed, and a former intravenous narcotic user. The 18-year-old mother left high school when she became pregnant at age 15. Both parents have been informed of their own HIV status as a necessary condition for their child's infection. They have also known of the deaths of several friends and relatives from AIDS. The community health nurse visits regularly to care for the child, to instruct the parents in his care and in matters of their own health. The nurse has achieved a warm positive relationship with this young couple who seem to be very much in love. On one of the nurse's visits to the family for follow-up care following the child's hospital discharge, Mary announces that she is now 4 months pregnant. The stunned nurse attempts to explain the possible adverse effects of pregnancy on Mary's HIV status, the 25% to 30% chances of the infant becoming infected with HIV, and the need for parenting of the children should they survive. The young couple argue that they are in love, and want a child to outlive them should the 2-year-old son and themselves die from AIDS. They view the 70% to 75% chance for survival of a healthy child to be favorable. They believe the decision to be their right and solely their own to make.

What are the liberty rights of HIV-infected parents to bear children at will? What of the parents' primary obligation to care for the seriously ill 2-year-old? Is carrying the fetus in the current pregnancy to term a case of wrongful life or harm to the potential child? What are the rights of members of society who provide complete support for the food, clothing, shelter, and costly long-term medical care for this family to prohibit further child-bearing and to require termination of this pregnancy?

C. H. Foreman, a research associate at the Brookings Institution, writes of the unsolved issues of AIDS. He cites the limited knowledge of people who resist behavior change when short-term gratification so inclines them and that the change may be short-lived or uneven. ". . . AIDS has never been just about disease control. It is also about rights and confidentiality . . . unavoidably bound up with sex. . . ."[19]

One argument holds that it is cruel and unjust to bear a child who must then suffer poverty, hunger, disease, and neglect of their human capacities because there are more mouths to feed than there is food. A new trend of voluntary sterilization is emerging in the United States, with an estimated three million couples undergoing vasectomy or tubal ligation. Voluntary efforts here and abroad are insufficient to control the world's increasing population and limited resources however.

Family Planning

Former Surgeon General Joycelyn Elders stated in a congressional committee hearing that the overpricing of long-term contraceptives, such as Norplant and Depo-Provera, has deprived poor women of two of the most effective means of avoiding unintended pregnancies.[20] These contraceptives could significantly expand women's contraceptive options if they were more reasonably priced. Norplant provides 5 years of protection from pregnancy and costs $500 to $600 for the medical exam, the implants, and the insertion. Depo-Provera injections provide 12 weeks of protection from pregnancy and cost $30.00 per injection in addition to the medical exam. Dr. Elders testified that

> If reproductive choice is to be a reality . . . (it) must include access to the latest, most effective means of contraception. . . . The fundamental problem remains—the price of Norplant and Depo-Provera is too high in this country for a large portion of working poor women to realize contraceptive equality . . . with 57% of all births . . . considered unplanned or unwanted, we need to insure that the newest, most highly effective methods of contraception are not priced beyond the reach of American women."[21]

Some insurance plans or Medicaid will cover these costs.

Forty two million women are of reproductive age; seven in 10 are sexually active and also do not wish to become pregnant. Unintended pregnancies result in over a million abortions annually, as well as over a million births that women did not want until later if at all. A total of 80% of teen pregnancies are unintended, and each year one in nine women aged 15 to 19 become pregnant, and more than half become mothers. "Widespread use of emergency contraception (increased doses of oral conctraceptives) could prevent an estimated million or more unintended pregnancies, and 800,000 abortions each year. These emergency kits are widely available.[22]

Policy proposals recommend that American aid to emerging countries should be tied to population control. The counterargument is that food and aid should be given solely on the basis of human need. Thus, the ethical controversy continues regarding individual liberty to produce as many children as desired and the duty of parents, and ultimately society, to provide children with the necessities of life, including health care.

Critics of population control say that separating nurture from procreation creates a dualism that downgrades the body as an inseparable element in all human events. A counterargument is that nurture is a significant human commitment to the welfare of another. In contrast, procreation is biological, without commitment to the care of the life generated. Thus, the supporters of family planning say that nurture is ultimately the more significant act.

Reproductive Technology

Artificial Insemination.   The ethical arguments for and against artificial insemination are related to the differing definitions of the meaning of marriage, parenthood, and the family system, and to the rightness or wrongness of reproductive interventions. The Roman Catholic position views artificial inseminations by either donor or husband for reasons of sterility or of fallopian tube closure as morally wrong. A recent Vatican speaker said ". . . artificial procreation is an act of production rather than communion between two people. [It] reduces human beings to objects and degrades their being, value, and dignity. Married couples have no right to children, only the right to perform the procreative act."[23]

The ethical arguments in favor of artificial insemination are based on a definition of marriage of mutuality and happiness. In Joseph Fletcher's conception, "marriage is not a physical monopoly."[24] Agreement to an anonymous donor by husband and wife is necessary for informed consent to the donation. Donation of sperm by the husband to the wife is free of problems to supporters of artificial insemination. The issues become more involved, however, when an anonymous ovum is needed to implant in the wife's uterus, or a uterus is needed in which to implant the wife's ovum to carry the fetus to term for a couple unable to have children.

The argument supporting artificial insemination by donor or by husband is that the human acts of sexual intimacy and procreation are different and separate. The main argument is that parenthood is not primarily a matter of biology but rather of broadly human function of commitment to the care and rearing of a child.

In Vitro Fertilization and Implantation.   Similar ethical arguments are used either to justify or denounce in vitro fertilization of the mother's ovum, or one purchased, by the father's sperm in a glass dish in the laboratory, followed by implantation of the embryo in the mother's body. Critics of the act say it is unnatural and undermines the marriage covenant of sexual love for procreation. It treats the procreative dimension of sexuality "as a mere biological function and defines parenthood in terms of nurturing life, not generating life."[25] Utilitarian advocates of the procedure point to the happiness achieved by the couples who are finally able to bear their own child. Others point to the great benefits to genetics and obstetrics coming from this research, which will be of benefit to future generations.

In vitro fertilization experimentation raises ethical issues in policy formation. Should this costly research, which ultimately benefits a few, be financed by scarce public funds that are needed for the benefit of the many? Is a child conceived in this manner subject to public curiosity, stigma, and rejection as a subhuman being?

A related issue that raises an ethical debate is that of "granny pregnancies." By means of sophisticated embryo donation techniques and fertility drugs, a 62-year-old Italian woman gave birth to a healthy, seven-pound son by caesarean section on July 18, 1994. In 1993, under similar circumstances, a 59-year-old British woman gave birth to twins.[26] Advocates of older women's pregnancies proclaimed these events as providing older women with the same rights and liberties as older men to parent children. Critics of granny pregnancies regard them as unfair to the child, who may be orphaned when young; possibly dangerous to the woman's health; and unfair to society that may ultimately pay for the procedure and care of the child.

Fetal Therapy.   The pregnant woman undergoes lifestyle changes, risks, and discomforts for the sake of her fetus. With technological advances in perinatal medicine and surgery, the fetus is accessible to in utero diagnostic procedures and treatment. New embryos in the first trimester that are less than an inch long can be seen so clearly through the viewing scope that the embryo's toes and fingers can be counted.[27] The technique is used experimentally to look at fetuses at high risk for abnormality. This technique is an advancement of fetoscopy, "done in the second and third trimester with a much larger scope and with a higher risk of the loss of pregnancy."[28] The aim is to identify deformities that signal severe birth defects early in the pregnancy so as to cure or correct them.[29]

CASE 9.2: Screening of an Eight-Cell Embryo for Tay-Sachs Gene.   Renee and David both carry the Tay-Sachs disease gene. Their first child died of Tay-Sachs at age 3. They long for a child of their own. However, they have a one in four chance of having another child with the disease.[30] They are offered the opportunity to be the first in the world to have four eight-cell embryos, fertilized in a test tube 3 days earlier, screened for Tay-Sachs disease. Any embryo found to be free of the genetic defect is to be implanted in Renee's uterus. The procedure is completely experimental and free of cost.

According to Lenon, "The pregnant woman and her fetus are increasingly viewed as two treatable patients."[31] Caesarean delivery and intrauterine transfusions are effective, standard treatments for fetal distress. "Shunt diversions for hydro-cephalus or obstructive uropathy are . . . research procedures."[32] These deci-sions, to treat or not to treat, involve the woman's autonomy and her rights to her own body. The moral conflict is "between the pregnant woman's own health, inter-ests, and desires and her perception of the best interests of her fetus."[33] This poses moral conflicts for the procreative family that must choose to either risk the mother's or the fetus's health. It poses conflicts for the health providers as well. In-forming the parents regarding the range of possible outcomes, including the birth of a defective infant despite treatment, is the basis for fully informed consent or rejection of the treatment.

Surrogate Motherhood.   Individual cases of surrogate motherhood in which the biological father and the artificially inseminated mother have waged bitter, prolonged lawsuits for possession of the contracted infant have been national news sensations. In the Baby M case, the surrogate mother, Mary Beth Whitehead, car-ried the pregnancy to full term on the basis of a financial contract with the biolog-ical father and his wife, then refused to give up the newborn. In still another ex-ample, the infant born to the surrogate mother supposedly fathered through artificial insemination turned out to be grossly deformed and retarded. The iden-tity of the father of this newborn became a legal and moral issue. Neither the contracting sperm-donating man nor the surrogate mother desired the defective newborn. A legal suit settled the identity of the father based on scientific evidence as the husband of the surrogate mother. He too rejected the infant.

The exercise of liberty rights of the participating adults illustrates the possible harms to the infant, as well as to the surrogate mother, her spouse, and her family. An issue arises as to whether the love-based model of ethics provides the surrogate mother justification to keep or to regain her infant and to break her promises to the contracting couple? There are several important ethical issues in surrogate motherhood. One is the woman's right to her own body to reproduce a baby for another person. Opposed to this is the idea that the product of a pregnancy, a healthy infant, is not for sale. A group of surrogate mothers demanded the return of their babies and the outlawing of the practice they called "an institutionalized form of slavery."[34]

The New York Task Force on Life and the Law sought legislation in the eight-ies to forbid surrogate parenting that makes money from human reproduction; the New Jersey Superior Court did likewise.[35] The New York State Task Force con-demned the characterization of pregnancy as a service like any other in the mar-ketplace. They rejected a price tag on pregnancy for all women. They reasoned that the purchase of another human being is in violation of the "inherent dignity and equality of all persons."[36]

The counterarguments are that the decision shows a lack of compassion for childless couples who want to use the technology to hire a surrogate mother. Theirs is a human need for which they are willing to pay. Some surrogate mothers desire the income and feel compensated for their labor. These are private affairs involving informed consenting adults who can change the conditions of the con-tract at any time including after the birth of the infant.[37]

Surrogate motherhood evokes conflicts of altruism, justice, rights, duty, subjectivism, and egoism among the participants. Each position has merits, but a decision was reached in the case of Baby M to award the child to the contracting couple with visitation rights permitted the surrogate mother—this was supposedly in the best interest of the child. Meanwhile the legal battle for custody continues.

The Nurse's Role in Reproductive Technology

The nurse's role is to identify her or his own attitude clearly so as to differentiate those values from the values of the prospective parents and the pregnant woman. This may require consultation and deliberation with colleagues until the nurse is clear on basic ethical values. If the nurse disapproves of artificial insemination, in vitro fertilization and implantation, or surrogate motherhood, then the nurse had best withdraw from participation, because such decisions and technology are generally legal and are clearly the right of consenting adults implementing the principle of moral autonomy.

GENETICS

The success of genetic testing in identifying defective genes creates ethical conflicts and dilemmas for individuals, families, institutions, health professionals, and society. For example, some Americans have lost their health insurance and others their jobs because of information obtained through genetic screening.[38] Thousands more will face similar discrimination as the number of tests for identifying persons at high risk for genetic diseases, mental disorders, and heart disease, for example, increases.

Eventually, the US Human Genome Project, a 13-year project (1990–2003), expects to identify most or all of the important genes that cause or contribute to disease.[39] There will be commercial pressure to use these tests as soon as they are available.[40] At present there are no standards for the safety and the accuracy of such tests; nor are there laws or regulations that forbid employers from collecting genetic information and discriminating against current or prospective employees.[41] The National Academy of Sciences panel recommended laws that prohibit consideration of genetic risk when making health insurance decisions.[42] In its broad guidelines, the panel cited the ethical principles of individual rights to consent and confidentiality as essential to the tested person's control of the information. The panel urged that extensive information about the disease and the options faced if carrying the gene (i.e., cystic fibrosis, Tay-Sachs disease, Huntington's disease) be provided to the carrier to reduce ethical conflicts between family and care providers.

CASE 9.3: Is There a Right to Bear Children Despite the Consequences?

Danny and Deborah are an Ashkenazi Jewish couple of strict Orthodox religious beliefs who marry with the intent of having children. The nephew of one of the spouses is born with Tay-Sachs disease, characterized by mental and physical retardation, blindness, deafness, convulsions, and death in the early years of life.

Tay-Sachs disease is 100 times more prevalent in Jewish children, especially in Ashkenazi Jews. There is a genetic test for the presence of an essential enzyme. During pregnancy, amniocentesis will reveal the presence of the required enzyme; if the enzyme is absent, the child will be born with Tay-Sachs disease.[43] The alternative is abortion, an unacceptable practice to this religious group and to the couple. What counsel should the nurse offer?

Prospective parents from vulnerable groups may experience considerable difficulty in even considering themselves as other than young, healthy parents who are competent to deliver a perfectly normal child. Yet some people, such as the couple in the case study, have a high familial probability of carrying the gene for disease. Genetic screening is a simple, effective way of determining their transmission status regarding Tay-Sachs disease. Genes are the way we project ourselves into the future through our children and their children. The ethical issue is the parents' liberty right to produce children without regard for genetic consequences. The counterargument to reproductive freedom is the parents' duties to the potentially afflicted child, other family members, and to society for the emotional, social, and financial cost of treatment and care.

As tragic as the circumstances surrounding the Tay-Sachs child are to the parents, perhaps the traits for sickle-cell anemia present more difficult decisions. There may be

> . . . no evidence to show that health disabilities are associated with carrying a sickle cell gene, except under extraordinary environmental conditions. The gene for hemoglobin S, even when present in a double dose . . . is remarkable for its variability of expression, and decisions about eugenic interventions to reduce its frequency are fraught with difficulty.[44]

This poses ethical problems for African American or Mediterranean American couples regarding screening of a prospective spouse so as to avoid transmitting a two gene sets for a disease that may be benign, debilitating, or lethal. It also involves the issue of truth-telling to a prospective mate if one has the trait, with the possibility of ending the relationship. There is also the question of the availability of health and life insurance or job security if the truth is told. For a short time, New York required non-caucasian, non-indian, and non-asiatic individuals to take a blood test for the sickle-cell trait before issue of a marriage license. This caused public outrage on the basis of its discriminatory effect on African Americans. The effect was to stigmatize them, imperiling their employment, health insurance, and loss of privacy. This law was repealed quickly on grounds that it was ineffective in reducing the frequency of persons in the sickle-cell gene pool.[45]

The case of retinoblastoma is even more complex and requires policy decisions. Retinoblastoma is a malignant glioma of the retina of the eye that occurs in young children and shows a hereditary pattern.[46] The disease incidence was once no more than 1 in 30,000 people. It now occurs in England in as many as 1 in every 18,000 births. This exponential increase took place roughly between 1930 and 1960 and [is] almost entirely the result of physicians' being able to detect the tumor, treat it, and allow the individuals to survive and go on to reproduce. . . . Between 60% to 90% of the individuals actually manifest the tumor . . . develop it in both eyes and would be blinded or die except for new developments in surgery and radiation therapy. Now 70% are saved from blindness and at least four out of five survive.[47]

Thus, the disease is costly to treat, requiring highly specialized eye surgery and treatment; is genetically transmitted; and leads to blindness in some cases. Because this is a dominant gene, it will be passed on by the survivors to ever-increasing numbers of offspring, who will in turn require costly treatment and care. The ethical issue then becomes the right of individuals at risk to pass on retinoblastoma to half their offspring, who must then be treated at public expense, versus the right of the state to refuse treatment based on scarce resources and priorities of prevention. Private insurance carriers may also refuse the risk because of its unfairness to other policyholders who bear the burden of cost.

The argument then extends to preferential treatment of retinoblastoma patients, who tend to have above average intelligence. In reality, most states practice preferential treatment. Patients receiving kidney dialysis three times weekly, for example, cost the state much more than a mentally ill or retarded person living in either a custodial public institution or substandard community facility.

THE ETHICAL ISSUES OF GENETIC SCREENING: MANDATORY VERSUS VOLUNTARY

Individuals and society have choices regarding genetic screening. For example, individuals whose parent or grandparent had Huntington's disease, a degenerative brain ailment that appears around 40 years of age, have a 50% chance of developing it. An estimated 200,000 such persons are at risk.[48] The director of the Huntington's predictive testing project at Johns Hopkins Medical School says that "nearly two thirds of young adults at risk of inheriting the gene say they would like to know if they have it . . . and many couples are testing fetuses early in pregnancy and aborting those that test positive."[49] Some individuals at risk prefer not to know, whereas others have committed suicide after learning that they have the gene.[50] The individual at risk faces further moral conflicts. Should the potential marriage partner be told of the risk for both developing and transmitting the Huntington's disease, or sickle-cell anemia, or Tay-Sachs disease? What is the duty of the nurse or physician to inform the potential spouse if the person at risk does not do so? Can the spouse and the children receive compensation from health providers for not forewarning them of the harm of genetic disease? Does the individual with the defective gene have the duty to inform close relatives as well?

Experts predict that employers and insurers will soon require genetic information unless states restrict testing of employees, as some states now do in the case of AIDS. The possibilities for discriminating against individuals known to carry a defective gene are enormous. The problems will multiply as genetic screening identifies persons with predispositions for atherosclerosis, cancer, arthritis, diabetes, Alzheimer's disease, bipolar disorder, and other common ailments. Will the pregnant woman then have a conflict of aborting a fetus who has the potential for heart disease in 50 years?

Mandatory testing, whether done in the premarital, prenatal, or postnatal period, has potential for moral dilemmas and tragic consequences. Mandatory prenatal screening presents women with terrible burdens and tragic choices if the fetus carries a defective gene. Prenatal screening is not morally neutral since the customary intent is to abort a defective fetus. The alternative, that of bearing the child with a known prognosis of disability, suffering, and death from Tay-Sachs disease, sickle-cell anemia, Huntington's disease, cystic fibrosis, or muscular dystrophy, for example, is equally tragic and possibly more threatening to the survival of the family.

A positive consequence of mandatory testing is that of phenylketonuria (PKU) detection in newborns and the prevention of neurologic damage, delayed psychomotor development, seizures, hypersensitivity, and mental retardation through restricting phenylalanine in the diet.[51] A pregnant woman with high serum phenylalanine is required to consume a low-phenylalamine diet to protect the fetus.[52]

Another response to known hereditary defects, one that violates individual's liberty rights, is compulsory sterilization. Sixteen states still have compulsory sterilization laws.[53] Historically, . . . by 1931, 30 states had passed compulsory sterilization measures, some of which applied to a very wide range of "hereditary defectives" in cluding "sexual perverts," "drug fiends," "drunkards," and "diseased and degenerate persons."[54] The parallels to Hitler's program of purifying the race by the elimination of non-Aryans is inescapable. Such a view mistakenly emphasizes biological fitness and denies the negative and positive contributions of the environment to individual worth and capacity.

A third option for the state requiring mandatory genetic screening is illustrated by the case of retinoblastoma, a tumor that leads to blindness or death if untreated. Because retinoblastoma is generally associated with an intelligence quotient of 116 to 128 and each case costs (conservatively) an average of $100,000 to treat, there is a conflict between costs, benefits, and risks, sometimes called cost-benefit analysis. A question is whether society can afford to finance each case of retinoblastoma. A converse issue is that, given their relatively high intelligence levels, society cannot afford to deny treatment to such persons in view of their social, economic, and cultural contributions. A related question, aptly put by Lappe is: "What are our obligations to those children who are at risk for genetic disease and what are their parents' duties to society?"[55] What if a genetic disease was correlated with lower-than-average intelligence levels; would society still have an obligation to care for this population? Lappe asks what obligations a society has to the less fortunate. He also asks, "How do these obligations change when there are scarce medical resources to be distributed?"[56] Are individuals measured by their contribution to the social good? What role do parents have in bearing the cost of treating genetic diseases? Should affected individuals or their families pay for their own treatment? If society as a whole pays, does society have a right to constrain individuals from procreating "by withholding marriage licenses entirely from individuals with a heritable form of retinoblastoma?"[57]

These questions present moral and political issues for the relation of individuals and society, including issues of support and control. To give society a role in deciding who procreates may set a dangerous precedent in imposing restrictions that may not be rational or free from encouragement of selective breeding, a practice once championed by the Nazis. An immediate practical difficulty of any program of selective breeding involving either negative or positive eugenics is that restricting human variety lessens the chances for good as well as bad species modifications. We are left with moral dilemmas that have no satisfactory answers. Each answer implies some serious negative consequences.

These questions involve the issue of libertarianism in opposition to legal paternalism and legal moralism. Libertarianism holds that a society is made up of individuals whose most important value is freedom from interference. According to legal paternalism, there are some common interests in society that call for justified interferences with individual liberties. These include a lifeguard at public beaches, safe drinking water (presently available to only a small fraction of the earth's population), requirements to wear seat belts in automobiles and helmets on motorcycles, rules providing for safe production and use of foods and drugs, and rules restricting underaged people from voting and drinking. According to a third position, legal moralism, society is viewed as a "seamless web," with individuals regarded as parts of a larger whole. Each individual's place depends on compliance with the requirements of a centralized decision-making group. On this view, the antithesis of libertarianism, individuals have diminished private lives. Every social virtue becomes a law, and every sin becomes a crime. Free will is at a minimum. Such a society is somewhat like the order found in the ownership model of family ethics.

THE NURSE'S ROLE IN GENETIC COUNSELING

We apply these positions, then, to the role of the nurse in genetic counseling. In this connection, Lappe opposes any restrictions "constraining individuals from procreation," and the "intrusion into the privacy of reproductive decision making by the state, which . . . constitutes a greater harm than leaving such decisions to the couples at risk."[58] The nurse, on Lappe's view, does not constrain a retinoblastoma couple against procreation but leaves the decision to them. Lappe prefers "voluntary genetic counseling," which he regards "as superior to compulsory counseling in both outcome and compliance."[59] He is concerned about some state restraints. Blindness is a major health problem in the state; the costs of surgical care are escalating.[60] Lappe proposes a principle consistent with our moral traditions. First, recognize that virtually every prospective parent who puts a child at risk for retinoblastoma will have had the same tumor and will have experienced the pain, suffering and other burdens of that condition. Lappe assigns primacy to this unique experiential basis for judging over and against rules imposed by society from outside the family.[61]

Families at risk decide, even though Lappe concedes that "society" rather than the average individual family "has the financial resources to cope with the surgical cost of treatment."[62] At any rate, Lappe sides . . . with Montaigne who said, "I have never seen a father who failed to claim his son, however mangy or hunchbacked he was. Not that [the father] does not perceive his son's defects . . . but the fact remains, the boy is his. . . . Love and parental bond establish the grounding for a procreative decision, one which works to the best interests of the child."[63] Lappe concludes that

> . . . the right to decide [therefore] must be vested exclusively with parents that are involved. We would be best investing the moral authority for making this decision not with the state but with these individuals who primarily bear the burdens of perpetuating their own genes. [Lappe sees the alternatives as] placing the state over the individual [which denies] the deepest feelings that parents have for their children.[64]

Lappe's message is to trust the parent who has had similar experiences. There is something inherently good and wise in parents. With a little care, one hears the refrain "Parents know best."

One may note the love-based ethics that provides an important moral premise for Lappe. The bond of love between parent and child suggests an innate wisdom and goodness, which parents, following Montaigne's reasoning, show in their decisions. Thus, procreative decisions should be left to parents. Lappe's advice to nurses may be regarded as a form of love-based ethics. His hypothetical advice to nurses is that in their genetic counseling they leave the option rights concerning procreation basically to prospective parents, rather than to the state in either a legal paternalist or legal moralist form. This view is also identified as a moral-sentiment view, expressed alternatively by Jean Jacques Rousseau (1712–1778) and Leo Tolstoy, both of whom valued the moral sentiments that are found among ordinary people, including peasants, who are viewed as "noble savages." This innate moral folk wisdom is the love parents have for their children. It reveals wise and untutored forms of public and private decency.

But is there evidence to support this view of the goodness and wisdom of parents? One has only to look at public institutions, such as those for the retarded, abandoned, rejected, or abused children, to learn of all the despised and rejected physical, emotional, and mental "hunchbacks" who are unwanted by parents. The parent does not always know best. Persons in authority, such as physicians, judges, nurses, and other representatives of society, have a role in sustaining good family relations even on the basis of paternalistic interference.

SUMMARY

A family can be positive if it enables individuals in the family to flourish separately and together. If the relationships are destructive or unwise, intervention by nurses and other relevant persons is appropriate. The nurse can help by supporting positive human relationships. One reason for nursing intervention is that in relations between spouses or parents and children, the stronger does not always know best.

Current knowledge of genetic traits expressed in serious, debilitating or fatal diseases such as Tay-Sachs, sickle-cell anemia, cystic fibrosis, retinoblastoma or Huntington's raise profound moral issues of the liberty and rights of individuals such as parents to procreate at will versus the rights of society to limit the use of resources to maintain a non-contributing member whose birth could have been avoided. The nursing role in genetic counseling is one of helping parents to secure relevant information concerning the incidence and course of a disease, its predicted progression, and the experience of other parents with similarly afflicted children. A further moral question is that of parental responsibility in the decision to conceive and bear a child whose life experience may be painful, tragic, and short due to the disease progression. The nurse can be helpful to the parents in considering the effects of the disease on the afflicted child as well as on the well-being of the whole family. As the Genome Project unfolds with the identification of more harmful genes, the decisions facing the procreative family will become ever more complex and difficult.

Discussion Questions

1. How would you examine four moral views such as paternalism, libertarianism, agapism, and utilitarianism in their approaches toward counseling the family with a sickle-cell trait?
2. What differences are there among agapism, utilitarianism, and Kantian ethics in relation to the use of reproductive technology?
3. In the relation between the state, the individual at risk or one who has a costly hereditary disease, or the procreative couple with a known genetic abnormality who bear children, who bears the major responsibility for providing for treatment? Who, if any has rights to treatment?
4. Which of the ethical theories discussed is most (least) helpful in justifying the wish to procreate in parents with AIDS or genetically transmitted diseases.
5. Do members of society have a right to restrict reproduction among AIDS patients or those with genetically transmitted diseases? For what moral reasons?

REFERENCES

1. Burgess EW, Locke HJ, Thomas MM. *The family* (4th ed). New York: Van Nostrand Reinhold. 1971;1.
2. ibid, p. 2.
3. Thomson J. In defense of abortion. *Philosophy and Public Affairs* 1971;1(1):47–66.
4. Goldman A. *The moral foundations of professional ethics.* Totowa, NJ: Littlefield, Adams. 1980;2–8, 20–22, 34–37, 49, 58–61, 65–69, 88–91, 109, 113, 273, 277–278, 281, 282.
5. Robbins M, Schacht T. Family hierarchies. *Am J Nursing* 1982,82(2):285.
6. ibid.
7. Feinberg J. The child's right to an open future. In: Aiken W, LaFollette H (eds). *Whose child? Children's rights, parental authority and state power.* Totowa, NJ: Littlefield, Adams. 1980;125–153.
8. Benoliel JQ. The nurse-family relationship. In: Curtin L, Flaherty MJ (eds). *Nursing ethics: theories and pragmatics.* Bowie, Md: Brady. 1982;121.
9. Mill JS. *Utilitarianism, liberty and representative government.* London, England: Dent. 1948;79.

10. Benoliel JQ. The nurse-family relationship. In: Curtin L, Flaherty MJ (eds). *Nursing ethics: theories and pragmatics.* Bowie, Md: Brady. 1982;121.
11. Toulmin S. The tyranny of principles. *Hastings Center Report.* 1981;11(6):31–39.
12. ibid.
13. Burns C et al. New diagnosis: Caregivers' role strain. *Nursing Diag* 1993;4(2):73–76.
14. Harding GJ. What about the family? *Hastings Center Report* 1990;20(2):5–10.
15. ibid.
16. Confronting domestic violence. *Report: Official Newsletter of the New York State Nurses* 1998;29(9):4.
17. Feldman J. Divorce and the children. In: Getty C, Humphreys W (eds). *Understanding the family: Stress and change in the American family.* East Norwalk, Conn: Appleton-Century-Crofts. 1981;336.
18. ibid, p. 333.
19. Foreman CH Jr. What the AIDS czar can't do. *The New York Times.* July 14, 1993;A19.
20. Leary WE. Long-term contraceptives cost called excessive. *The New York Times.* March 19, 1994;10.
21. ibid.
22. Planned Parenthood. *The future of birth control.* October 18, 1999.
23. Berger J. Vatican official assails method of fertilization. *The New York Times.* October 8, 1987;B6.
24. McCormick RA. Reproductive technologies: Ethical issues. In: Reich WT (ed). *Encyclopedia of bioethics.* (Vol. 5) New York: Free Press. 1978;456.
25. ibid, p. 1463.
26. Italian oldest to give birth. *Daily Hampshire Gazette.* July 19, 1994;5.
27. Kolata G. New scope examines embryos in first trimester. *The New York Times.* July 11, 1993;32.
28. ibid.
29. ibid.
30. Healthy baby born after test for deadly gene. *The New York Times.* January 28, 1994;17.
31. Lenon JL. The fetus as a patient: Emerging rights as a person? *Am J Law Med* 1983;9:1–29.
32. American Academy of Pediatrics Committee on Bioethics. Fetal therapy: Ethical considerations. *Pediatrics* 1988;81(6):898–9.
33. ibid.
34. Schneider K. Mothers urge ban on surrogacy as form of slavery. *The New York Times.* September 1, 1986;A13.
35. Editorial. *The New York Times.* June 4, 1988;A26.
36. ibid.
37. D'Amato A. Letter to the editor. *The New York Times.* February 18, 1988;A26.
38. Hilts PJ. Panel reports genetic screening has cost some their health plans. *The New York Times.* November 5, 1993;A20.
39. ibid.
40. ibid.
41. ibid.
42. ibid, p. 19.
43. *Taber's Cyclopedic Medical Dictionary* (14th ed) Philadelphia: FA Davis, 1981;1427.
44. Lappe M. Genetics and our obligations to the future. In: Bandman EL, Bandman B (eds). *Bioethics and human rights: A reader for health professionals.* Lanham, Md: University Press of America. 1986;86.
45. ibid.

46. *Taber's Cyclopedic Medical Dictionary,* 1246.

47. Lappe M. Genetics and our obligation to the future. In: Bandman EL, Bandman B (eds). *Bioethics and human rights: A reader for health professionals.* Boston: Little, Brown. 1978;87.

48. Blakesle S. Genetic discoveries raise painful questions. *The New York Times.* April 21, 1987;C1.

49. ibid.

50. ibid.

51. Bullock BL, Rosendal PP. *Pathophysiology* (3rd ed). Philadelphia: JB Lippincott. 1992;53–54.

52. ibid.

53. Lappe M. Genetics and our obligations to the future. In: Bandman EL, Bandman B (eds). *Bioethics and human rights: A reader for health professionals.* Lanham, Md: University Press of America. 1986;91.

54. Ludmerer KM. Eugenics: History. In: Reich WT (ed). *Encylcopedia of bioethics.* (Vol. 1) New York: Free Press. 1978;459.

55. Lappe M. Genetics and our obligations to the future. In: Bandman EL, Bandman B (eds). *Bioethics and human rights: A reader for health professionals.* Lanham, Md: University Press of America. 1986;86.

56. ibid.

57. ibid, p. 91.

58. ibid.

59. ibid, p. 92.

60. ibid.

61. ibid, p. 92.

62. ibid.

63. ibid, p. 93.

64. ibid.

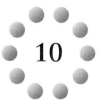

10

Nursing Ethics
and the Problem of Abortion

Study of this chapter enables the learner to:

1. Appreciate the moral significance of a woman's decision regarding procreative choice.
2. Understand the Supreme Court's and legislative decisions regarding abortion.
3. Identify the uses of reproductive technology in relation to abortion.
4. Use the ethical arguments in opposition to and in support of abortion as the basis for forming an individual position regarding this problem.
5. Apply moral reasoning to the formulation of abortion policy.

OVERVIEW

A sexually active woman has a most important decision to make. As Shakespeare's Hamlet asked, "To be or not to be?" To begin or not to begin a new life? Several moral arguments provide justifying reasons in deciding whether to initiate or to continue a new life, a decision surrounded by enormous responsibility. The power of life and death is in the hands of those who decide. For this reason, all problems in bioethics, in ethicist Willard Gaylin's view, keep coming back to abortion. Moral principles are designed to answer the question whether to terminate a life or not. As we shall see, these principles, while helpful, do not always work. One principle, expressed by St. Thomas Aquinas (discussed in Chapter 4), is that life is a gift given by Him who alone gives life and therefore no human is to take that life. But this principle is occasionally in conflict with a utilitarian principle—which holds that the good for human beings is the greatest happiness of the greatest number—and may require the deliberate termination of a fetus, such as when amniocentesis shows serious physical or mental anomalies (see Chapter 5). Moreover, a feminist rights principle holds that a woman who has a major role in the upbringing of a child must be free to decide whether to bring a fetus to term or to abort it (see Chapter 7). For these reasons, abortion continues to be controversial.

LEGAL STATUS OF ABORTION

In the landmark case of *Roe v. Wade,* 410 US 113 (1973) and *Doe v. Bolton,* 410 US 179 (1973), the Supreme Court established the right of every woman to have an abortion legally. *Roe v. Wade* reversed the Texas statute restricting abortion to instances necessary to save a woman's life. *Doe v. Bolton* overturned the Georgia statute permitting abortions only if necesssary to the woman's health, to prevent the birth of a malformed child, or to terminate pregnancy from rape. The Court's decision invalidated similar laws in other states that restricted abortion.

In the decision favoring abortion, the Court recognized the right of personal privacy in the Constitution, with roots in the First, Fourth, Fifth, Ninth, and Four-teenth Amendments, as well as in the Bill of Rights; and with reference to *Gris-wold v. Connecticut,* 381 US 479 (1965).[1] The majority of justices said that only fundamental personal rights extending to marriage, procreation, contraception, child rearing, and education can be included in the right to personal privacy.[2] Based on these amendments, a woman's absolute, unrestricted right to terminate pregnancy was argued. The Court, however, could not agree to the woman's ab-solute right to privacy without the state asserting its interests in safeguarding health through maintaining standards of medical practice and "in protecting potential life."[3] The Court refused to accept the fetus as a person because of sub-stantial disagreement on the concept of personhood and the omission of the un-born from consideration in the Fourteenth Amendment. "The unborn have never been recognized in the law as persons in the whole sense."[4]

Without resolving the question of when life begins—whether at birth, con-ception, quickening, or viability—the Court recognized states' interests in the woman's health and the potential human life approaching term as compelling. The Court summarized its decision in the following provisions:

1. Any state criminal abortion laws such as the Texas type, which "excepts from criminality only a lifesaving procedure on behalf of the mother, without re-gard to pregnancy state and without recognition of the other interests in-volved," violate the due process clause of the Fourteenth Amendment."[5]
   a. The abortion decision in the first trimester is between the woman and her physician.
   b. The state may regulate the abortion procedure to protect the mother's health after the first trimester.
   c. Following the stage of viability (a fetus usually 28 weeks or older, capa-ble of living outside the uterus), a state may regulate, or even prohibit, abortion except where medically necessary to preserve the life or health of the mother.
2. Only licensed physicians are permitted to perform abortions.

One might consider this decision from the highest court of the land to be au-thoritative and final. Not so. The controversy over abortion continues, and two more Supreme Court decisions affect the implementation of the *Roe v. Wade* decision.

In two cases (*Beal v. Doe* 432 US 438 [1977], *Maher v. Roe* 432 US 464 [1977]) the Supreme Court ruled that states are not required to spend Medicaid funds for elective, nontherapeutic abortion. Congress then promptly banned the use of federal funds for abortions, with some exceptions. Thus, quite effectively, the Supreme Court's 1973 decision permitting abortion was seriously restricted by withholding funds for abortions from poor women, the recipients of Medicaid funds for health care, as unnecessary medical service. Thus, one social class, the poor, is singled out for the restriction of the fundamental right to abortion because of the inability to pay. Moreover, the justices' majority opinion argued for the states' "valid and important interest in emergency normal childbirth."[6] On the grounds of the state's significant interest in a woman's pregnancy, the state funds childbirth but need not fund elective abortions. The Court said that while the state may not prevent abortions, it need not help poor women obtain them as a remedy for social and economic ills.[7] The Court left the federal government and the states free to provide or withhold funding for abortions.

Assaults on *Roe v. Wade* reach the Supreme Court each year. Cases involving the consent of both parents for abortion in underage women, or the consent of the supposed responsible male for abortion in an adult pregnant woman, or an imposed waiting period of at least 24 hours before the procedure, have all been heard by the Supreme Court. Each of these requirements interferes with the reproductive choices and rights of women. An enforced waiting period is especially detrimental to poor women from outlying areas who cannot afford overnight lodging and transportation costs.

In *Planned Parenthood v. Casey* (1992), the Supreme Court recognized a woman's right "to choose an abortion before fetal viability."[8] The Court, however, replaced the trimester system of *Roe v. Wade* with the "undue burden" standard. According to *Roe v. Wade*, a woman had a right to decide whether to abort within the first trimester. In the second trimester, the state may regulate an abortion in relation to maternal health. In the third trimester of "fetal viability, the state may regulate and even prohibit abortion, except where it is necessary to preserve the life or health of the mother."[9] The "undue burden" standard means that the burden is shifted to the woman to establish that giving birth would be too heavy a burden to bear. A reason the Court gave for the "undue burden" standard was that the "state has legitimate interests from the onset of pregnancy [for] protecting a woman's health and the life of the fetus that may become a child."[10]

The Court declared its reasoning as follows: The State's "substantial interest in potential life" implies that "not all regulations" (that interfere with a woman's liberty to decide) are "deemed unwarranted. Not all burdens on the right to decide whether to terminate a pregnancy will be undue."[11] Therefore, the Court concludes that "the undue burden standard is the appropriate means of reconciling the State's interest with the woman's constitutionally protected liberty."[12] The Court distinguished an appropriate burden from an "undue burden" by regarding spousal notification of the intended abortion as "an undue burden."[13]

The Court ruled that a woman has a liberty to choose to have an abortion in accordance with *Roe v. Wade*, but "a woman's liberty is not so unlimited . . . that the Court cannot show its concern for the life of the unborn."[14] In effect, the Court ruled that a woman has the liberty to decide to have an abortion, provided that her liberty is not in conflict with the State's interest in caring for potential life after fetal viability. Of course, it is necessary to recognize the law even if one disagrees with it. Yet, we view *Casey's* replacement of the trimester system as too stringent a requirement on women to prove that their pregnancy is an "undue burden."

The most recent legislative controversy centers around late-term abortion, so-called partial birth abortion, despite its occurrence in less than 6,000 cases. Late-term abortions are defined as those in which the fetus is allegedly able to live outside the womb after 22 weeks following conception. There are bans on late-term abortion in 30 states, with some imposing severe penalties on the practitioner; however, in other states the ban was found unconstitutional.[15] These attempts to ban late-term abortions are regarded as attempts to ban all abortion by misrepresentation of their number and circumstances.

In *Madsen v. Women's Health Center* (1994), the U.S. Supreme Court upheld parts of an injunction against protesters at a Florida abortion clinic.[16] The Florida Court had previously found that abortion protesters hindered access to the clinic by blocking the driveway and harassing the cars' occupants as they slowed down to avoid hitting the protesters.[17] As many as 400 protestors sang and chanted into loudspeakers and bullhorns "causing stress to patients during the surgical procedure and in the recovery room."[18] Women seeking an abortion who turned away because of the crowd delayed the procedure and thus increased their health risks.[19] Physicians, nurses, clinic workers, and volunteer escorts were also harassed at work and at home, as were their families, children, and neighbors. Two physicians and one volunteer escort were killed in Florida in the course of these demonstrations.

The Supreme Court also supported restraints on "singing, chanting, whistling, shouting, yelling, use of bullhorns, auto horns, sound amplification equipment or other sounds or images observable to or within earshot of the patients inside the clinic."[20] This case is significant because the federal Freedom of Access to Clinic Entrance Act (1994) was passed, designed to provide federal remedies, injunctions, and criminal penalties for violent protests at abortion clinics.

REPRODUCTIVE TECHNOLOGY AND ABORTION

Abortion Technology

Theoretically, mifepristone (also known as RU-486), which was approved by the FDA in September 2000, will eliminate the need for the nearly 1.6 million surgical abortions performed in the United States each year.[21] In 1994, the drug's developer donated the US rights to a nonprofit contraceptive research organization, the Population Council.[22] RU-486 can be used within 49 days of the first day of the last menstrual period. The abortion can take several days, but it can be done on an outpatient basis and monitored by a physician with access of a hospital.[23] A leader of abortion rights groups, Mary Wilder, sees the "end of the tyranny of anti-choice extremists who for too long have held science hostage to their religious and ideological views."[24] Opponents of abortion called RU-486 "a human pesticide. . . . (They) warned that any company making the pill would be subject to boycotts and other economic attacks."[25] The so called "morning after" pill consisting of increased doses of oral contraceptives, are widely available, and could prevent a very large number of unintended pregnancies and consequent abortions.

Prenatal Tests of Fetal Health

The possibilities for choosing abortion to end an unwanted pregnancy are growing explosively as a consequence of three new prenatal tests for fetal health.[26]

Chorionic Villus Sampling.

This test may be used as early as the ninth week of pregnancy. Cells are taken from the villi, the gestational sac that surrounds the fetus in early pregnancy. In a few days, the results "disclose birth defects like Down syndrome, Tay-Sachs disease, or other genetic disorders."[27] The experts believe that the time advantage will result in this test replacing most amniocentesis procedures.

Alpha-fetoprotein Screening.

This is a blood test that California physicians are required by law to offer their patients. It is given at 16 weeks of pregnancy to women of all ages. The test measures levels of alpha-fetoprotein that the fetus excretes into the amniotic sac and the mother's bloodstream. The test is used to detect neural tube defects. If the neural tube fails to close at the top, the baby is born anencephalic and dies at birth or soon after.[28] If the neural tube is open at the spine and the spinal cord is exposed, then the infant is born with spina bifida and probably hydrocephalus and mental retardation.[29] The test also detects risk of Down syndrome. Neural tube defects occur about 1 in every 1,000 births to women without a family history of birth defects. This test is the only way to detect such affected fetuses.[30]

Amniocentesis.

Amniocentesis is used to obtain cells from the amniotic fluid surrounding the fetus. This procedure can be done only at about the fourth month of pregnancy and the result takes two weeks to develop. At four-and-a-half months of pregnancy, abortion is physically and emotionally more difficult for the woman. This test detects such genetic defects as Down syndrome and Tay-Sachs disease.

Benefits, Harms, and Risks of Prenatal Tests

The benefits of the alpha-fetoprotein screening test are that women younger than age 35 with high levels of alpha-fetoprotein are informed of the increased risk of carrying a fetus with Down syndrome or neural tube defects and are then offered amniocentesis.[31] Women over age 35 with normal levels of alpha-fetoprotein are at low risk for having a fetus with Down syndrome and on this basis can choose to reject amniocentesis.[32]

The harms and risks of amniocentesis and the chorionic villus sampling tests lie in the 0.5% to 1.5% of abortions induced by the test.[33] The harm of the alpha-fetoprotein test lies in the suggestiveness of the results and the need for follow-up tests that can be hazardous to the fetus. However, these tests offer the pregnant woman data regarding the health of the fetus as the basis for exercising her right to abortion.

Fetal Reduction

Some infertile women have resorted to the use of fertility drugs or to in vitro fertilization and implantation. Consequently, some women have had multiple pregnancies of as many as eight fetuses, all of whom have little chance of survival. One approach to this problem is selective abortion of the most accessible fetuses (seen through the sonogram) by injection with a lethal dose of potassium during the first trimester of pregnancy.[34] Most pregnancy reductions leave the woman with twins as a margin of safety or, in some cases, with the healthiest single fetus. Some of the decisions to reduce the number of pregnancies were made for the woman's convenience. Other abortions were made solely to ensure the survival of at least one or two of the multiple fetuses.

Arguments for and against this experimental procedure have ranged from support for a woman's absolute right to her body to a total rejection of abortion in any form. Richard McCormick, an ethicist, argued that the procedure could be justified when all the fetuses would otherwise die. "It is against the abortion position of the Catholic Church, (but) . . . I just don't think that the abortion position of the Church was formulated and designed with any circumstances like these in mind."[35] John Fletcher, another ethicist, said that the reduction did the "least harm for the most potential good."[36]

The Use of Embryonic Tissue

Another moral dilemma has arisen from the growing clinical need for human fetal tissue. Fetal grafts from human embryos are considered to be a major advance in treating degenerative disorders such as Parkinson's disease, radiation disorders, and juvenile diabetes, and in repair of damaged hearts.[37] Fetal tissue reportedly integrates and survives longer in the host and resists rejection better than adult tissue grafts.[38] Research using embryonic cardiac cells for cardiac repair is more feasible than total heart transplants according to Regelson. A moral dilemma arises from the massive need for human embryonic cells, and the current inability to grow them without using fetuses for "personal or commercial exploitation."[39] An aging society with increasingly prevalent degenerative diseases and growing demand for their treatment by the best means available will "further polarize attitudes toward abortion."[40]

ETHICAL AND RELIGIOUS ISSUES IN ABORTION

Even if there were a clamor for legalization of abortion, the controversy continues as to whether abortion is morally permissible.

Positions on abortion are largely justified by opinions held on the status of the product of pregnancy. At one end of the spectrum, the Catholic Church, through its popes Pius XII and now John Paul II, views life as sacred and to be preserved from the moment of its conception. All abortions, even for therapeutic reasons or for reasons of socioeconomic distress, are illicit.[41] This view holds that a human being emerges at conception through the parental combination of genetic packages with all of the potentialities of a person in the zygote, including a fundamental right to life.

An argument favoring abortion is that, because the embryo lacks electrical activity in the brain, it is simply living tissue, which may be eliminated like other unwanted tissue, such as the appendix or tonsils. The counterargument of those opposing abortion is that reflexes are present in the embryo and, although lacking in brain activity, "its potentialities for full human life and personhood set it apart as quite different from a being whose permanently nonfunctioning brain signals that he is dead."[42] The counterargument is that, as Dedek and the Supreme Court decision point out, the fetus is a potential person and not actual, "Just as the acorn is potential but far from the actuality of an oak tree. Acorns are not oak trees."[43] Thus, the counterargument against abortion rests on the potential personhood of the fetus, who has the same right to life as any other person.

Judith Thomson, a philosopher who defends abortion under certain circumstances, confronts the premise of the fetus as a human being from the moment of conception. She acknowledges that human development is continuous and to draw a line of personhood at any point, whether at conception, quickening, viability, "understanding," "reasoning," or "life projects," is to make an arbitrary choice. The same kind of thing might be said about the relation of the acorn to the oak tree but, she argues, "it does not follow that acorns are oak trees."[44] Arguments of this sort are notorious examples of the slippery-slope fallacy (discussed in Chapter 8).

For the sake of developing both sides of the argument, Thomson grants that if the fetus is a person from the moment of conception, then, like every other person, it has a right to life. Likewise, the mother is a person and has a right to her life and to decisions determining what is allowed to happen in and to her body. At this point, the anti-abortionists believe that a person's right to life, in this case the fetus's, outweighs "the mother's right to decide what happens in and to her body. . . . So the fetus may not be killed; an abortion may not be performed."[45]

Thomson responds to this point with her well-known analogy of waking up back-to-back with a famous unconscious violinist. The violinist has a lethal kidney ailment and is plugged into your compatible circulatory system. To unplug him would be to kill him. The hospital director soothingly tells you, "But it's only for 9 months." But do you have to agree to it? Thomson asks. And what if it were 9 years or your lifetime? The hospital director says, "Too bad. Everyone has a right to life, and this violinist is a person. His right to life outweighs your right to your own body. Therefore, you cannot be unplugged from him ever."

This is an outrageous argument, in Thomson's view. It is especially outrageous in instances of pregnancy through rape or when the pregnancy threatens the mother's life. If, on this view, the mother and the fetus have an equal right to life, why not flip a coin, or grant that the mother's right to life as well as her right to what happens in and to her body outweighs the fetus's right to life?

The anti-abortionist view is that performing an abortion is direct killing, whereas not doing anything is only letting the mother die and not killing an innocent person, namely the fetus. The direct killing of an innocent person, such as the fetus, is regarded as murder and therefore is not permitted as preferable to letting either the mother, the fetus, or both die. Thomson responds that it cannot be murder for the mother to save her life by performing an abortion. No woman need sit by passively waiting for her death. Using the violinist analogy, she has only to unplug herself. Thomson believes that to refuse an abortion to such a mother "is to refuse to grant to the mother the very status of person which is so firmly insisted on for the fetus."[46]

Thomson sees this situation as analogous to that of a mother trapped in a very tiny house with a rapidly growing child; she will be crushed to death by the lack of space. Thomson argues that third parties, such as health care providers, may refuse to choose between the mother's life and the fetus's life, but the mother, who is the person housing the child, has the right of self-defense against threats to her life; she owns the house. Thomson likens the houseowner analogy to that of two people freezing to death, with one the owner of a coat that will save his life—the coat owner has the right to the coat. Likewise does the pregnant woman own her body, which houses the fetus. Therefore, the health care provider can refuse to act in performing an abortion, but someone needs to protect the rights of individuals both to their own bodies and to their own coats.

Thomson then considers the case for abortion when the mother's life is not at stake. She sees the anti-abortionist argument here as resting on the fetus's claim to a right to life. This view regards the right to life as unproblematic. Thomson says that life is not unproblematic. In her view, the right to life includes the right to the "bare minimum . . . for continued life."[47] But what if the bare minimum is something to which the person has no right, such as continuous free food, clothing, shelter, health care services, and loving care?

Thomson raises the counterargument to this position, which is that even if no one has a right to be given anything, there is a right not to be killed by anyone, by unplugging, shooting, or knifing. But to refrain from unplugging the previously mentioned violinist is to allow him to continue the use of your kidney. Although he has no right to the original use of your kidneys, the anti-abortionist argument says that the violinist has the right against you "not now to intervene and deprive him of the use of your kidneys."[48] Contrary to the anti-abortion position, the right to life, in Thomson's view, does not guarantee the use of another's body even if such use is lifesaving. To illustrate her case, Thomson uses the example of a gift box of chocolates to two brothers. If the gift was given to both jointly and the older brother eats the whole box without giving any to his brother, he is unjust, for the younger brother was given half. Contrariwise, unplugging the violinist is not unjust, because you gave neither him nor anyone else the right to the use of your kidneys. Unplugging him would surely kill him, but not unjustly and without violation of his right to life, because the use of another's body is not guaranteed in the right to life.

Thomson then responds to the charge of abortion as unjust killing. Certainly the rape victim has not given the fetus "a right to the use of her body for food and shelter."[49] But isn't there some sense in which a woman engaging in intercourse who then becomes pregnant is at least partly responsible for the life within, even if she did not invite it in? (It is a statistical fact that not all contraceptives are 100% effective.) Does the woman's partial responsibility then give the fetus the right to the woman's body, and can the woman now kill it even to save her own life? Thomson points to the argument that a fetus's right to life as an independent person is fallacious because, in fact, the fetus is dependent on the mother and the mother has a special kind of responsibility for its well-being. Nurses know the significance of the mother's nutrition, health habits, and lifestyle in supporting the fetus's proper growth and development. Thomson uses other analogies to support her arguments in defense of abortion. If, for example, I open the window of my home and a burglar climbs in, it would be incorrect to say, "Ah, but you opened the window and now he's in, and therefore you're partly responsible and must let him stay."[50] Or, for example

> People seeds drift about in the air like pollen, and if you open your windows, one may drift in and take root in your carpets or upholstery. You don't want children, so you fix your windows with fine mesh screens, the very best you can buy. As can happen . . . one of the screens is defective; and a seed drifts in and takes root. Does the person plant who now develops have a right to the use of your house?[51]

The required move might be to seal your windows and doors and to live with bare floors and without furniture. Surely a person plant who enters your house does not have a right to a place in the house, any more than a burglar has who came into your house without permission. A woman could have a hysterectomy to avoid unwanted pregnancies, but like the person who keeps the person plants out of her home, a woman who wishes to avoid rape would never leave home without an army. Because this is virtually impossible for most persons, abortions of unwanted pregnancies are justified.

Thomson concludes with a distinction between concepts of a Good Samaritan and a Minimally Decent Samaritan. She recounts the parable of the Good Samaritan.

> "A certain man" going from Jerusalem to Jericho was attacked by thieves and left half dead. A priest walked by where the wounded man lay in the road and went to the other side. A Levite also passed by. Both ignored the wounded man. "But a certain Samaritan" on seeing the man "had compassion . . . " and "bound up his wounds." Before leaving, the Samaritan asked others to care for him and said he would repay them when he came by again[52] (Luke 10:30–35).

Although we are all oriented by the Good Samaritan example, there is another kind of Samaritan called the Minimally Decent Samaritan. These are the nurses, mothers, and other people who recognize that caring for patients, children, and others, even if it is at times inconvenient to themselves, is the right thing to do. To fail to help someone in dire need, when the cost of helping is quite small, is "monstrous." Thomson cites the example of Kitty Genovese being murdered in an apartment house parking lot in New York City while 38 apartment residents looked on from adjoining windows and did nothing to help her. Not one person called the emergency police number, a very small effort.

Another example of the failure to be a Minimally Decent Samaritan is that of the onlookers of the Holocaust, both inside and outside of Germany, failing to help Jews and other victims from being exterminated by the Nazis. A further example is that of a woman in her eighth month of pregnancy who decides to compete for a tennis match; to do so she will need an abortion. Thomson regards such a decision as morally indecent. A woman does not have a right to do anything she desires and not consider the moral requirement to be a Minimally Decent Samaritan. A person's rights are limited by the requirement to be a Minimally Decent Samaritan. On this view, nurses have a moral responsibility to care for their patients and not treat them like the 38 onlookers who treated Kitty Genovese passively, indifferently, and without caring.

Some difficulties arise for several aspects of Thomson's argument. One is that to have a right in and to one's body, compared to owning a house, is not absolute. There are exceptions to one's rights in and to one's body. If one has a contagious disease, such as typhoid or smallpox, one cannot go anywhere one pleases. Nor can one use one's body to swim in the community drinking water supply. The "landlord" analogy, to use a metaphor of Toulmin's about certain abortion arguments,[53] implies that a pregnant woman has the right to decide whether to evict her "tenant," and it presupposes that a woman owns her offspring. Some writers even go so far as to assert that a "pregnant woman makes a baby, presumably like a carpenter, sculptor, or architect."[54] Viewing a pregnant woman as a landlady, factory owner, or sculptor begs the question and gives the case away to those who argue that a pregnant woman may do with her body as she pleases. A criticism of the property or artifact metaphor is that a life growing within another person is not quite like somebody's property or a factory or simply clay in someone's hands, contrary to the claim of those who write that a mother makes a baby.

A mother does not make a baby, because there are factors outside a mother's control that affect the development of the fetus. A mother's contribution to the fetus's physical development is largely involuntary, unlike a carpenter's, sculptor's, or architect's, whose will and design has more to do with shaping the outcome. The mother cannot decide the sex, size, color, or genetics of her offspring, for example. Opposed to the landlady, factory-owner, or sculptor metaphor of a mother-fetus relationship is the comparison of a pregnant women to a passive receptacle, such as a flower or an oven, who does not create the life within her. On this view, God alone makes or creates a baby, and the mother is only the one who will help it grow, like a plant growing with the help of water and sunlight. A woman's role is to receive male sperm, which then develops inside her womb. On another view, there are scientific accounts of fetal development which do not invoke God. But "the gift of life," to use St. Thomas Aquinas's metaphor, is not any human being's to take or to destroy under any circumstances. According to Aquinas, "Life is God's gift to man and is subject to His power who kills and who makes to live."[55]

The analogy that compares a woman to a flower also has weaknesses. How could one test the assertion that God makes a baby, for example? What kind of gift is life that it cannot be refused or destroyed by anyone else? Is life necessarily or always a gift, even for an infant or older person with multiple physical or mental deformities such as spina bifida, myelomeningocele, or cancer? Another view denies the essentially passive role of women in pregnancy and child rearing. A woman, on this view, has a role and a stake in the outcome. She is no mere receptacle to be filled at will by a man who owns and controls her nature and destiny. To compel a woman to bring to term an unwanted pregnancy is regarded by one writer as "forced labor."[56]

But whether a given practice counts as forced labor may be philosophically debatable. For example, Nozick argues that taxation beyond that which is necessary for a minimal state—one that protects individuals against one another—is "forced labor."[57] Ingenious as is Nozick's idea of forced labor, there is room for debate. His argument does not present us with a fixed truth. For example, taxation for libraries, museums, parks, colleges, or public preservation of the wilderness, as Feinberg points out,[58] hardly constitutes forced labor.

We can distinguish two senses of forced labor. Most of us must work to make a living. A woman who wants a child exerts labor and force to bring a fetus through the birth canal. A second sense of forced labor, akin to slave labor that is morally impermissible, imposes the duty to bring a fetus to term. In this negative sense of forced labor, if there are any a priori truths in morals, they include the statement that "forced labor," slave labor, is morally wrong. But this principle conflicts with another principle that murder is wrong. Abortion in certain circumstances is murder and is therefore wrong.

The use of the property and flower metaphors attempts to answer the question, "When does life begin and end?" This question presupposes an answer to the metaphysical question, "Is a pregnant woman one being or two?"[59] To individuate the fetus very early in pregnancy or at the moment of conception is to regard a pregnant woman as two persons, each with equal rights. A conflict then develops between the rights of each, calling for a settlement by a third party such as the church or state. To individuate later in the pregnancy or near the time a woman gives birth is to regard a pregnant woman as one person and, therefore, as the only rightholder. Against this one pregnant person, a growing fetus may be conceived of as an intrusive invader if that fetus is unwanted. The mother decides who to let into her house or body, as one chooses who to invite to one's party. On this view, the decision is hers to make. She owns her body and everything in it. The force of the ownership model, is again an intuitively powerful source of appeal when it comes to a woman claiming her rights; for if she owns anything, it is her body. But this argument has a conceptual drawback, namely that a woman or a man does not own her or his body. Women and men are their bodies, but do not own them in the way they own their belongings or their property, about which they may justifiably exercise control. In the case of a woman's body, however, a moral question arises as to whether she may sell blood, for example, to someone in need. Therefore, a conception of a woman being identified as her body puts other people on notice that they may not enter or do anything to her body without her consent.

In opposition, Brody argues that humanity begins with a fetus. A human fetus has the same moral status as a mother and, therefore, the same right to live. This means abortion is not morally justifiable, even in cases that threaten a mother's life. By analogy, a bigger, stronger person has no right to kill a weaker one. To Brody, Thomson's self-defense argument does not work, because the fetus is not the mother's pursuer.[60] Instead, the fetus is a miniature human in the sense that it has an essential property of being human, namely a brain,[61] which it develops sometime between the second and twelfth week after conception.[62]

There are strengths and weaknesses in Brody's argument. His argument does refute one version of Thomson's self-defense argument: A pregnant woman is not opposed and pursued by her fetus. Another strength is his appeal to the obvious resemblances between a fetus and an infant human being. A third strength is the respect Brody engenders for the living and the moral wrongness of killing. Brody's argument, however, is nowhere able to equate human life as a set of conscious acts with the undeveloped fetus's state of mind. This discrepancy between ordinary humans and fetuses undermines his claim that fetuses are human.

The philosophical point is that, while each side has its proponents and opponents, neither side has as yet delivered a decisive refutation of the other. There is not sufficient evidence to show that either God or a mother makes a baby. Neither the receptacle nor the property metaphor answer the objections raised by the other side. An acorn may not be an oak tree, and a fetus may not be a person, but without acorns and fetuses it is unlikely that there will be oak trees or persons. Appeal to the principle of potentiality cannot be lightly dismissed.

Nor, however, can one dismiss the woman's role in our culture in caring for and carrying the burden of bringing up her offspring long after its birth. Therefore, she ought to have a large role in deciding whether to foster or terminate the life inside her. For if the mother cannot sustain the life once it is born and promote the child's actualization of its potential for full personhood, then she might do better to terminate such a being earlier in its development rather than later.

A recent variation on the pro-choice argument claims that in our culture only the female parent and not the male parent, physician, nurse, or any other person has a right to decide whether to abort. The decision is the woman's, the argument goes, not because of her right to her body, but rather, according to a view recently put forward by Jaggar, on the basis of two other principles.[63] The first principle is that the right to life means "the right to a full human life." Jaggar contends that a newborn has the right to a full human life, and if the woman is unable or unwilling to provide such a life, she has a right to terminate her pregnancy. The right to life of a fetus is not merely a right to be born. A person's right to life is a right to the means necessary to a full life, such as adequate nutrition, shelter, clothing, education, health care, love, and affection. A newborn being's right to a full life and to all the means necessary to achieve it leads to Jaggar's second principle, "decisions should be made . . . only by those importantly affected by them."[64] Since in our culture the main onus and responsibility of parenting rests on a woman, she, being most importantly affected, is the one to decide. "This principle provides the fundamental justification for democracy."[65] A woman's role in giving birth terminates approximately 20 or more years after birth, after a mother has provided the major conditions for the child's being on the way to achieving the right to a life of fulfillment and decency.

To Jaggar's argument we would add this further post-Malthusian point. (Thomas Malthus [1766–1834], an economist, argued that while the earth's food supply increases in an arithmetical progression, the population increases in a geometric progression.) Abortion is regrettable and may well be a serious trauma to a woman. To abort goes against the drive to support life. Contraception is preferable to abortion in controlling population growth. However, abortion is morally more desirable than serious overpopulation, in which each individual cannot be given an opportunity and the conditions for "a decent and fulfilling human life." A family that has more members than it can amply provide for has to give each individual fewer resources, including love. A consequence of placing no restrictions on reproduction is to have too many people struggling over meager resources, with a resulting increase in violence.

There are several serious conceptual difficulties for anti-abortionists evident in the syllogisms they use to defend their position. For example:

- Killing an innocent person is wrong.
- A fetus is an unborn, innocent person.
- Therefore, it is wrong to kill a fetus.

The question at issue is not with the top line, the major premise, but with the second line, the minor premise, which defines a fetus as an unborn, innocent person. The claim is that an unborn, innocent person is identical to a person, which begs the question whether a fetus is a person. The result of begging the question with the second, minor premise is the commission of the fallacy of equivocation—of shifting from "innocent person" to an "unborn innocent person" to describe the fetus. If one notices the second, minor premise, "A fetus is an unborn, innocent person," a fetus or so-called unborn child is not yet a person. It may become one after viability, but its route from potentiality or viability to the actual birth of a person depends on a number of conditions—physical, nutritional, environmental, and developmental—that, if unfulfilled, do not result in the actual birth of a baby.

Warren defends the moral permissibility of abortion on the grounds that a fetus is not a person and, therefore, abortion is not murder.[66] She defines the traits central to personhood as consciousness and the ability to feel pain; reasoning; self-motivated activity; communication; and self-awareness.[67] A fetus satisfies none of these conditions. As an example of genetic humanity, a fetus does not have full moral rights.[68] According to Sherwin, the fact that the fetus is a potential person does not outweigh the right of an actual person to protect her life by terminating an unwanted pregnancy.[69]

Sherwin, a feminist, views personhood as a social category. On her view, no human or fetus can exist apart from relationships. Because the fetus is within and dependent on a particular woman, the responsibility for determining the value and social status of a fetus belongs to that woman alone.[70] Sherwin maintains that to free women from having abortions out of economic necessity, vast changes are necessary in health care and legal policy, housing, employment, and child care.[71]

THE NURSE'S ROLE IN ABORTION

CASE 10.1: A College Freshman's Unintended Pregnancy. Jane Smith, a 17-year-old freshman student at a large state university, graduated from a small-town high school in a rural county, sexually inexperienced and socially naive. She becomes pregnant and is rejected by her lover as "irresponsible and dumb." She does not inform her parents, who are against premarital sex and abortion. She cannot provide for a baby, has never worked, and is without skills. She comes to the college health service for advice. What kinds of moral justification could you provide for and against abortion?

In response to the unhappy situation just depicted, the first step might be for the nurse to help the young woman give careful consideration to the alternatives of aborting or continuing the pregnancy. What are the main arguments relevant to the issue of abortion on a personal and a social policy scale? What arguments for and against abortion are useful to the nurse as a counselor?

The nurse primary-care practitioner has at least three positions he or she may take regarding the college student's request for advice regarding an unwanted pregnancy cited in Case Study 10.1. The nurse should have reflected earlier on the ethical issues so that he or she has thoughtful, deliberate, ethical justifications and not scattered reasons for counsel to the troubled young student. If the nurse assumes that human life begins at conception and that this person has a right to live that overrides the unwed woman's right to rid herself of an unintended pregnancy, then the nurse concludes that abortion is wrong. The nurse's conviction that abortion is morally wrong does not, however, mean that abortion is legally wrong. Abortion is now legal in all states, according to the Supreme Court's decision in *Roe v. Wade,* along with added restrictions cited by *Planned Parenthood v. Casey.* However, not all states fund abortion for poor women through Medicaid. Nor does the nurse's belief that abortion is morally wrong free him or her of professional obligations to advise the young woman. The nurse's responsibility is to give the patient objective information and referrals to appropriate resources before, during, and after an abortion.[72] The Division on Maternal and Child Health Nursing Practice of the American Nurses Association (ANA) recognizes the woman's right to seek a legal abortion free from the imposition of anyone else's judgments or beliefs. This position is consistent with the ANA's *Code for Nurses,* which says that

> Each client has the moral right to determine what will be done with his/her person; to be given the information necessary for making informed judgements; to be told the possible effects of care; and to accept, refuse, or terminate treatment. These same rights apply to minors . . .[73]

Clearly, then, the young woman with the unintended pregnancy has the right to information and counseling, with consideration given to all the alternatives to abortion as the basis of informed consent. The patient who chooses abortion has the right to information and counseling in an environment of mutual respect, trust, privacy, and confidentiality. Referrals are expected to be made to facilities where expert nursing and medical care is provided.

Nurses also have rights to their own moral and religious values. However, these values and beliefs do not give the nurse license to impose or to influence an already frightened, worried, and vulnerable client to accept the nurse's value preferences. Nor should the client's self-esteem be lowered by implication that her decision is less than morally acceptable. The nurse in any situation, except an emergency where the patient's well-being is at stake, has the

> . . . right to refuse to participate in a voluntary interruption of pregnancy . . . and . . . a right not to be subjected to coercion, censure or to discipline for reasons of such refusal.[74]

Beverly Jazelik, a New Jersey nurse who was assigned to the obstetric floor, refused to participate in procedures related to abortion. The state's law supported her refusal. The hospital then transferred her to another unit where she would have no contact with patients undergoing abortion. Ms. Jazelik objected to the transfer and sued the hospital. The Court ruled in favor of the hospital's right to transfer Ms. Jazelik to a nonabortion area.[75] Thus, the patient's right to interrupt pregnancy and the nurse's right to refuse to participate are both upheld. But moral questions arise if the nurse who opposes abortion is the only nurse available and a patient decides to have an abortion.

Nurses who defend or oppose abortion have similar responsibilities to provide information concerning the alternatives as the basis for informed consent and appropriate referral to resources. Alternatives include prenatal care, adoption, or keeping the baby and seeking financial aid.

Clearly, abortion in the case of the college student in Case Study 10.1, as in so many others, is a concern and responsibility primarily for women in our culture. Tragic choices such as this require the utmost kindness and consideration from the nurse in support of the patient's struggle with the decision. Providing conditions of calmness, free from pressures of time and place, in which the alternatives can be thoroughly explored is helpful to the process of deliberation and decision. Few women ordinarily prefer abortion. Some women are forced into securing abortions because of socioeconomic, psychological, or physiological circumstances that are unsupportive to a minimum decent life for themselves and a child. For them, there is no alternative. Other abortions are performed because of contraceptive failure. The intent was not to have a child. Increasingly, humans have exercised control of their procreative functions. Much remains to be done in the way of medical research to enable each couple to bring each new life into the world by deliberate choice and design, and as a consequence of mutual love, respect, and desire for a family.

The nurse who assists with abortions on a regular basis may understandably be saddened by the loss of so much potential life; yet the nurse's concern properly belongs with the woman who, in the last analysis, must part with a potential life in which she is deeply invested. In most cases of abortion, the woman is the victim of her biological and social vulnerability and deserves the respect and help accorded all human beings by reason of their humanity. Unlimited procreation without controls implies massive starvation, malnutrition, pain, and suffering—all due to the refusal to accept the moral permissibility of abortion and contraception.

Beyond the individual level, the nursing profession has the collective responsibility in policy formulation. An example of how this may be done is the New York State Nurses Association's support of the repeal of a restrictive state abortion law. The Association cited two reasons for liberalizing the law. First the law "encourages poor health practices,"[76] because women are forced to resort to illegal and hazardous abortions. Second, the restrictive law "deprives certain segments of the population of adequate medical care."[77] Poor women are simply unable to pay for safe and legal abortions. The Association stated unequivocally that it "takes no position on the moral aspects of abortion"[78] and supports the law that protects the rights of individuals refusing to participate in any procedure "contrary to their religious beliefs or conscience."[79]

Rights to Initiate, Sustain, and Terminate Life

In Chapter 7, reference was made to a rights-based view of nursing ethics. One may note that the problem of abortion may be expressed in the form of three basic rights: to initiate, to sustain, and to terminate life. Rights help to connect abortion arguments to justifiable moral principles. Three different positions on abortion reflect the search for principles[80]: 1) If a woman carries a fetus and if a fetus is a person at all stages of pregnancy, then abortion is murder, and therefore a violation of a person's right to life; 2) If a woman carries a fetus and if a fetus is not a person, then abortion is not murder, and therefore is not a violation of a right to life; 3) If a woman carries a fetus after L stage and if the fetus after L is judged to be a person, then abortion after L is murder, but not before L.[81] No. 1 expresses an essentially pro-life position, No. 2 expresses an essentially pro-choice position, and No. 3 expresses a compromise, one that is morally the least contestable, and therefore the least objectionable.[82] For although all three positions attempt to draw a morally justifiable line between abortions that are morally permissible and those that are morally impermissible, No. 3, as the least contestable of these positions, appears to provide the closest approximation toward a morally justifiable position on abortion.

SUMMARY

The opposing positions of pro-life and pro-choice, and a spectrum of views between these extremes, reveal the complexity of the issue of abortion. Competing ethical models and metaphors are at work. Pro-life supporters claim the principle of the sanctity of life. Pro-choice supporters base their arguments on the human rights to one's own body and the utilitarian principle of maximizing happiness and minimizing harm. Meanwhile, reproductive technology advances increase the significance of abortion to the individual and to society.

Legal restraints on abortion or a lack of them reveal deep moral differences on the abortion issue. On some issues, one or the other side tends to be or is right. On other issues, there is a stalemate. On still other issues, both sides may be "talking past each other." The abortion issue seems to us to be either a stalemate or a case of communicating on different levels. Perhaps when anti-abortionists speak of the beginning of life, they refer to the moment of conception, whereas pro-choice supporters refer to newborns.

In saying this, however, we do not wish to hide behind the banner of neutrality; we have supported the argument on behalf of a woman's right to choose. But we also think it only circumspect to point out that the issue of abortion has not been resolved with a conclusively justifiable or morally compelling answer. The reason is that, on such questions, no such answer is forthcoming. But we have tried to provide an answer that is least unsatisfactory, one that is morally least contestable. We have tried to whittle down the unreasonable aspects of both the pro-life and the pro-choice positions.

Discussion Questions

1. What conditions make abortion legally permissible or impermissible? According to what Supreme Court decisions?
2. What conditions make abortion morally permissible or impermissible, and for what reasons?
3. If abortion were universally regarded as murder and there were no contraceptives, or using them was universally regarded as immoral, what consequences would there be to the human race?
4. How does the presence of multiple anomalies among some newborns affect the abortion issue?
5. How does overpopulation affect the attempt to justify a pro-life argument?

REFERENCES

1. *Roe v. Wade,* 410 US 113 (1973).
2. ibid.
3. ibid.
4. ibid.
5. ibid.
6. Segers MC. Abortion and the Supreme Court: Some more equal than others. *Hastings Center Report.* 1977;7(4):5.
7. ibid.
8. *Planned Parenthood of Southeastern Pennsylvania v. R.P. Casey,* 112 S.Ct., 2791 (1992).
9. Munson R. *Intervention and reflection: Basic issues in medical ethics* (4th ed). Belmont, Calif: Wadsworth. 1992;61–62.
10. *Planned Parenthood of Southeastern Pennsylvania v. Casey,* 505 US 833 (1992).
11. ibid, p. 2820.
12. ibid.
13. ibid.
14. ibid, p. 2816.
15. Appeals Court Upholds Bans on a Type of Late Abortion. *The New York Times.* October 27, 1999;A18.
16. The Supreme Court: Balancing free speech and government interests: Excerpts from ruling backing limits on abortion protest. *The New York Times.* July 1, 1994;A16.
17. ibid.
18. ibid.
19. ibid.
20. ibid.
21. Seelye KQ. Accord opens way for abortion pill in the U.S. *The New York Times.* May 17, 1994;1, A16.
22. ibid.
23. ibid.
24. ibid.

25. ibid.
26. Kolata G. Tests of fetuses rise sharply amid doubts. *The New York Times.* September 22, 1987;C1.
27. ibid, p. C10.
28. ibid.
29. ibid.
30. ibid.
31. ibid.
32. ibid.
33. ibid.
34. Kolata G. Multiple fetuses raise new issues tied to abortion. *The New York Times.* January 25, 1988;1, A17.
35. ibid.
36. ibid.
37. Regelson W. Letter to the editor. *The New York Times.* October 8, 1987;A38.
38. ibid.
39. ibid.
40. ibid.
41. Dedek JF. Abortion. In: *Ethical issues in nursing—A proceeding.* St. Louis, Mo: The Catholic Hospital Association. 1976;77–78.
42. ibid, p. 81.
43. ibid, p. 82.
44. Thomson J. A defense of abortion. *Philosophy and Public Affairs* 1971;1(1):47–66.
45. ibid.
46. ibid.
47. ibid.
48. ibid.
49. ibid.
50. ibid.
51. ibid.
52. Thomson J. A defense of abortion. In: Munson R (ed). *Intervention and reflection* (4th ed). Belmont, Calif: Wadsworth. 1992;79.
53. Toulmin S. The tyranny of principles. *Hastings Center Report* 1981;11(6):31–39.
54. Held V. Abortion and the rights to life. In: Bandman EL, Bandman B (eds). *Bioethics and human rights: A reader for health professionals.* Lanham, Md: University Press of America. 1986;108.
55. St. Thomas Aquinas. *The sin of suicide.* In: Abelson R, Friquegnon ML (eds). *Ethics for modern life* (2nd ed). New York: St. Martin's. 1982;25.
56. Held V. Abortion and the rights to life. In: Bandman EL, Bandman B (eds). *Bioethics and human rights: A reader for health professionals.* Lanham, Md: University Press of America. 1986;105–107.
57. Nozick R. *Anarchy, state and utopia.* New York: Basic Books. 1974;169.
58. Feinberg J. *Social philosophy.* Englewood Cliffs, NJ: Prentice-Hall. 1973;54.
59. Ruddick W. Parents, children and medical decisions. In: Bandman EL, Bandman B (eds). *Bioethics and human rights: A reader for health professionals.* Lanham, Md: University Press of America. 1986;165.
60. Brody B. Opposition to abortion: A human rights approach. In: Arthur J (ed). *Morality and moral controversies.* Englewood-Cliffs, NJ: Prentice-Hall. 1981;200–213.
61. ibid, p. 211.
62. ibid, p. 212–213.

63. Jaggar A. Abortion and a woman's right to decide. *Philosophical Forum* 1973–1974; 5:351.

64. ibid.

65. Warren MA. On the moral and legal status of abortion. In: Munson R (ed). *Intervention and reflection: An introduction to medical ethics* (6th ed). Belmont, Calif: Wadsworth. 2000;103.

66. ibid, p. 102.

67. ibid.

68. ibid, p. 70.

69. Sherwin S. Abortion through a feminist ethics lens. In: Munson R (ed). *Intervention and reflection* (6th ed).

70. ibid.

71. Executive Committee on the Division of Maternal and Child Health Nursing Practice. *Statement on abortion.* Kansas City, Mo; June 12, 1978.

73. American Nurses Association. *Code for nurses with interpretive statements.* Kansas City, Mo. 1976;4.

74. Executive Committee on the Division on Maternal and Child Health Nursing Practice. *Statement on Abortion.*

75. Curtin L, Flaherty MJ. *Nursing ethics: Theories and pragmatics.* Bowie, Md: Brady. 1982;254.

76. Legislative Bulletin No. 14. Albany, NY: New York State Nurses Association. April 27, 1972.

77. ibid.

78. ibid.

79. ibid.

80. Dwyer S. Understanding the abortion problem. In: Dwyer S, Feinberg J (eds). *The problem of abortion* (3rd ed). Belmont, Calif: Wadsworth. 1997;1–20.

81. Sumner LW. A Third Way. In: Dwyer Feinberg (eds). *The problem of abortion* (3rd ed). Belmont, Calif: Wadsworth. 1997;98–113.

82. Gallie WB. Moral Concepts. In: *Proceedings of the Aristotelian Society.* 1980;80:139.

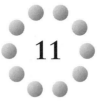

11

Ethical Issues in the Nursing Care of Infants

Study of this chapter enables the learner to:

1. Use ethical arguments to facilitate the family's decisions concerned with underweight, premature, and deformed babies.
2. Formulate the nurse's role as patient advocate for protecting the infant's right to care and safety and the family's well-being.
3. Understand the significance of such moral issues as quorum features and the potentiality/actuality distinction.
4. Discriminate among relevant principles of utilitarian, deontological, love-based, ego-based, and justice-based and rights based ethics in relation to each problem infant.

● **OVERVIEW: DEVELOPMENTAL HIGHLIGHTS**

A tiny helpless infant appeals to the strength and benevolence of adults. The newborn's total dependency on a supportive environment and a loving family matrix for its growth and development evokes adult nurturing and protective responses. The newborn child needs a healthy and friendly environment. Some newborns are premature, underweight, or defective. For them, one of the best friends is a good nurse—one who cares for them, who can identify and respond to feelings of discomfort from wetness, hunger, and thirst and to the infants' desire for warmth, closeness, and gratification.

Appreciation of the feelings of another with the desire to help that person is necessary to be an effective nurse. Infants, young children, and sometimes even older children and adolescents are unable to express feelings and needs effectively. They are often defenseless against imposition of painful treatments or the withholding of treatment by parents and health professionals.[1] Research studies show that newborns do feel pain and circumcision does hurt, as demonstrated in neonates' high-pitched cries, breath holding, apnea, cynosis, gagging, vomiting, and increased glucose consumption. Pain medication by injection or cream application appears to reduce the pain.[2] These are opportunities for implementing the nurse's role as an advocate of the patient's rights to respect and to receive treatment. These young patients are the most vulnerable to neglect, indifference, rejection, or manipulation and abuse. Equally serious may be the moral conflicts that arise when the child is either physically or mentally abnormal.

Ethical problems and dilemmas arise when the parents want a normal child and the newborn is severely retarded or has physical abnormalities, such as trisomy 18 syndrome, myelomeningocele, or Down syndrome. Does the nurse comply with the parents' wishes if they refuse treatment for the child, or does the nurse exert initiative to save the infant's life based on the child's right to live?

If family and community resources are scarce, competing moral values may call for other moral values to be given priority over the interests of preserving the life of a severely abnormal newborn. Some people call the failure to save a life "murder." Others condemn the practice of preserving infants that show few or no prospects of becoming independent, self-sufficient persons. The question is: How to decide who lives and who dies, and who is given quality care and who is not?

The issue of treatment for the abnormal infant is filled with moral concerns and conflicts as well as numerous possibilities for good or harm. This is another example of the quantity versus quality of life issue.

The pediatric nurse has a special role in evaluating the viability of the infant. Systematic assessments of the infant's functional assets and deficits as well as responsiveness are useful data in the final decisions of whether to care for, treat, or place the infant with the family or in an institution. Each nurse caring for the infant is a vital link in compiling the data to be considered in making that ultimate decision. Nurses' interactions with parents provide data regarding parental perceptions of their ability and desire to cope with the problematic situation. Despair may be profound. Parents may be overwhelmed, guilty, angry, and ambivalent about what to do. Their moral conflicts may be acute. The advice given to them may be conflict-ridden, and the time for decision may be short and pressured. Parents may turn to the nurse for advice, support, and help.

One form of help a nurse may give is to show awareness of ethical theories that affect nursing practice. Every ethical theory has its principles that reveal its major aspects. For example, the greatest happiness principle is derivable from utilitarianism.

The nurse's role as advocate of the child's right to live and to be treated under all conditions may conflict with other moral principles holding that the happiness of

What if you were the nurse caring for the pre-term, extremely low-birth-weight infant of a 39-year-old primipara who is overjoyed about her baby? The infant weighs less than 160 g, the gestational age is less than 26 weeks, and the parents urge the neonatologist to "do everything" despite the physician's explanations of possible brain damage, cerebral palsy, retardation, and other serious future disabilities. The parents simply view the baby as tiny but with the potential to become normal through their loving care. What would your advice be to the parents?

the greatest number, in this case the family, may be in direct contradiction to saving the child. Careful consideration of all the variables relevant to the infant's capacities and potential, as well as those of the family's abilities and willingness to cope with a painful, problematic situation of an abnormal child, are determining factors in the final decision. In some situations, with which some nurses are in agreement, the principle of the sanctity of life may prevail over all other considerations.

However, the sanctity of life principle—that human life is to be preserved under all conditions—conflicts with another principle, "the quality of life." This principle holds that there are conditions, sometimes referred to as quorum features, such as the presence of consciousness, that define a worthwhile human life. Thus, not all life is to be preserved if it fails to comply with quality of life standards. Consequently, five sometimes conflicting principles govern health professionals' first encounters with newborn infants. One principle is to save human life under all conditions (sanctity of life principle), developed from love-based ethics. A second principle is to promote worthwhile human life with the implication of productivity and independence (quality of life principle). A third principle is to prevent or minimize harm (nonmaleficence principle). A fourth principle is to alleviate suffering. A fifth principle is to seek to do good, as by giving skilled nursing care (beneficence principle). The last three principles are outgrowths of utilitarian ethics. These principles will be considered in relation to examples of moral dilemmas in the nursing of infants.

ARGUMENTS FOR AND AGAINST SAVING PREMATURE AND DEFORMED INFANTS

Infanticide of deformed and even normal female babies was an ancient practice for controlling population. High infant mortality rates were accepted. The death of a deformed baby was often welcomed and perhaps assisted by midwives sympathetic to women's destiny of uncontrolled pregnancies.

The contrary principle, that life is the highest good, is supported by the Judeo-Christian tradition prohibiting abortion, infanticide, and euthanasia. Significantly, medical technology has now advanced to a level of saving an increasing number of premature, underweight, and underdeveloped infants by means of neonatal intensive care units. The most sophisticated forms of monitoring vital signs and regulating electrolytes, food, and fluid are keeping premature and deformed infants alive at an astonishing rate.

Catlin interviewed 54 physicians in five perinatal sub-specialties who resuscitated extremely low-birth-weight pre-term infants, 54,400 of whom are born each year; half of the infants weighing less than 1,500 g survived, with up to 40% of those expected to suffer severe long-term neurologic and developmental impairments.[3] Some of these extremely low-birth-weight, pre-term infants face long hospitalizations, surgeries, extensive treatments, troublesome long-term outcomes, or death. Yet resuscitative measures are standard, with some 20- to 23-week old fetuses being "saved."[4] Physicians surveyed admitted to many ethical problems, including their refusal to resuscitate if presented with such an infant of their own.[5]

Most neonatologists surveyed recognized the need for rational guidelines because neither the legal system or cost considerations affected their decisions, which they regarded as burdensome and with regret that the funds spent were not used for better prenatal and child care. Among the burdens identified were physicians' ambivalence and indecision in resuscitating neonates who did not die immediately. Other burdens included the suffering experienced by the children, the families, the nurses, and the workers in the intensive care units, and the disagreements caused among physicians and nurses.[6] Despite their discomfort, the neonatologists did not discuss hospice or comfort care that employed warmth, holding, and pain control while enabling neonates to die. The researchers concluded that physicians chose not to limit a fetus's potential, but to support and wait until after evidence of immaturity, suffering, or lack of response was presented.[7] The principle of saving all life is respected through routine application of extraordinary means to continue the living processes of these infants. The cost of continuous professional care, high-level technological equipment and supplies, and prolonged hospitalization is more than $2,000 per day per child in some neonatal intensive care units. In these fully lighted, windowed enclosures, nurses adjust flow rates of fluids and gases in response to readings of the monitoring devices attached to each infant. The operating principle and the goal are identical: To save all life with no regard for the quality of life saved or the costs to parents and society. The infant is given care, in most instances, without regard for the present and later burden that may be imposed on families and society or even the suffering of the infant itself from necessary injections and intubations. Once the infant is received in the neonatal intensive care unit, the decision has already been made to treat fully and intensively, with no regard for such long-term consequences as brain damage or chronic cardiopulmonary disease.

However, not all premature or deformed infants are immediately transferred to intensive care units. Three examples of frequently occurring problems in newborn infants illustrate the scope and depth of the moral issues involved in decisions of treatment or nontreatment. These cases point to the usefulness of identifying short-term and long-term goals and consequences to the individual affected as well as to the family and society.

The first example of a neonatal problem is the birth of very premature, underweight, underdeveloped babies as a result of spontaneous or induced abortion. On one view, the gasping infant is left to die in a surgical pail. On another view, that infant is admitted to an intensive care unit. On one view, the decision to seek an abortion is an automatic death sentence for the fetus; on another view, the abortion decision is one of ending the pregnancy. On one view, the viable fetus has the right to live and the nurse, as patient advocate, has the duty to protect the fetus's life above all other values. Questions arise as to who decides, and by what criteria, either to save or not to save the infant. Other questions arise as to what difference voluntary versus involuntary abortion makes. Related questions concern the effect of socioeconomic status, race, age, and the mother's marital status on decisions to resuscitate and treat, or not to resuscitate and treat.

The second example is that of the infant born with multiple life-threatening defects, such as the baby who was placed on a respirator due to respiratory difficulty with diagnostic evidence pointing to trisomy 18 syndrome. This genetic disorder leads to severe mental retardation, failure to thrive, and many other abnormalities.[8] Adapting the case somewhat, suppose one parent insists that the chief of pediatrics does nothing to keep a 4-day-old trisomy 18 infant alive. A pediatric resident points out that another infant who has a respiratory difficulty cannot be put on a respirator because the trisomy 18 infant is using the only available machine. Without the respirator, the other infant, "who is otherwise healthy, has a 50% risk for some brain damage."[9] The fact is that 87% of trisomy 18 infants die in their first year. At this point, two nurses who are directly responsible for the infant's care interrupt. Nurse A insists that the trisomy 18 infant "has every right to live and should not be allowed to die by human hands." Nurse B disagrees and says that those beings with a meaningful life have the right to be given health care resources, that an otherwise healthy infant with a respiratory difficulty should not be sacrificed for the trisomy 18 infant. Nurse A supports the principle of "the sanctity of life" under all conditions. Nurse B believes in the principle of "the quality of life"; she believes that the trisomy 18 infant has a poor prognosis. If you are Nurse C, what do you advise the parents and Nurses A and B to do: Save the trisomy 18 infant or leave it to die? Further questions arise as to the original decision to start a life support system and to continue it. Considering the evidence of multiple defects, a poor quality of life, and an expected span of less than a year, questions arise as to what criteria for decision making are relevant, who the decision makers are, and what the role of the nurse is in facilitating the decision.

A third example involves a baby girl who had Down syndrome and also had a surgically repairable duodenal obstruction. The parents, by not consenting to surgery, contributed to the death of their 6-day-old Down syndrome child.[10] One writer, who adds a fictionalized scenario to the actual case, points out that "many nurses and physicians thought it was wrong that the baby was forced to die[11]. . . . The burden of caring for the dying baby fell on the nurses in the obstetrics ward. The physicians avoided the child entirely, and it was the nurses who had to see to it that she received her water and was turned in her bed. This was the source of much resentment among the nursing staff, and a few nurses refused to have anything to do with the dying child. . . . But one nurse . . . was determined to make . . . [the baby's] last days as comfortable as possible. She held the baby, rocked her, and talked soothingly to her when she cried. . . . But even [this nurse] was glad when the baby died. 'It was a relief to me,' she said. 'I almost couldn't bear the frustration of just sitting there day after day and doing nothing that could really help her.'"[12] But there was this actual case.

Dr. Milton Heifitz writes of an actual case in which "the world press in 1971 condemned the 'inhumanity' of a husband and wife and the staff of a major American medical center. A mongoloid baby was born with an intestinal obstruction at Johns Hopkins Hospital in Baltimore. The parents, who had two normal children, refused to give consent to correct the obstruction. The infant could not be fed and died within fifteen days."[13] According to Heifitz, "the child's death caused a furor in medical and lay circles. It was a major topic at an international symposium concerning medical ethics. Panelists disagreed with the parents. They suggested the child's right to life, to the limit of happiness possible, was more important than the years of anguish and burden the child would bring the family."[14] Thus, "the sanctity of life" overrides all other principles on this view. However, arguments for the sanctity of life principle do not respond to the opposing view of parents' preference for a life of quality for themselves and their offspring. Nevertheless, proponents of the sanctity of life principle can raise the spector of the Nazi policy and practice of exterminating population groups that were regarded as "unfit."

NEWBORN HIV TESTING

This country is experiencing a new wave of people infected with HIV: The infants and children born of infected women.[15] An HIV-positive woman may transmit the virus to her offspring during pregnancy, during labor and delivery, or through breast-feeding.[16] The virus crosses the placental barrier. Because the rate of HIV infection through caesarean section does not significantly differ from that of vaginal delivery, it appears that most infections occur during pregnancy.[17] Projections for 1991 were that HIV will be one of the five leading causes of death among childbearing women. Current projections are that 3 million people are infected, 600,000 of whom are newly infected newborns.[18] Because 80% of the infected children received the virus from their infected mothers, women of child-bearing age should reasonably be the targets of major educational efforts.[19] In this connection, one may appreciate Plato's principle that knowledge is a virtue and that ignorance is evil.

Proponents of HIV testing point to a recent federal study showing that pregnant women with HIV can drastically reduce the transmission of the virus in utero by taking AZT.[20] On almost any moral grounds, including utilitarian ethics, these women thus are justifiably identified and treated during pregnancy.

In 1997, New York hospitals began the open, mandatory testing of newborns for HIV as the debate over its value continued. The heretofore anonymous testing of newborns for statistical reasons has now changed to mandatory disclosure of results to mothers after they leave the hospital. Because one fourth of the exposed babies contract HIV and only the mother's antibodies can be detected at birth, the mother's HIV status is revealed. Since the likelihood of infection transmission is dramatically reduced, mandatory prenatal testing and treatment is preferable. Patients have generally been cooperative when informed of the mandatory testing. Most HIV mothers know their status before delivery, but a few previously unknown HIV positive babies are discovered and treated. Tracking down these mothers after hospital discharge is a challenge, as is persuading them to return for help. Some are never found. Some women requested notification of results. Some HIV-positive women accepted notification of their results.[21]

The ethical issues are clearly drawn in this legislative battle. The conflict is between the mother's right to confidentiality regarding her positive HIV status and the negative consequences of disclosure, and the newborn's right to appropriate health care in the event that the HIV test is positive. One could cite the ethical principle of love for the vulnerable newborn as the basis for disclosing the baby's positive HIV status. One may regard the HIV-positive mother who refuses to be identified as using the principle of egoism by placing her own interests first, above those of the infant. One can cite the need for Rawls's second principle of justice, specifically the HIV-positive status of the newborn as disadvantaged, to justify disclosure and treatment of child and mother. The second part of Rawls's second principle—that positions and offices are open to all on the basis of equality of opportunity—is violated here by the newborn's lack of equal opportunity to develop normally. The utilitarian approach is one of securing the greatest happiness for the greatest number. Identification of HIV mothers and their offspring, followed by prompt treatment, may help them directly and indirectly reduce the possibility of transmission to more people and to more pregnancies.

ETHICAL CONSIDERATIONS IN THE NURSING CARE OF INFANTS

Nursing Interventions

Nurses working with infants, like nurses working with any other age group, have a number of roles. Pediatric nurses, however, may perceive themselves as primarily patient advocates for the rights of the helpless, vulnerable infants in their care. They may see advocacy responsibilities as a significant feature in the delivery of quality care to each baby. The American Nurses Association *Code for Nurses* defines the role of client advocate in sweeping terms.

> The nurse's primary commitment is to the client's care and safety. Hence, in the role of client advocate, the nurse must be alert to and take appropriate action regarding any instances of incompetent, unethical, or illegal practice(s) by any member of the health care team or the health care system itself, or any action on the part of others that is prejudicial to the client's best interests.[22]

This definition of the role of client advocate is tantamount to a mandate or command to safeguard the infant's life against those who would not treat or feed the infant because of a decision using a quality of life argument. But a question arises as to whether a nurse is an advocate of the infant client or the infant's parents. This becomes crucial if the infant's parents have conflicting interests between themselves or if their interests are not those of their infant. Pediatric nurses who are most often in contact with the infant may feel that the parent's decision to terminate an infant's life to be unfair or to be tantamount to an act of murder. These nurses perceive themselves to be advocates for the infant's right to life.

Patient advocacy may be expressed in a variety of ways. One way is to marshal the facts based on careful, systematic assessment of the infant's status as the basis for arguments favoring the continuation or termination of life based on quorum features. The arguments may then be presented to the physician and family for consideration. Through contact with the parents, pediatric nurses may exert considerable influence on their decision. Sharing of nurses' knowledge of this child's estimated needs for care through the life span and the experience of other parents facing similar demands may be useful information in the parents' process of decision. In some cases, nurses as patient advocates comply with the directive of the *Code for Nurses* for being fully aware of institutional policies and procedures as well as state laws regarding unethical, incompetent, or illegal practices by taking necessary steps to initiate action through appropriate channels. It is important to provide careful documentation and to use established mechanisms for appeal so as to avoid reprisals. There have been instances in which the courts have directed that an infant be fed and treated where the parents have refused treatment. Sometimes, custody of infants is taken from parents at the instigation of a family agency on grounds of neglect when the parents refuse treatment. A counterexample occurred in 1982 in Bloomington, Indiana, where two Monroe County courts and the state Supreme Court all declined to force parents to feed or treat a baby born with Down syndrome and an incomplete esophagus. The Monroe County prosecutor said he would not file charges in the death of the week-old baby despite plans for an appeal to the Supreme Court.[23] Those nurse advocates who participate in securing legal advocacy for this and similar babies to whom nourishment, treatment, and life itself were denied are committed to the sanctity of life principle.

Other nurses may support the quality of life principle. Nurses committed to this principle may believe it is cruel and unjust both to the child and the family to prolong the suffering of a severely handicapped child. Such nurses may support parental decisions not to treat the deformed infant while giving compassionate care to the hungry infant. Such babies can be kept sedated and comfortable until they die. Parents need the support of nurses and physicians in handling the inevitable guilt feelings concerning their decision not to treat or feed.

In still other examples, parents may not consent to treatment for correction of a minor deformity that will not interfere with the full potential of the infant. The nurse as patient advocate may in this instance be in the best position to protect the "client's care and safety"[24] by persuading parents to permit treatment on the grounds of the child's right to a full human life. Nurses and physicians, in advocating infant's rights, may consider in extreme cases openly disagreeing with the parents by presenting morally cogent reasons and arguments. Nurses and physicians may also appeal to the courts, if necessary, to protect the right of a minimally deformed child to be fed and treated.

Another issue for the nurse advocate to consider is the principle to do no harm. Such a principle is as relevant for the physician as it is for the nurse. Some research involving infants may be justified in terms of benefit to the immature client. Other research may be done for the social benefit of others at some indefinite time without any benefit to the infant subject. We have all benefited, after all, from research done on others at an earlier time or at some other place. On a reciprocity basis between generations and places, we owe it to others to submit to research, but not as our primary duty. The nurse who secures consent from the parents for research or experimentation involving their child needs to make the clear distinction between benefit to the parents, benefit to the individual, and social benefit. A truthful account would distinguish research for the benefit of one's child and research for the benefit of other children. Some opponents argue that research that is of no benefit to the infant is solely an assault against its tiny body. A counterargument is that donation of an anencephalic infant's organs to other babies is an act of generosity by the parents for the benefit of other children.

Those nurses who agree with the quality of life argument and the need to minimize the suffering of the affected infant and family appreciate the integrity of the study by Duff and Campbell, who found that in a 30-month period, 43 infants judged by parents and staff to have little or no hope of achieving personhood were left to die by withholding essential medical treatment.[25]

The role of patient advocate for handicapped infants became a national issue in April 1982 when 6-day-old "Baby Doe" of Bloomington, Indiana, died from lack of food and water. Treatment of the infant's tracheoesophageal fistula was denied by the parents, who were supported in their decision by the Indiana courts. Presumably the parents refused surgical repair of the condition because the infant also had Down syndrome.

In the same year, in response to the public outcry of indignation, the US Department of Health and Human Services issued a notice based on section 504 of the Rehabilitation Act of 1973 to health care providers that no otherwise qualified handicapped person should be deprived of nutrition or medical treatment necessary to correct a life-threatening condition under the threat of legal prosecution. Considerable resistence from national organizations followed, with charges of undue regulatory intrusion into the parents' privacy and the high potential for futile therapy. The Supreme Court struck down the regulations, and responsibility and consent was returned to families and physicians. The American Academy of Pediatrics agreed that the person's medical condition should be the sole focus of decision.[26] The Americans With Disabilities Act (1990) protects citizens, including those with AIDS, against discrimination with as yet unresolved applications to congenitally impaired newborns.

If the potential for human relationships or the capacity to survive infancy and participate in human experience is significant, then nurses play an important role in these decisions[27] through their participation in both the assessment and the judgment process. If open-ended moral dialogue is regarded as an essential condition of the decision-making process, then that process is one of mutual respect. Mutual respect in this context means that the negotiation process is open and encourages reasoned arguments until some approximation of consensus is reached about the infant's right to live versus the benefit to the child, as well as to the family and society, which bear the cost. As a caregiver with understandable feelings of deep compassion for the short and tragic life of the tiny, defenseless patient, the nurse provides for the comfort of the dying infant to whom food and treatment are denied. If the nurse disagrees with this order or is unable to give skilled care and comfort to the infant because of resentment of the family's "dumping of their responsibility," then the nurse may refuse to provide care.

Before the nurse takes individual action, he or she might benefit from institutional review. There is a need for the development of institutional policies and review processes that apply broad rules to specific cases, such as the priority given to the best interests of the infant, with care not withheld solely because of mental retardation.

When the parents of a seriously ill newborn are disqualified from making decisions because of incapacity, disagreement between them, or choices that are clearly against the infant's best interests, there are currently civil courts, state laws, child protection agencies, and even criminal penalties available to respond to the presumed neglect of the handicapped infant. Until such policies and processes are developed in each caregiving institution, the nurse is the best interim advocate protecting the interests of these infants.

ETHICAL AND PHILOSOPHICAL CONSIDERATIONS

Several Philosophical Moves

Moral and philosophical questions arise about these cases, such as: Whose rights are to be taken most seriously? Because decisions concerning these cases involve values, either the sanctity of or the quality of life, these questions cannot be settled by science, by evidence, or by verifying only what is true or false. Nor can one settle these questions by considering sociological factors, such as: "What do most people favor?" These are philosophical value questions, which if they are settled at all, are done so by showing that one moral value is more justifiable than another. One way to justify a moral argument that an anencephalic infant (congenital absence of the cranial vault and cerebral hemispheres of the brain) has less justification to live than a normal infant or one with mild Down syndrome is to show that the consequences clearly favor one side over the other. Another way to justify a value preference is to show that one belief has fewer conceptual and practical difficulties than any other.

Quorum Features.   Several philosophical moves have recently been developed in an attempt to clarify the right to life and parental, health professional, and nursing responsibilities. One move consists in applying the idea of "quorum features"[28] to the question, "When does a person's life begin and end?" A quorum at a meeting means that a previously agreed-upon number of persons is required to be present for the meeting to take place. Thus, as one applies the idea of a quorum feature to the question, "What is a person?", a being who lacks the quorum or majority of essential features of an ordinary person (i.e., an individual with multiple deformities, or an individual who lacks consciousness, such as a trisomy 18 infant) does not satisfy the quorum features of being a person. What makes the refusal to save the life of the Down syndrome infant morally questionable to some people and an outrage on the border of "murder" to others is that the Down syndrome patient is more clearly a person than the infant with trisomy 18 syndrome. Some might say that the Down syndrome infant has some prospects for a meaningful human life, whereas the trisomy 18 infant does not.

Tracing and Examining for Appropriate Metaphors and Models.   A second philosophical move consists of considering a viewpoint that purports to provide an answer to the question, "What is a person?" One then traces that viewpoint to some deeply acknowledged metaphor, word picture, or pictorial analogy on which defense of the viewpoint depends philosophically. One then examines the metaphor to determine how it applies or breaks down in practical discourse. One may next consider whether supplementary or alternative metaphorical analogies aid in the defense of a given viewpoint. For example, one may regard any being born to be unconditionally worth preserving on the ground that "life is a gift,"[29] to cite St. Thomas Aquinas's insightful metaphor. One thus traces a viewpoint to a metaphor on which its philosophical defense partly rests. But one may next examine the metaphor to note what conceptual or practical limits or difficulties it implies. A difficulty immediately becomes apparent. Is life always a gift? Is it necessarily a gift, so that there could be no instance of life that was not a gift? One has only to consider some terminally ill patients or a seriously maimed or wounded person to note that there are exceptions to life always being a gift. Furthermore, in ordinary language, if one gets a gift, one may keep it, give it to someone else, or discard it. But the gift of which St. Thomas Aquinas speaks, because it is given, may not be taken. This is a strange requirement for any gift. And yet one can appreciate that the recognition that life is a gift spurs health professionals to save it. A metaphor may thus be examined for its illumination as well as for its implied difficulties. Life is not always a gift, as the trisomy 18 syndrome example amply shows.

The Potentiality-Actuality Distinction

A related effort to answer "What is a person?" is to regard any potential person as a person. Thus, an acorn is potentially an oak tree and therefore is to be accorded the recognition that someday it will be an oak tree. Similarly, a girl is a potential woman. Because a rock, a stamp, or an oak tree is not a potential person, one need not confer personhood status to these entities. But even a seriously deformed person enjoys the status of being a person, according to the potentiality principle. This is not true, however, if one shows that the potentiality principle has limits. According to philosopher Stanley Benn, "A potential president of the United States is not on that account Commander in Chief of the US Army and Navy."[30] According to another philosopher, Joel Feinberg, "A dog is closer to personhood than a jellyfish, but that is not the same thing as being 'more of a person.' . . . In 1930, when he was 6 years old, Jimmy Carter didn't know it, but he was a potential president of the United States. That gave him no claim then, not even a weak claim, to give commands to the US Army and Navy. Franklin Roosevelt in 1930 was only two years away from the presidency, so he was a potential president in a much stronger way . . . than was Jimmy Carter. Nevertheless, he was not actually president and he had no more of a claim to the prerogatives of the office than did Carter."[31] One could, however, criticize this analogy by pointing out that a fetus's becoming a person is a biological process rather than a social or political process, unlike a presidential candidate's becoming president. Nevertheless, the point remains that potentiality does not imply actuality; and the potential person may be discounted from being regarded as an actual person. Although a trisomy 18 infant who has multiple deformities is potentially a person, it is not actually a person. The analogy one appeals to is to show that a presidential candidate, who is a potential president, while closer to being a president than a potential candidate who is 6 years old and therefore underage, is not an actual president, who alone has the rights and responsibilities associated with being a president. The analogy of president to person shows that a potential president is not an actual president, and thus a potential person is not an actual person. Concerning Aristotle's and Aquinas's Potentiality Principle, Engelhardt says,

> If X is a potential Y, it follows that X is not a Y. If fetuses are potential persons (X), it follows clearly that fetuses are not persons (Y). . . . The language of potentiality is . . . misleading for it is often taken to suggest that an X that is a potential Y in some mysterious fashion already possesses the being and significance of Y.[32]

To avoid the mystery of "potentiality," Engelhardt prefers to speak not of X being a potential Y, but that X has a probability of being a Y.

Traditional Ethical Viewpoints Applied to Infant Cases
A fourth and last philosophical move one might consider is to examine how the ethical principles previously discussed apply to resolving the question of what to do about infants with abnormalities. A utilitarian, for example, would adopt the quality of life principle. In relation to competing demands for the available respirator, the utilitarian ethicist would say that considering "the greatest happiness of the greatest number," one ought to give preferential treatment to the normal infant with respiratory difficulties over the infant with trisomy 18. A utilitarian might even defend the refusal to consent to surgical repair of a duodenal atresia in the case of a Down syndrome infant. However, on a Christian or agapist or love-based ethical view, which favors the sanctity of life, one does all one can to save the life of a trisomy 18 or Down syndrome infant on the ground that such infants "are all God's children," to cite another metaphor.

One may think that Kantian deontological ethics commits one to a similar ethical conclusion, but Kant confines his ethics to rational beings. The point about Kant's deontological ethics is that appeal to universal principles requires the same treatment for all individuals within a given group without exception, except when relevant differences are shown.

From a rights point of view, if persons alone have rights, and a seriously deformed being is not regarded as a person, then such a being, including an anencephalic infant, is not a person and hence is not a subject of rights. The infant with mild Down syndrome who falls within the quorum feature of being human—that is, it satisfies the requirements of personhood—does have rights, including the right to live. The violation of such an infant's right to live is an indication of its moral wrongness.

Because one cannot always reconcile these alternative moral points of view, one has to consider the place both of tragedy in human life and of stalemate in the effort to resolve sometimes unresolvable problems.

Application of Philosophical Moves to Infants With Handicaps
We have seen that the federal regulation issued as a "Notice to Health Providers" on May 18, 1982, required health providers "to meet the immediate needs that can arise when a handicapped infant is discriminatingly denied food or other medical care."[33]

In regard to this handicapped infant ruling, goal-based ethics (see Chapter 4) says: Consider the consequences. A consequence to future generations may be borne in mind. For every pregnancy, two questions are relevant: Who will provide? and How will it be provided for? On an aggregate macrolevel, there are enough people with the capacity to develop into persons of adequate achievement to contribute to advancing levels of knowledge, science, and technology for everyone. One might refer to the principle to reproduce no more people than there are resources for them as the principle of proportionate resources to people. The need to provide persons of social and economic merit is basic to the dictum that people generally have to pay their way in the world. Future health care and human service providers will be decreasingly able to cope effectively with excessive numbers of essentially dependent people.

Consequently, infant health care policies cannot be oriented solely toward the principle of saving every infant, no matter how handicapped. Nor, however, can health care policies be oriented toward saving only those people who are deemed as fit to lead a high-quality life.

A problem for both those who strive to save everyone and those who exclude individuals with less than optimum human qualities is analogous to having either too many or too few people at the world's dinner table. If there are too many at the table, then everyone will not have enough to eat. If one excludes too many, then those excluded will have nothing to eat. Moreover, the principle of selection and the basis for excluding are likely to be arbitrary. A difficulty of including or excluding too many beings is illustrated by having to decide whether to treat infants with myelomeningocele, hydrocephalus, severe mental retardation, and unalterable anomalies.

One can picture this dilemma of distributing resources to people labeled P and R by drawing two circles. One circle represents limited available Resources and the other circle represents People and their needs and desires. The larger the People circle is made in relation to the Resources circle by having to thin out the resources, the smaller will be the shares for each person, or some people will be excluded. One possible resolution of the dilemma of having too many people is to limit the number of people, keeping the circle representing Resources as close in size to the Person circle as possible. A dynamic equilibrium between the world's population and available resources calls for such a plan.

On this ground, utilitarianism or goal-based ethics seems to have a claim on future societal needs. Decisions have to be made employing fair, rational, and relevant criteria as to whom to help and whom to save. To save blue-eyed infants, for example, seems to be irrelevant or unfair. It is fairer to save those who have the best chance of leading socially useful lives. In addition to observing this dictum, one works to achieve a balance between extreme positions: regard for merit and regard for the equal distribution of socially useful resources.

The appeal to the achievement of merit calls for exclusions of those who show little or no merit. Exclusions of this or that group may be painful. Such exclusions may also be unjust. Including everyone, however, means resources may be too thinly distributed to do much good. A policy, like section 504 of the Rehabilitation Act, may tip the scale in favor of attempting to save too many infants, and also more infants than can be provided for throughout the life span, because of their continuous requirements of medical care, special education, and housing and financial assistance.

One strikes a balance not by ignoring the claims of each position, but by attending to both claims, prevention of harm and caring for quality of life.

There is no innate obligation to favor either the prevention of harm or quality of life principle. Both are good because of the good they bring, in the estimation of people who have good reasons for judiciously applying both these principles. According to Aristotle, the good is "that at which all things aim."[34] One may amend this to read: The good is that which attempts to reconcile the good at which people aim. One aim that is believed to be good is the prevention of harm. Another is fostering quality of life. One route is to realize that, as with life, there are moral polarities, intermediate positions, priorities, and criteria for selection. Appeal to rational criteria, such as impartiality and consistency, helps resolve disputes between goals. A health care policy, for example, may take the form, "Every baby having features A, B, C . . . is regarded as a person and every baby with D, E, F . . . (medically untreatable) does not qualify as a person. Every person shall be adequately cared for and treated. Therefore, babies having features A, B, C, . . . being persons, shall be treated; and babies with D, E, F (and medically untreatable), not being regarded as persons, shall not be treated." Invoking a Kantian appeal to a universal moral principle minimizes (but may not eliminate) arbitrariness as to what counts as a person. Specifying features, such as A, B, and C (drawing a justifiable and useful distinction between these features of a "person" and those without such features), may reduce arbitrariness somewhat.

On this view, a health care policy would be a guideline to health providers. Details of the features of persons and nonpersons would be worked out in health care ethics committees by appropriate professionals, including nurses, with input from public policymakers, parents, and other representatives of society. A so-called hotline would go, not to a centralized bureaucratic government agency, but to an appropriate impartial patient-advocacy group. Its functions would be to guide present and future decisions effectively, rather than to blame or punish health providers for past decisions.

SUMMARY

Ordinarily, the wonder and joy of human life begins with the birth of an infant. The mother of the new infant is likely to feel the emotion of participating in the creative process of life. But the infant is fragile, helpless, and dependent. It requires the highest quality of nurture parents are prepared to give it in order to grow into childhood, adolescence, and responsible adulthood. Not all newborns, however, are normal at birth. Some are born with minor deviations from health, others are born with gross abnormalities. Nurses are involved in the health care activities and processes of decision making for all infants. Therefore, nurses contribute their observations regarding the infant's health status when decisions are to be made regarding who lives, who receives special consideration, and who is left to die.

The quorum feature or majority feature of a human life, including evidence of consciousness, helps parents and health professionals, including nurses, to make ethically justifiable decisions. The sanctity of life principle, in which life is regarded as sacred under all conditions, may conflict with the quality of life principle in those instances when not all can be effectively helped to live decent, fulfilling lives. If resources are scarce and not all can be saved, the sanctity of life principle may appear impractical, inflexible, and unworkable. If the quality of life principle is then invoked, then questions of arbitrariness arise. How one decides on just grounds who lives and dies is the question continuously considered by morally reflective people. Therefore, while both principles, the sanctity of life and the quality of life, have a claim on nurses, neither principle is satisfactory in every case. Nor is either one quite free from fault or able to withstand further questions.

Discussion Questions

1. What is the cutoff point for determining the human viability of an infant's life? For example, are lines drawn at mild, moderate, or severe retardation? What physical and mental attributes are criteria of a viable infant?
2. How do changes in technology affect standards for justly deciding the viability of an infant's life?
3. If an infant is denied all surgery necessary to save its life, is it being discriminated against and are its rights being violated?
4. Are rights attributable only to conscious human beings? Why is it appropriate or inappropriate to attribute rights to an infant with multiple mental and physical anomalies?

REFERENCES

1. Pasero CL. Pain control: Pain during circumcision. *Am J Nursing* 1997;97(10):21.
2. ibid.
3. Catlin AJ. Physicians' neonatal resuscitation of extremely low birth weight preterm infants. *Image J Nursing Scholar* 1999;31(3):269.
4. ibid.
5. ibid.
6. ibid.
7. ibid.
8. Body H. *Ethical decisions in medicine* (2nd ed). Boston: Little, Brown. 1981;116.
9. ibid.
10. Shaw A. Dilemmas of "informed consent" in children. In: Hunt R, Arras J (eds). *Ethical issues in modern medicine.* (2nd ed). Palo Alto, Calif: Mayfield. 1983;252–258.
11. Munson R. *Intervention and reflection: Basic issues in medical ethics* (3rd ed). Belmont, Calif: Wadsworth. 1988;114.
12. ibid, p. 114–115.
13. Heifitz MD, Mangel C. *The right to die.* New York: Berkley. 1975;59–60.
14. ibid, p. 60.
15. Bulloch BL, Rosendahl PP. *Pathophysiology* (3rd ed). Philadelphia: JB Lippincott. 1992;318.
16. ibid.

17. ibid.
18. *The New York Times.* September 8, 1999;A15. (Advertisement: The Elizabeth Glaser Pediatric Foundation.)
19. ibid.
20. Sack K. Battle lines drawn over newborn HIV disclosure. *The New York Times.* June 26, 1994;23.
21. Sontag D. HIV testing for newborns dated ANSW. In: Beauchamp TL, Walters L. *Contemporary issues in bioethics* (5th ed). Belmont, Calif: Wadsworth. 1999;763–765.
22. American Nurses Association. *Code for nurses with interpretive statements.* Kansas City, Mo. 1985;8.
23. Munson R. *Social context: The baby Doe cases intervention and reflection* (6th ed). Belmont, Calif: Wadsworth. 2000;139–143.
24. American Nurses Association. *Code for nurses with interpretive statements.* Kansas City, Mo. 1985;8.
25. Duff RS, Campbell AGM. Moral and ethical dilemmas in the special care nursery. *N Eng J Med* 1973;289:885.
26. American Academy of Pediatrics. Joint Policy Statement. Principles of Treatment of Disabled Infants. *Pediatrics* 1984;73(4):559–560.
27. ibid.
28. Hospers J. *An introduction to philosophical analysis* (3rd ed). Englewood Cliffs, NJ: Prentice-Hall. 1988;122–124.
29. St. Thomas Aquinas. *The sin of suicide.* In: Abelson R, Friquegnon ML (eds). *Ethics for modern life* (3rd ed). New York: St. Martin's. 1986;25.
30. Benn S. Abortion, infanticide and respect for persons. In: Feinberg J (ed). *The problem of abortion.* Belmont, Calif: Wadsworth. 1973;102.
31. Feinberg J. The problem of personhood. In: Beauchamp T, Walters L (eds). *Contemporary issues in bioethics* (2nd ed). Belmont, Calif: Wadsworth. 1982;113–114.
32. Engelhardt HT. *Foundations of bioethics.* New York: Oxford University Press. 1986;111.
33. Federal Register. March 7, 1983. 48(45):9630–9632.
34. Aristotle. *Nichomachean ethics.* Ostwald M (trans). Indianapolis: Bobbs-Merrill. 1962;3.

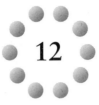

12

Ethical Issues in the Nursing Care of Children

Study of this chapter enables the learner to:

1. Identify the ethical issues involving children's rights to health care, safety, and well-being in problematic situations.
2. Facilitate the parents' participation in shared decision making regarding the well-being of the child in relation to the whole family.
3. Distinguish between a biological and a biographical life as a criterion for personhood.
4. Clarify the role of children's rights in relation to parental rights and duties and societal rights and duties owed to dependent children.
5. Recognize the state's interests and duties owed to dependent children.
6. Evaluate the role of the nurse as patient advocate in nursing practice with children.

OVERVIEW: DEVELOPMENTAL HIGHLIGHTS

Children are almost universally regarded as the hope of the future for a better world. Yet in some parts of the world, large numbers of children are ill fed, inadequately clothed, housed, and educated, and in dire need of curative, preventive, and rehabilitative health care. Children may be neglected and abused even in affluent cultures. Children are perceived in the light of cultural values and mores. It is the culture that defines "the length of childhood, the essential nature of childhood, and the meaning of childhood."[1] At least one writer claims that childhood is a European invention of the 16th century. This means that from that time on, children were taken more seriously as distinct beings.[2] But this assertion is debatable in view of child labor laws and the cruelty and abuses that have been inflicted on children since then.

The pluralistic culture of the United States presently supports a wide range of values reflected in child-rearing practices. Children are incorporated into various family models. One model of parent-child relations is that of ownership. According to this model, children are perceived as being possessions of their parents. A second model, which is widely practiced, especially in remarriages, is that of club membership. Here, the members of the family are not cared for very much as individuals. They are essentially left on their own. A third model, partnership, implies that children are more approximately equal with their parents.

Family socioeconomic differences are usually reflected in the prevalence or absence of family planning, number of children, and the desirability of the birth of each child. Middle- and upper-class families in the United States are usually child-centered, attempting to meet each need and to foster individuality. Poor families may struggle to provide basic necessities of life with little concern for the special needs of each child. Nevertheless, both affluent and poor families may have difficulty meeting their children's rights owing to the parental tendency to prefer either the ownership or club membership models over the partnership model.

In response to the largely dependent and vulnerable status of children all over the world, several declarations of rights have been developed. The *Declaration of the Rights of the Child,* developed by the United Nations in 1959, recognizes the worth and dignity of each human being. The *Declaration* recognizes the special protection needed for enabling the immature child's physical, mental, moral, social, and cultural growth and development to proceed. Humankind "owes to the child the best it has to give . . . to the end that he may have a happy childhood and enjoy for his own good and for the good of society, the rights and freedom . . . set forth."[3] The *Declaration* calls for nondiscriminatory entitlement to rights that recognize the interests of the child. At birth, the child has a right to a name and a nationality. The child has the right to adequate food, shelter, recreation, and health care. The handicapped child shall be given special care, treatment, and education. Every child's need for love and understanding, parents, and security will be supported by state assistance to families and care of children without families. The child has a right to education, at least through the elementary grades, free of cost but on the condition of compulsory attendance. This requirement is purportedly justified by the need for the child to develop his or her abilities and to contribute to society. The child has the right to special protection from neglect, cruelty, and exploitation in the form of traffic or employment that is detrimental to health and development. Lastly, the child will be protected from discriminatory practices and be reared in "peace and universal brotherhood."[4]

According to Wieczorek and Natapoff, the *Declaration* omits rights "to love from a significant adult . . . to a safe environment . . . to reach individual potential . . . to be a wanted child in a situation that has resources . . . to respect the individual autonomy of the child, and . . . to personal space that may include sexual expression."[5] All of the rights listed have the dual function of enhancing the child's personhood and protecting the child's fundamental needs in its growth and development toward humanity.

ETHICAL ISSUES RELATED TO CHILDREN, WITH RELEVANT CASES

Some major ethical issues concerned with children between 1 and 12 years of age involve the principle of informed consent, its scope, and its limits when applied to children. Other issues concern parental control versus the child's growing autonomy. Another moral concern is that of the abuse of children directly and through neglect or denial of the child's rights to the truth, proper health care, education, and a safe environment, as well as by direct infliction of harm and injury. A particularly heart-wrenching case involving a parental decision that probably contributed to a 3-year-old's avoidable death is that of Chad Green.

CASE 12.1: Parent's Decision to Withhold Life-Saving Drugs. According to A. Holder, a legal expert on children, Chad, age 3, had leukemia with, according to his physician, a 50% to 75% chance of 5-year survival. Although at first Chad's parents agreed to chemotherapy, they soon decided to add laetrile and vitamins. When the physician warned the parents that laetrile could be toxic, the Greens removed Chad from all treatment and the Massachusetts Department of Public Welfare, on behalf of the hospital and the physician, prevailed in a request to the court for an order to treat Chad. . . . The Department of Public Welfare presented testimony by five physicians that laetrile was not only worthless but could be harmful. The court found that the child had a high probability of long-term remission with chemotherapy and that laetrile might cause cyanide poisoning. The parents were ordered to keep Chad on chemotherapy and to stop their home remedies. The Greens then fled to Mexico to escape the court order and Chad died there.[6] This case illustrates the relation between a child's best interests, parental authority, and state power. It revealed the tragedy and harm that may be caused by ignorance of dubious drugs.

Selective cases will illustrate the importance of these issues to the child's survival as a person. As these cases illustrate, there is a continuum of decision regarding children's rights. At one end there is absolute parental control, with complete child autonomy at the other end. This gives rise to conflict in making health care decisions when there is disagreement between parent and child or parent and health care provider regarding the child's so-called best interests. The process of making decisions for and by the child is also related to the quality of child-parent relationships and family values, the age and maturity of the child, the diagnosis, and the significance of the treatment to the future of the child.

Some decisions to treat or not treat are uncomplicated. For example, a pediatrician does not prescribe drugs for a hyperactive child at the request of the teacher or school nurse without parental consent. One might also expect that the decision for tonsillectomy in a 6-year-old would be the sole decision of the parents. On the other hand, one would expect sensitive parents to seek the informed consent of a 10-, 11-, or 12-year-old child to the same surgery. Where parents are divorced, the parent with legal custody of the child is legally responsible for informed consent to treatment.[7] Moral considerations, however, are complex when parents, whether married or divorced, have an honest difference of opinion regarding the desirability of treatment, such as tonsillectomy or amputation for a malignant tumor. Here the principle of beneficence (to do good) directly collides with the principle of "do no harm," or nonmaleficence. This is a common problem in the example of tonsillectomy, where the tonsils are not a focus of infection but where frequent colds and sore throats occur. The evidence for tonsil removal or retention is inconclusive.

The situation becomes even more complex when the child disagrees with the parents. Holder says that when a genuine emergency occurs, the child is to be treated even without parental consent.[8] In a nonemergency, for example, when a 10-year-old wearing glasses requests contact glasses from the ophthalmologist to participate in sports, parental consent is morally indicated. The parents and the child need information regarding the benefits, risks, and costs of the procedure as the basis for informed and judicious consent. In contrast, a 12-year-old with venereal disease seeking treatment who refuses to name or to notify her parents has the moral and legal right to receive treatment, because the consequences of nontreatment to the child and to society override the rights of the parents to know of the infection and to agree to its treatment. Generally, any communicable disease is an emergency to be treated without parental consent if necessary.[9] Holder maintains that the physician who will not treat a drug-addicted child who will refuse treatment if his parents are notified is "himself guilty of contributing to the delinquency of his patients."[10] The trend appears to favor the consent of the minor to health services. This is reflected in the Statement on Consent by the American Academy of Pediatrics (AAP) Task Force on Pediatric Research, Informed Consent, and Medical Ethics, which permits the self-supporting and separated minor to consent to treatment. The statement also calls for treatment of any pregnant, infected, or addicted minor without parental consent.[11]

The AAP's statement provides that any minor with physical or emotional problems who is capable of rational decisions and who refuses help if parents are notified may consent to treatment. The health professional may legally thereafter tell parents or guardians, unless it jeopardizes the patient's life or treatment results.[12] If serious health care procedures are to be given without parental consent, approval is sought from another physician. Thus, the AAP statement seeks to protect the minor's rights to treatment, the parents' right to be informed of the health of their child, and the physician's right to provide treatment without legal consequences.[13] The AAP statement strives to protect the child's right to privacy and confidentiality. The following cases present moral dilemmas.

CASE 12.2: A Mass Screening Program of Children Based on Coercion of Mothers.

A mass screening program for iron-deficiency anemia in children requires the direct participation of nurses. The focus of concern is for the nutritional status of lower socioeconomic class children whose mothers use food stamps to purchase foods that are less nutritious and contribute to dietary deficiencies. The plan is to assess hematocrit levels using finger-prick blood samples from the children by requiring the child's blood test as a prerequisite for the mother to secure food stamps. Anemic children would be immediately provided with free iron supplements.[14] Nurse A argues in favor of the test, pointing to the inadequacy of current detection of iron deficiency of children, the free treatment, and each child's right to health care. A signed consent form will be requested of each mother. Nurses are the only available health professionals to do this test.

Nurse B argues against the compulsory nature of the screening and invokes other moral arguments favoring truth-telling and the client's moral right to self-determination, in this case the mother's deciding for her child. The issue is whether the coercion used in this screening program is ever morally justifiable, even though the predicted consequences are beneficial to the child.

CASE 12.3: The Nurse Decides an Issue of Life or Death.   Another case adapted from Brody is that of 10-year-old Janie, who was admitted for routine observation following a fall against the corner of the fireplace. Her head wound was superficial; no skull fracture was found. On a routine check, the nurse discovered the girl was not breathing, and was cyanotic with fixed, dilated pupils. She was immediately intubated, given drugs, and placed on a cardiac monitor. The heartbeat returned in 30 minutes but the pupils remained fixed and dilated. The evidence points to a considerable period of anoxia of the brain "with irreversible damage, but you cannot be sure."[15] The issue becomes one of treating or not treating by transferring Janie to a respirator in the intensive care unit where tests will be performed to diagnose brain death or irreversible brain damage. Supposedly, this diagnosis will be followed by turning off the respirator. The counterargument is that once Janie is on the respirator and treatment is started, it will be continued regardless of Janie's diagnosis or condition. Nurse A argues in favor of pronouncing the child dead for the sake of the greater good of the family and society. Nurse B argues for giving the child every help and every chance regardless of the consequences to Janie, the family, or society. Nurse B favors the sanctity of life, while Nurse A favors the greater happiness

CASE 12.4: May an 8-Year-Old Give Informed Consent to Kidney Donation?   A further case illustrates the ethical problems of organ donation of one sibling to another, and raises the issue of whether one sibling or child should be used to help another when there is no benefit to the donor. An 8-year-old girl suffered from a life-threatening kidney disease which necessitated the removal of both kidneys. Her identical twin sister was the ideal donor. She appeared to understand and to agree with the procedure. The issue for the nurse as a member of the transplant team is on what grounds should the healthy sibling be permitted or denied the donation of her kidney to her sick sister while placing herself at some risk.

Nurse A argues for donation on grounds of the greatest happiness of the greatest number, the utilitarian position. Nurse B argues against the donation on egoistic grounds of no benefit to the donor, but certain risk and pain. Nurse C argues for donation on the grounds of the child's autonomy and self-determination. Nurse D argues for donation on grounds of love-based ethics, (i.e., the golden rule principle). The 8-year-old donor appears to understand the issues and to be closely identified with her sister. The moral dilemma is whether to permit or deny the kidney donation.

Abuse of young children is a frequent problem of deep concern to nurses in emergency departments, crisis centers, hospitals, schools, and public health agencies. The abuse may be physical, sexual, or emotional.

CASE 12.5: Shall the Nurse Expose Incest?   One not infrequent example of abuse is that of an intimidated wife and a sexually abused 9-year-old daughter with whom the husband/father is having intercourse. In a routine examination, the school nurse discovers signs of penetration, and upon questioning, the child admits to intimacy. She begs the nurse not to tell anyone of her secret, because the father has threatened to kill mother and child if he is exposed. The child fears her father and is convinced that he will carry out his threats. The nurse is horrified at the exploitation of this child and all other defenseless, vulnerable children who are abused and neglected. She views her role as that of patient advocate with her "primary commitment . . . to the client's care and safety."[16] The nurse is aware of the laws protecting children from abuse and the sad lack of implementation by child and family welfare agencies and child placement facilities. The incest is clearly "prejudicial to the client's best interests" by interfering with the child's normal psychosocial growth and development. The father-daughter relationship will undermine the child's perception of the security and trust expected of parents and other authority figures. The incest may seriously warp the child's future relationships with intimates. Despite these serious misgivings, the nurse weighs the child's present security against an uncertain future in a foster home, separated from the family. The nurse is filled with doubt regarding the pledge of confidentiality to the child and the moral problem she faces.

Abuse

In most states, registered professional nurses are legally required to make a report whenever there is a reasonable cause to suspect child abuse or neglect of either a physical, emotional, verbal, or sexual nature. There are child abuse hotlines in every state.

Signs and symptoms of abuse include bruises; burns; fractures; genital, vaginal, or anal injuries; abandonment; extreme fearfulness of parents or other adults; delinquency; running away; truancy; self-destructive acts or suicide attempts; hysteria; phobias; sleep disorders; inhibited play; parents's contradictory explanations of child injuries; over- or under-reaction to the child's condition; and use of many different health care facilities or practitioners.[17]

ETHICAL ISSUES IN THE CARE OF CHILDREN WITH HIV/AIDS

CASE 12.6: Can Robert Go to School?   Robert, a 5-year-old hemophiliac who acquired HIV through blood products, is ready to enter kindergarten in the local public school. However, his attendance is opposed by parents who fear that Robert would spread the disease to their children. The school board, the school principal, and the parent-teacher association asks the school nurse, Ms. Brown, to advise them on all aspects of HIV and AIDS in children as the basis for both a discussion about Robert and for policy formulation.

The question posed to Ms. Brown is: Should we allow Robert and other children with HIV or AIDS to attend public school? Ms. Brown, BS, RN, compiles an extensive survey of the practices and regulations of other states and calls the Centers for Disease Control and Prevention (CDC) for its recommendations. Ms. Brown finds that the CDC's recommendation is to allow most children with HIV/AIDS to attend school while protecting their privacy.[18] This recommendation is followed by most school districts. Most states, she finds, allow children with HIV/AIDS to attend regular classes. New York City, with a large proportion of the HIV/AIDS cases in the United States, set up a panel to review each child with the disease. . . . Children with open sores, those who lack control over their bodily functions, or those who show a tendency to bite are dealt with under special programs and not allowed to enter ordinary classrooms.[19]

Ms. Brown learned that no child yet has transmitted HIV/AIDS to anyone else. Nevertheless, some parents see any risk to their child from the disease as unacceptable.[20] Ms. Brown concludes that a case for general contagion and quarantine, like measles, mumps, or chickenpox, cannot be made for HIV/AIDS. The virus is transmitted by blood or semen or other body fluids directly into the bloodstream of another person.

Ms. Brown, a committed nurse, reflects and analyzes the controversial ethical issues surrounding Robert's case. After visiting the mother and Robert at home, she has no doubt that at this time the child is not infectious to other children. She believes that the greatest happiness for the greatest number would be served by allowing this child to learn to play and to become friends with the other children in his class. Ms. Brown, moreover, believes that appeal to Kant's principle of respect, the altruistic principle of loving others, and the Rawlsian principle of caring for the least advantaged are best served by including Robert. She also believes that Robert has a legal right to have free, public school education as long as his health permits, and to have that education in "the least restrictive environment."

Issues of Truth-Telling: AIDS and Children
In a family where both child and mother, solely the mother, or solely the child are HIV positive, the burden of secrecy is very heavy. "One mother described the complexity of maintaining this secrecy and its impact on her relationship with her son" to nurse researchers.[21]

CASE 12.7: A Mother's Deception.   I won't tell anyone at school about Louis (7-year-old son). I don't want him made fun of or anything. When I went to the parent-teacher conference, the teacher wanted to refer Louis to a psychiatrist. She said Louis keeps say, 'My mom's going to die.' Then he misses a lot of school because of his appointments, and I have to write notes about why he missed. I hate lying . . . it's like I'm back on the street conning again. I tell Louis he has anemia. He even asked me, 'Mommy, do I have AIDS?' I said, 'Do you see the word AIDS when you go to the doctor? Why do you think you have AIDS?' Then he won't ask for awhile.[22]

Clearly, the mother's motivation is that of love for her son and her wish to protect him. However, a question must be raised regarding the child's right to know the truth. According to Kant's theory of duty-based ethics, the mother is violating the principle to "Always tell the truth." There are several possible reasons underlying the mother's deception. She may believe that the child will unwittingly disclose his AIDS status to outsiders, who may then stigmatize and discriminate against him. The mother may not wish to jeopardize her relationship with the child by admitting that she is a causal factor in his disease.

Nurse researchers Andrews, Williams, and Neil identified mechanisms by which children provide support to a seropositive mother. Children help decrease their mother's feelings of isolation that come with the disease. The children need care and affection, which the children sometimes seek to return.[23] These children provide a means of strong attachment to the world because the mothers are forced to engage with others in whatever support networks will increase the well-being of their children.[24] Another mechanism that binds the seropositive mother and child is the necessity for secrecy to avoid the stigma and discrimination of HIV and AIDS.[25] Mothers in the study struggled with the issue of whether or not to tell their young children of the diagnosis.[26] Most did not disclose on grounds of young children's inability to understand or deal with the implications of their mother's forthcoming early death.[27] The nurse researchers regard this dilemma as stressful to the mothers, but not as stressful as having to deal with the worries of their young children.[28] The very presence of children can force these mothers to face life positively, according to these researchers. When the mothers were asked to identify those factors that contribute to their current health, they responded in terms of their children's needs to be cared for by their very own mothers, themselves.

The researchers concluded that for the mothers in this study, "children are inevitably partners in the dance between life and death" as the mothers search constantly for "balance between attachment and loss, hope and despair, engagement and withdrawal. . . . It seems clear . . . that children are central forces in the lives of many HIV-positive women. These women . . . cannot be treated in isolation from their children and families."[29]

Lipson views health professionals as relatively open to repeated discussions of HIV with infected children. In studies of children with cancer, ". . . positive results of disclosure were reductions of anxiety, improved family function, and (for survivors to adulthood), long-term gains in pschyosocial judgment."[30] The question then becomes how, rather than whether, to speak with the child about disease. Most pediatric nurses have had patients who talk with them about the disease and the possibility of death in the attempt to gain some control over their bodies and lives. Recognition of the child's autonomy, self-awareness, and rationality supports nurses' and health professionals' bias toward disclosure.[31] The concept changes from that of a disclosure moment into that of a dialogue . . . around the process of sharing information, fears, and pleasures in which all parties participate.[32]

MORAL IMPLICATIONS IN THE NURSING CARE OF CHILDREN

In working with children, the nurse's role involves consideration of the parents' significant contribution to the child's well-being. It is the parents who generally carry the lifelong burden of caring for a seriously handicapped child. Parental responsibilities include investment of their energies, emotions, time, and finances in the care of the disabled child. Continuous health care, frequent hospitalizations, and special education are usually indicated throughout the life of the child. Some parents may fear the birth of another defective child and so devote the rest of their lives to the care of this one. Siblings may be deeply hurt and resentful of the disproportionate share of parental involvement and family resources taken up by the afflicted child. Mothers in particular may be forced to give up career aspirations in order to provide continuous care to the child. Parental conflict and even divorce may occur as a consequence of spousal guilt, frustration, and rage in this troubled situation.

Thus, in the *Code for Nurses,* the description of the nurse as advocate "with primary commitment . . . to the client's care and safety"[33] may be in conflict with other moral principles, such as the greatest good of the greatest number of family members. The nurse may be in a genuine dilemma regarding the conflicts of the infant's right to life and the family's right to a full human life without the lifelong burden of a child who has little potential for personhood. The sensitive nurse ponders the identity of the client: Is it primarily the child, the family system, or the interests of society? The nurse can muster persuasive arguments favoring the family system and still other arguments favoring the individual child as the client in need of advocacy. If the nurse gives serious and primary consideration to the children's bill of rights previously discussed, then the role of advocate as "primary commitment . . . to the client's care and safety"[34] is the only morally permissible alternative.

If the statement in the *Code* is to be taken literally, then all deformed children will be treated and no respirators will be turned off. Moreover, no thought will be given to the burdens of the handicapped child to the parents and the negative consequences to the family. No child will be deprived of the chance to live in the state to which he or she is restored, whatever that may be. Much more can be done by official and voluntary agencies to help families care for the retarded and the handicapped at home. The mother deserves compensation for her care. Allowances are needed for special foods, special clothing, and extra transportation to clinics and schools for the child. The overburdened family would thereby be helped in concrete ways, with considerable savings to the state. Most important, life will be saved, and each child will live to the extent of its potential.

A difficult situation for nurses occurs when the parents have opposing opinions about whether or not to treat. The tendency is for deeply troubled parents to turn to nurses caring for their child with such questions as, "What would you do if this were your child?" The child does not belong to the nurse, of course. Nor can the nurse put himself or herself in the parents' shoes. The nurse does not know the parents' circumstances, their values, commitments, feelings, or relationships as they do.

However, the nurse can facilitate parents' careful assessment of the relevant facts of the case, the parents' values, family resources, and the deep concern of each parent. Identification of the problem, facts, values, and concerns are useful steps in helping parents resolve ambiguities and ambivalence in problem situations. Parents can be encouraged to talk together alone and with pediatric or family-practice nurses, physicians, clergy, lawyers, children, and relatives. Other families who have experienced similar problems may be consulted regarding their experiences with a handicapped child. Nevertheless, after all possible help is given parents, there remains the difficult choice of sustaining the fragile life with the utmost commitment to the child's right to life or denying that right based on the principle of the greatest happiness for the greatest number. Although some physicians and nurses tend to make that decision to treat or not treat for others, it may be viewed as the parents' rightful decision, since they bear the lifelong burden. However, if the parents' decision is seen as improper, inappropriate, ethically unjustifiable, or illegal, then the nurse as patient advocate has the duty to appeal that decision in the most effective way possible.

The nurse who works with families in which there is abuse seeks information concerning laws that protect children, local regulations surrounding reporting of abuse, law enforcement agencies, child and family welfare agencies, and measures for protection of the child. A nurse may view her or his role as primarily one of patient advocate committed to the child's care and safety. In that case, the regulatory and child-caring resources can be used to the utmost on behalf of the child. If the nurse views himself or herself as an advocate of the family, he or she can then secure the resources of community family agencies in enlisting the family's participation in family therapy or counseling.

As the child's advocate, the nurse has an important role in facilitating the child's participation in ethical decision making regarding its own health care. The partnership model of relationship (discussed in Chapter 7) recognizes children as full human beings who are owed respect for their thoughts, feelings, interests, and desires in relation to their own health care. Ideally, the partnership model of relationships is based on an open, shared decision-making process, in which children's growing autonomy is supported to the extent of each child's cognitive maturation, personality, and thought processes. This model recognizes children's rights to information about their health status and to truthful answers concerning diagnosis, hospitalization, treatment, intensive procedures, chronic disease, and even impending death. Such knowledge is shared in words and at times by persons appropriate to the child's age, understanding, emotional state, and relationship with the nurse and significant others. Wieczorek and Natapoff recommend interviewing children regarding their health status. Some children will readily respond; a few will not. The process reveals whether the parents use the ownership, club membership, or partnership models of family relationships. Some parents answer for the child. Other parents qualify the child's answers. Parental interference is consistent with the ownership model. The ownership model may shield parents who evoke religious or philosophical beliefs to rationalize withholding medical care from their children. For example, a 2½-year-old Boston boy died from bowel obstruction in 1986 after 5 days of "treatment" by a Christian Science practitioner and nurse. His parents were exempted from legal blame on the basis of religious belief. If you were a judge, would you agree with this decision? (Putting oneself in the place of another person or role is known in philosophy as a counterfactual judgment.)

Some parents support the child's expression of his or her thoughts regarding the health problem; this is consistent with the partnership model. The nurse who practices within this model believes it important to find out what children think is causing their health problem, as well as the nature and source of their worries.[35] The child's sense of autonomy is enhanced by responsibility for providing information and sharing thoughts and feelings with the nurse and the physician about the health problem. In turn, the stress for the hospitalized child can be reduced by the warm and sympathetic nurse who supports the school-age child's ability to reason, to generalize, and to understand cause and effect in relation to the illness and treatment. The nurse as partner and child advocate is willing to support the child's autonomy by giving simplified scientific explanations for bodily changes, functions, diagnostic procedures, treatments, and the workings of the various hospital machines. Likewise, the nurse who respects the child gives truthful explanations for illness and treatment appropriate to the child's understanding. Such explanations are significant to children, especially younger children, who may believe that their illness is related to their being bad in some way or that it is causing their parents considerable distress. Other misconceptions can be clarified.

The process of nurse-parent-child shared decision making assumes that all three have the capacity to understand essentials of cause-and-effect disease processes, as well as stages and principles of human growth and development, and that they are oriented toward a partnership model.

The nurse who perceives the role of advocate as a meaningful one can then move into shared decision making with the child. The nurse's alliance with the child is supportive of the child's participation in health care decisions. Concretely, the nurse permits as much freedom as possible and encourages independence. Some hospitalized or sick children may be astute observers, with heightened awareness of their bodily changes, and they may want to be in control of themselves. Enabling children to participate in developing their health care plans, such as making choices about sites of injection, days and times of scheduled visits, or going home to die, is a manifestation of deep respect for children's right to participate in health care decisions.

In England, the Royal College of Pediatric Health Ethics Advisory Committee stressed the importance of listening to children and respecting the decisions of competent children of any age. An example is that of a 7-year-old girl whose second liver transplant failed and who persuaded her parents, the transplant team and consultants that she did not want a third transplant and that she fully understood the consequences. Her decision was accepted without court hearings, and she went home and died soon after.[36] In the United Kingdom, several children 7 to 10 years of age refused transplantation and other major surgery that was supported by parents and the medical team.[37]

The nurse can assist parents in helping the child express fears associated with dying, such as pain and abandonment, and in providing the necessary comfort, freedom from pain, and security. The nurse supports the child's participation in his or her own health care until the very end by respecting the child's determination of the need for pain medication, privacy, and peer, sibling, and parental visits. Children are respected throughout their illnesses as persons of worth who are intensely concerned with what is happening to their bodies and their lives, with nurses perceiving themselves as allies to dying young patients. Despite the overwhelmingly tragic outcome to the child, when the nurse and child interact in shared decision making together on a mutually benevolent basis, a morally significant human relationship may occur that serves as an example for other human relationships.

ETHICAL-PHILOSOPHICAL APPROACHES TO NURSE-CHILD-PARENT RELATIONSHIPS: RIGHTS, DEPENDENCY, PATERNALISM, AND FREEDOM

Several Philosophical Moves

There are several ethical considerations that function as an ethical checklist for evaluating nurse-parent-child relationships. In addition to the quorum feature notion discussed in Chapter 9, there is a further philosophical move by four contemporary philosophers, Sartre, Rawls, Rachels, and Ruddick. This move consists in distinguishing biological or zoological life from biographical life. Human beings live anatomically and physiologically biological lives. Those who fulfill the majority features of being human also give evidence of being conscious. A person with hopes, projects, history, joys, frustrations, and expectations for the future with plans and prospects—all of which presuppose consciousness—is said to have a biographical life, and is not just living a biological life.[38]

Joseph Fletcher, a prominent Protestant theologian, restates the biological/biographical distinction by citing several conditions for being regarded as a person, including a minimum intelligence quotient of 20 to 40, self-awareness, a sense of past and future time, the ability to have human relationships and to show caring and concern for others, and the ability to exercise some self-control over material and psychological conditions of existence. Fletcher's criteria boil down to the presence of consciousness.[39]

Margot Fromer, an astute commentator and interpreter of Fletcher's view, argues for Fletcher's criteria of personhood. Fromer points out that Fletcher's criteria for personhood are the most commonly used, but she concedes that "many people disagree with them."[40] According to Fromer, for Fletcher "the one characteristic basic to all others is the presence of neocortical functioning, without which biologic life may exist but personhood does not. . . ."[41] To Fromer, "health professionals are concerned with the quality as well as the sanctity of life,"[42] but she thinks it is unlikely that human beings will agree about what is an acceptable quality of life.[43]

Whether one refers to the quality of life or to a biographical life, to one's rational life plan (as does Rawls), to one's projects (as Sartre does), or to consciousness, one uses these distinctions to refute the contention that the sanctity of life is unconditional, absolute, and undebatable. Although children cannot carry out all the cognitive functions of adults, normal children are expected to develop capacities that will enable them to fulfill more and more of these cognitive functions as they grow up.

There are advantages and drawbacks to the conception of biographical life. A strength of this distinction is its use as a practical basis, a cutoff point, for deciding who is a person to be helped and who may be medically ignored without public censure. For example, a long-time comatose child or a child with severe mental and physical anomalies may be given little or no medical attention without public recrimination.

A drawback to this distinction is that it can be used to decide that some types of humans, such as social deviants, cripples, and the comatose, are arbitrarily ruled out as persons. Therefore, no charge of genocide or homicide attaches to those who cause these unfortunate beings to be killed. This would be unjust.

However, the advocates of a biological/biographical distinction respond that the members of any society cannot afford to keep all breathing beings alive if they are not conscious and productive nor have they any hope of being so. Such a cut-off point, the advocates of this biological/biographical distinction claim, is not like the Nazi basis for eliminating unwanted human beings with mental illness and epilepsy or healthy Jews, Slavics, and blacks, because ethnic and religious factors are not relevant to the consciousness or social productivity of the person. Nazi claims about the inferiority of non-Aryan groups were false, but even if their claims were true, the mistreatment of these groups would not be morally justifiable on biographical grounds. The Nazi project of exterminating Jews was evil as is the selling or giving of addictive drugs to children or using children to sell or transport drugs.

The Concept of Rights Applied to the Nurse-Child-Parent Relationship

A further philosophical move consists in clarifying the concept of rights that apply to children in a health care context. The question of whether children have any rights has one of four responses and accompanying arguments. One view is that children have no rights at all. Parents, nurses, and other adults may have duties, but children have no rights. A second view is that children have the right to be cared for, fed, clothed, sheltered, given health care, and educated, but no liberty rights to make their own decisions. A third position is that children have limited subsistence rights and liberty rights in relation to their readiness to make responsible decisions. Children, for example, may walk across the street when they show that they are careful. But children do not have the liberty right to stay out all night and imbibe alcohol whenever they wish. A fourth position holds that children have unlimited liberty and subsistence rights that are shared equally with adults.

Each position has proponents and opponents. The customary philosophical moves consist in arguing on behalf of one of these views. In the process, one may make use of philosophical arguments to clarify the concept of rights applied to children. Several arguments for rights are worth noting. Rights imply liberties; they also imply corresponding duties imposed on other appropriate persons and groups, such as nurses, parents, and schoolteachers. The AIDS crisis imposes serious constraints on children's rights of sexual expression and imply the need for adults to restrain children's erotic pursuits. Unless a cure for AIDS is found, these constraints against sexual expression will become increasingly severe; and justifiably so, on utilitarian-consequentialist grounds and on a rights-based view.

Cranston, a prominent writer, points to three requirements of rights: practicability or feasibility, which means a right can be put into practice; universality, or the equal application of the right to all those to whom it applies without arbitrary exceptions; and "paramount importance," or the singling out of these needs deemed vitally urgent to individuals in society.[44] The third requirement confines rights to the most urgent conditions of social life, rather than fads and frills. The paramount requirement or value priority calls for a society to have "fire engines and ambulances," for example; "Fun fairs and holiday camps"[45] are luxuries rather than the rights of persons. If rights have no restraints, then rights become every-thing, and if they mean everything, as with any other term that has no exclusions, then rights become frivolous. Applying Cranston's criteria shows that whereas one can speak of a child's right to food, clothing, shelter, health care, and education, the child cannot have a right to be loved in the same way. For every child to be loved may be a desirable ideal, but to refer to a child's right to be loved is in Cranston's terms, "a utopian aspiration" or ideal, but not a right.[46]

Furthermore, morality may be separated into agent or character morality, act or decision-making morality, and the critics' or judges morality. The first concerns classical and contemporary virtues, such as wisdom, courage, compassion, love, generosity, kindness, devotion, and loyalty. The second, act or decision-making morality, is about decisions made or acts or actions that agents make. Act morality concerns declarations of rights, duties, justice, equality, and fairness. The third morality, that of the critics or judges, consists in applying critical canons in evalu-ating both agents and actions as being either courageous or cowardly, wise or un-wise, trustworthy or untrustworthy, and judging actions as fair or unfair, or as re-specting or violating rights.

Thus, there can be no right to love, because love belongs to agent morality rather than to act morality. Rights belong to the class of acts that are either just or fair; violations of rights are their opposite.

Dependency, Paternalism, and Freedom

One difference between adults and children that needs to be considered in ethical decision making and in ascribing rights to children is that children, while potential adults, are dependents. As dependents, children are not always able to make ef-fective decisions. There is a three-way child-health professional-parent relation-ship, in which parents or health professionals, including nurses, have the role of deciding on behalf of a helpless, dependent child what therapeutic intervention is presumably best for that child.

The point is that a child between 1 and 6 years of age may undergo health care measures, such as injections, vaccinations, prescribed drugs, and operations, such as tonsillectomy, often without asking his or her permission. The doctrine of in-formed consent does not apply to children in the earliest years of life. This general exemption is connected to the principle that to have rights presupposes conscious-ness or the capacity for rational behavior. Yet children are expected to become conscious adults who have the capacity to make decisions. The place of children falls between other sentient beings who are governed more by feelings and in-stincts and those beings who have a rational capacity.[47] This immature state of chil-dren presents a dilemma: How are children to be regarded?

One way out of this difficulty of either denying that children have rights, and thus treating them as inferiors with paternalistic intervention, or attributing the same rights to children as to adults, is to carve out a special class of rights for children. These are called "rights in trust," which are the rights they will have when they are sufficiently mature to exercise them. Rights in trust are held in safekeeping by relevant adults, who in the appropriate time will turn those rights over to the children to whom they properly belong.[48] Appropriate adults, including nurses, have the role of safeguarding children's rights. In that role, appropriate adults are guardians, protectors, trustees, and advocates of the children in their charge.

The question arises, however, as to whose rights nurses and other health professionals protect, the parents' rights or the child's. If parents are clearly abusive, then the nurse's role is to protect the child's rights. But if a parent, such as a Jehovah's Witness, intends no harm but refuses blood transfusion for a child who is seriously hurt and in need of blood, then nurses may feel they are in the middle of a conflict. One consideration for the nurse is to invoke the prevention of harm principle. The harm to the child from an unnecessary death gives the health professionals a strong reason to override the parents' right to decide to refuse a blood transfusion.

On the other hand, if a 10- or 11-year-old child has a form of cancer which only a leg amputation can arrest, and if the child refuses the operation, then the parent, invoking the principle of preventing the greater harm, has the moral right to override the child's refusal. The parents have the legal right to decide in favor of amputation as well; presumably they know better what is in the child's best interest. (See Chapter 7 for some counterexamples.)

There are fairly clear cases of benign versus malignant paternalism. The abusive parent falls into the latter category. The parent who consents to amputation to arrest cancer in the hope of preventing greater harm falls under the benign paternalism category. Because the term paternalism is used in succeeding pages, a definition of the term may be helpful. Paternalism comes from the Latin word *pater* (father) and refers to the idea that father knows best and has the authority to decide. Rational paternalism, developed by Plato (see Chapter 4), implies that the parents act on the basis of wisdom.

There are obviously cases and arguments in which paternalism is defensible, such as the parent who orders a stomach pump for a 3-year-old child who has just swallowed household cleaning fluid. The nurse's role in such a case is solely to aid the parent in saving the child's life, even if the procedure is painful to the child. There are other cases and arguments in which paternalism, exercised by parents more powerful than their children, is clearly indefensible. Examples are parents who abuse their children by putting them in scalding hot water, beating them senseless, or putting them into a hot oven. In such abuse cases, the nurse's role is to intervene on behalf of the child and secure legal protection to prevent further abuse.

Two sometimes complementary models of patient advocacy may be consulted. One is the model presented by the legendary figure of Robin Hood, who fights and overcomes oppressors. There are no conflicts between children and adults on this model. Considerations of justice and fairness determine whose rights the nurse protects. We identify this as the group confrontational model. An example of a second nurse-advocate model is presented by the protagonist in Sophocles' *Antigone*. Antigone directly confronts and defies Creon, king of Thebes, who has decreed that her brother Polynices is a traitor and to be left unburied, which is contrary to custom. Even though her power is no match for the king's, Antigone demands the right to bury her brother.[49] We may call this the *individual-confrontation* model of patient advocacy. Some nurses treat their patients in that way, doing what they regard as right, regardless of consequences to themselves. Other nurses use institutional channels to protect children who have been victimized. On a higher, macrolevel, professional organizations are also child advocates through sponsorship and support of legislation and social policy affecting children's rights and welfare.

SUMMARY

Children the proverbial hope of the future, are developing persons. To become mature persons, children need the nurture given by parents and health professionals to support their growth into adolescence and adulthood. The health and well-being of children places a pleasurable obligation on parents and health professionals to provide maximum resources.

One way to recognize the importance of children is to attribute health care rights to them. An advantage of attributing rights to children rather than imposing duties on parents alone is that rights give force to the duties imposed. But the kinds and quality of rights that children have also pose certain difficulties. The rights of children cannot include the right to drink alcohol, use illicit drugs, spend their parents' money without restrictions, or absent themselves from school. Children's rights call for constraints.

Most important, children do not have the capacity to decide what is in their own interests in health matters. Thus, children cannot have such rights as the right to informed consent until they reach an appropriate degree of maturity. To offset these difficulties, the concept of "rights in trust" is applicable to children. Such rights, however, presuppose that children are beings who have not only a biological but also a biographical life, one with plans, projects, hopes, expectations, and realizations as well as failures and disappointments. These aspects of one's biographical life give evidence of human consciousness, a necessary condition for being regarded as a person.

The challenge to the nurse working with children is to support the growing independence of the child. One way is by encouraging the child's responsibility for and participation in his or her own health care. The child's growing awareness of his or her bodily processes, recognition of the fragility of a state of wellness, and a relationship of trust with the nurse can all be strong forces in the sick child's return to health. This child can be an articulate participant in planning and implementing his or her health care.

The role of the nurse working with very young or abused and neglected children is largely that of patient advocate. Such children need protection and help. Sometimes, for the sake of the child's very survival, the child needs to be removed from the home in which the parents are abusive or incestuous. The nurse can effectively advocate for every kind of help available, such as the use of police and referral to child and family welfare agencies.

Discussion Questions

1. Parents are told by physicians that their 3-year-old child has a malignant form of leukemia that may respond to an experimental drug with highly unpleasant and possibly fatal adverse effects. All health professionals recommend the treatment to the parents in the "best interests" of the child. The parents refuse the drug in the "child's best interests" and to avoid needless suffering from the adverse effects. Who is right? What does this example show about appealing to the "best interests" doctrine?
2. Using the same case, how is appeal to the substitute judgment doctrine also begging the question? Can one reasonably speculate as to what the child would have wanted? (What the child would have wanted is an example of a counterfactual judgment.)

REFERENCES

1. Wieczorek RR, Natapoff, JN. *A conceptual approach to the nursing of children.* Philadelphia: JB Lippincott. 1981;31.
2. Aris P. *Centuries of childhood: A social history of family life.* New York: Vintage. 1962;128.
3. United Nations. *The declaration of the rights of the child.* New York: United Nations; 1959.
4. ibid.
5. Wieczorek RR, Natapoff JN. *A conceptual approach to the nursing of children.* Philadelphia: JB Lippincott. 1981;33.
6. Holder AR. *Legal issues in pediatrics and adolescent medicine.* New York: John Wiley & Sons. 1977;137.
7. ibid, p. 138.
8. ibid.
9. ibid, p. 143.
10. ibid.
11. Brown RH. Consent. *Pediatrics* 1976;57(3):414–416.
12. ibid.
13. ibid.
14. Brody H. *Ethical decisions in medicine.* (2nd ed) Boston: Little, Brown. 1981:253.
15. ibid.
16. American Nurses Association. *Code for nurses with interpretive statements.* Kansas City, Mo. 1985;8.
17. Report: NY State Nurses Association. Recognizing the signs and symptoms of child abuse/neglect. May, 1999;30(5):4–6.
18. Munson R. *Intervention and reflection: Basic issues in medical ethics.* (4th ed) Belmont, Calif: Wadsworth. 1992;223.
19. ibid.
20. ibid.
21. Andrews S, Williams AB, Neil K. The mother-child relationship in the HIV-1 positive family. *Image* 1993;25(3):193–198.
22. ibid.

23. ibid.
24. ibid.
25. ibid.
26. ibid.
27. ibid.
28. ibid.
29. ibid.
30. Lipson M. What do you say to a child with AIDS? *Hastings Center Report* 1993; 23(2):6–12.
31. ibid.
32. ibid.
33. ibid.
34. ibid.
35. Committee on Bioethics. American Academy of Pediatrics. *Pediatrics* 1988;81(1): 169–171.
36. Nicholson R. Letters. *Hastings Center Report* 1999;29(1):5.
37. ibid.
38. Ruddick W. Parents, children and moral decisions. In: Bandman EL, Bandman B (eds). *Bioethics and human rights: A reader for health professionals.* Lanham, Md: University Press of America. 1986;165–170.
39. Fletcher J. Four indicators of humanhood—the enquiry matures. *Hastings Center Report* 1974;4(6):5.
40. Fromer MJ. *Ethical issues in health care.* St. Louis: Mosby. 1981;12–14.
41. ibid.
42. ibid.
43. ibid, p. 32.
44. Cranston M. Human rights, real and supposed. In: Raphael DD (ed). *Political theory and the rights of man.* Bloomington, Ind: Indiana University Press; 1967,50–51.
45. ibid.
46. Cranston, M. *What are human rights?* New York: Taplinger. 1973;67.
47. Houlgate L. *The child and the state.* Baltimore: Johns Hopkins Press. 1980;50.
48. Feinberg J. A child's right to an open future. In: Aiken H, LaFollette H (eds). Totowa, NJ: Littlefield, Adams. 1980;125–126.
49. Cranston. *What are human rights?* New York: Taplinger. 1973;9–10.

13

Ethical Issues in the Nursing
Care of Adolescents

Study of this chapter enables the learner to:

1. Distinguish the rights and values of adolescents in relation to physiological, psychological, social, cultural, and legal dimensions of capacity and maturity.
2. Define the role of the nurse as patient advocate of adolescent clients seeking health care.
3. Develop the role of the nurse in controversies between parental control, state authority, and adolescent autonomy.
4. Recognize the adolescent's duties and responsibilities to themselves, their families, and society as dependent, independent, and interdependent persons in partnership family models.

OVERVIEW

Adolescents differ from children in the degree of autonomy they claim and exercise. Some middle- and upperclass segments of this society support adolescents in prolonged dependence on parents. These adolescents exercise decision-making rights as well as rights to receive care. These include decision-making rights (within reasonable, adult-considered limits that accord with adolescent "readiness") as well as rights to financial support, education, clothing, recreational allowances, and health care. In Chapter 10, we referred to a trilogy of rights: to initiate, to sustain, and to terminate life. In this chapter, we consider the rights to sustain and terminate life.

DEVELOPMENTAL HIGHLIGHTS: EARLY, MIDDLE, AND LATE ADOLESCENCE

In American culture, adolescence is currently regarded as a time of turmoil, and trial dreaded by parents, school teachers, law enforcement officials, and the community at large. Adolescence is generally thought of as a period of rebelliousness against parental and established authority and the norms of conventional society. Adolescents tend to test the most cherished rules and expectations of parents and adults groups. Thus, teenagers may succeed in frustrating the best intentions of nurses if they fail to listen carefully and respectfully to the adolescent's independent appraisal of the health care situation and its significance for them. Adolescents depend on the help and support of effective parents as well.

Adolescence is a developmental epoch divided into remarkably different phases. Early adolescence is characterized by ". . . wide, invisible mood swings without obvious predisposing factors."[1] At this stage, the peer group has influence, with disdain for parents and adults in general, and in adolescents' drive for independence, identity and their own values. They intensely seek privacy and companionship and perhaps intimacy of friends of the same sex.[2] As sexual feelings, curiosity, and interest increase, they become extremely conscious of their bodies and appearance compared with peers and celebrities whom they regard as models and objects of rapt admiration or love. They may live in a fantasy with unrealistic goals and role models.

Dependence and parental attachment are likely to be broken in heightened conflicts in the middle phase of adolescence.[3] These adolescents "consistently challenge rules and attempts to renegotiate them."[4] The adolescent drive for inclusion can lead to sexual behavior, with intercourse beginning at an early age. "Feelings of omnipotence and infallibility cause risk-taking behavior to peak and often lead to experimentation with drugs and dangerous activities, such as driving fast or engaging in unsafe sexual encounters."[5]

In late adolescence, peer relationships mature as sexual identity is reached and intimacy and responsibilities are understood. Relations with parents open up to reasoning processes and fewer simplistic judgments. The future becomes the dominant time perspective, with further education, marriage, or a career beckoning.

The spectrum of goods and services available to each adolescent passenger in the metaphorical lifeboat is driven by the concept of rights. Adolescents tend to claim rights and liberties that are regarded as prerogatives of adults. These rights include such activities as sexual freedom. This single issue raises many questions regarding parental responsibility for such adolescent problems as pregnancy and care of the ensuing child, abortion for unintended pregnancy, compliance with contraceptive measures, and medical care for sexually transmitted diseases, including AIDS. Thus, a central issue of adolescent health care is the extent of the autonomy of an adolescent in relation to the duties, responsibilities, and rights of parents and other significant adults, some of whom represent state power.

A related issue is the extent of adolescent rights and the duties of society to protect and to provide for those rights. The United Nations' *Declaration of Children's Rights* lists rights to be provided by society and parents. Despite its good intentions, the *Declaration* may be seen as either a paternalistic or utopian doctrine, because it places the fundamental responsibility of the child on his or her parents.[6] Moreover, its provisions are far-fetched, desirable ideals in some cases, but not practical or feasible. There is a doubtful presumption here that adolescents lack interests that they are able to identify, express, and evaluate independently of the interests and values of their parents, teachers, and others in authority.[7] Arguments can be put forth that adolescents generally are competent to defend their own interests. Other arguments show that adolescents are still immature and inexperienced. Therefore, in important matters of health, parents' concern for the best interests of their children may be in direct conflict with the values, moral principles, and autonomy of the adolescents. This may place nurses in the middle of adversarial camps, which they may seek to reconcile on behalf of continuing parent-child dialogue concerning rights, duties, responsibilities, trust, fairness, and other moral values.

ADOLESCENT HEALTH CARE ISSUES

Acute care (rather than preventive care) without a particular provider or source of routine medical care is the common practice of health care delivery to adolescents, resulting in lack of understanding of the health care experience or the decision making process.[8] Motor vehicle accidents involving drunken driving, a drunken pedestrian, and unused seat belts account for 75% of unintentional traumatic injuries. Homicide is the second leading cause of death among 15- to 24-year-olds; it is the leading cause in African American males in the same age group.[9] Suicide is the third leading cause of death among adolescents, with gay and lesbian youth accounting for almost 30% of completed suicides.[10] Eating disorders and disturbances in body concept lead to dietary abuses and use of steroids to increase body mass development with serious medical consequences. Use of tobacco and alcohol, and binge drinking have increased among youth with small decreases in the use of cocaine and heroin. High risk behaviors can lead to unprotected sex, exchange of dirty needles, direct injury to organ systems, (i.e., heart, brain), and disturbed interpersonal and social relationships.[11]

"Sexual abuse is estimated to occur in one fourth of girls and one tenth of boys before the age of sixteen,"[12] with risk of sexually transmitted disease and damage to self-esteem and trust. Sexually transmitted diseases facilitate HIV infection; younger female adolescents are more susceptible. AIDS is the sixth leading cause of death for young women aged 15 to 24 years . . . and young persons of color . . . represented more than their proportion in the general population.[13] New medications appear to help control, although not cure, AIDS. However, their cost and regimented use present serious challenges.

Teenage pregnancies have reently decreased with poorer outcomes related to late prenatal care, poor nutrition, and poor preparation and support for delivery, followed by necessary dependence on public assistance that often helps to continue the cycle of poverty.[14]

The resulting decline of social values affects adolescence in negative, destructive ways of alienation, nihilism, suicide, homicide, bigotry, casual sex, drug abuse, and abuse of themselves and others. These replace respect for "life, liberty, and the pursuit of happiness," civility, responsibility, duty, and obligation. This return to "a state of nature" is reminiscent of Hobbes's feared notion that life is "short, nasty, and brutish" in the absence of an enforceable social contract (discussed in Chapter 3). A sad example of this social deterioration occurs when a mother, often a single parent, tells her child to take his AIDS medication, and the child replies, "Why should I listen to you? You're dying of AIDS."

The use of condoms is the most effective barrier against the spread of AIDS and other sexually transmitted diseases. The proposed free distribution of condoms to adolescents in schools has provoked a storm of controversy among parents, school administrators, religious authorities, and the general public. The arguments center about adolescents' rights versus the rights and duties of parents in restraining or forbidding their children to be sexually active and knowledgeable. In New York City, a group challenged the "condom availability" part of the school system's "education" program on AIDS.[15] The group objected to the lack of prior parental consent or even a way for parents to prohibit their adolescents from receiving condoms (using an ownership model of a family, discussed in Chapter 7).[16] The New York State court stated that condom distribution is not "health education," but rather a "health service" program requiring parental consent.[17] "The court held that distributing condoms without parental consent violates the parents' constitutional rights, specifically Fourteenth Amendment due process rights construed to concern the rearing of their children."[18] The court held that there is no need for schools to act in the place of parents in creating an environment where adolescents will be permitted and encouraged to use contraceptive devices that may be contrary to the fervent beliefs of parents,[19] as well as offering "the means for students to engage in sexual activity."[20] The state court upheld the ownership model of a family. Meanwhile, despite the increase in morbidity and mortality from AIDS among adolescents, the opponents to free school condom distribution charge that such distribution is an attack on

> parental sovereignty . . . a tactic of ideological dissemination to democratize the public's perception of AIDS, . . . and to expand (the authority) of government. The agenda, critics charge, is to assert equal legitimacy for all 'life styles' (non-traditional) or 'preferences' (e.g., homosexuality) and to reduce personal responsibility under a therapeutic state, for the consequences of choices.[21]

On this view, people should suffer the consequences of their choices, in this case AIDS. This is a legal moralist point of view, and is punitive and exclusionary.

ETHICAL ISSUES IN THE LIFE AND DEATH OF ADOLESCENTS

Many other health care problems and tragedies exist for adolescents in addition to HIV and AIDS, such as substance abuse.

CASE 13.1: An Adolescent's Right to Exercise Autonomy by Refusing Life-Saving Treatment. Karen, age 16 and the second of seven siblings in a Catholic family, was hospitalized for chronic, active glomerulonephritis in 1968. Her kidneys were removed following 2 years of intense but unsuccessful treatment. A transplant of her father's kidney was unsuccessful. Hemodialysis before and following surgery caused her to have "chills, nausea, vomiting, severe headaches and weakness."[22] Psychiatric evaluation and treatment was provided for Karen and her parents before and following the transplant.

[Two years later] it was obvious that the transplanted kidney was not functioning. "Karen and her parents expressed the desire to stop treatment."[23] This decision was unacceptable to the medical staff. A psychiatrist and a social worker attempted guidance toward continuation of medical care. The family agreed to home care, which Karen found isolated and restricting. She was fatigued and uncomfortable. She was then hospitalized for high fever and removal of the transplant; the shunt became infected, clotted, and closed. At this point, Karen and her parents again refused dialysis and shunt revision. The staff was angry and frustrated and of the opinion that this was an unsound, immoral, and inappropriate decision for a 16-year-old. Karen discussed the decision with the hospital chaplain. She decided that hell and possibly heaven were nonexistent, but that "nothingness would be far better than the suffering which would continue if she lived."[24]

On consultation, the child psychiatrist found that Karen was not psychotic and that her decision was carefully reasoned and rational. The nephrologist agreed. The staff was then to make her life comfortable "with daily counseling in the event she changed her mind." The alternatives of taking the case to court to force treatment or requiring the parents to take Karen home to die so as to avoid the staff's assistance in what they thought to be a suicidal act were considered. A dialysis nurse visited Karen and insisted on further dialysis. Staff members who had witnessed Karen's prolonged suffering were more supportive.

Karen's spirits and appetite improved following her decision. She thanked the staff, picked a burial place near her home, wished her parents happiness, and supported them in their doubts about the decision. She died on June 2, 1971, suddenly and peacefully, with both parents at her side.[25]

Because there was no consistent parental opposition to Karen's decision, the issues appear to be her autonomy and right to die in conflict with the staff's view of this act as suicidal and immoral. Some staff members, such as the hemodialysis unit nurse, were strongly opposed to Karen's decision and in favor of intervention on a paternalistic basis. Other staff members supported Karen's right to decide to terminate treatment.

CASE 13.2: An Adolescent's Right to Life-Saving Treatment.   A case that complements that of Karen is the case of 12-year-old Phillip Becker, who had mild Down syndrome. He needed heart surgery, but his parents refused to consent. Phillip's parents said in court that in their opinion he was better off dead than alive. They appealed to the "best interests" doctrine. Fortunately, foster parents, following the lead of George Will,[26] came to his rescue and provided the needed surgery for Phillip. The parents regarded him as an "embarrassment."[27]

Less clear-cut are examples of 13- to 18-year-old adolescents living dependently under the parental roof who seek abortions without the knowledge and consent of their parents. These minors do not qualify for the status of emancipated minor, because they are not independent, self-supporting, or married. One moral stance is that the nurse must protect the privacy and confidentiality of these young patients on grounds of the adolescent's right to her own body. Another issue is that of the parents' rights to be informed of the health concern and to decide for the immature offspring.

ETHICAL ISSUES IN QUALITY-OF-LIFE CASES OF ADOLESCENTS

Although ethical issues in adolescent health care do not all involve life and death matters, they may nonetheless be serious to those affected.

CASE 13.3: Parent's Refusal to Consent to Surgery for an Adolescent on Grounds of Religious Belief. Martin Sieferth, age 14, and a cleft palate and harelip and was in need of surgery. According to a petition by the Health Department, the boy was declared to be neglected, and the Department ordered that surgery be performed. Martin's father, unlike Phillip Becker's father (Case Study 13.2), showed signs of parental affection. Martin's father believed, however, in "mental healing" and in letting "the natural forces of the universe work on the body."[28] Therefore, he refused surgery to repair his son's seriously deformed and unattractive jaw. Martin agreed with his father.[29] The court agreed with Martin on the grounds that he was old enough to give or withhold consent to surgery. Martin was consequently disfigured as an adolescent and will need physical and emotional relief if he is to flourish.

In three-way relations, parents, children, and the state do not always agree, as illustrated in Martin Sieferth's refusal of treatment for desirable cosmetic surgery, which was supported by the court.

CASE 13.4: Parental Refusal of Consent Versus the Adolescent's Surgery. A 14-year-old boy suffered from a serious neck and face deformity which could be alleviated by surgery. He wished to have the operation so that he could lead a normal life. His mother had no objections to the surgery, but she was a Jehovah's Witness and refused to consent to blood transfusions. The surgeon refused to perform the operation unless he could transfuse the patient. The court held that the child was neglected and ordered the surgery performed.[30]

CASE 13.5: Parental Refusal to Consent to Adolescents' Tonsillectomies. Four adolescents were removed from their home by court order on grounds of physical neglect and child abuse. Their father refused to allow necessary tonsillectomies, on religious grounds, but his objection was overruled by the court.[31] In a triangular relation between adolescents' rights, parental authority, and state power,[32] some courts, although not all, rule in favor of surgery.

THE NURSE'S ROLE IN ADOLESCENT CARE

Working with adolescents is particularly challenging. They tend to shift between determined independence and exercise of autonomy and the delayed recognition that the situation is fraught with problems and possibly peril. This developmental phase is characterized by the notion of omnipotence. High value is placed on acceptance by peers, with consequent behavioral and role experimentation within the peer group. Thus, the adolescent may experiment with drugs and sexual and criminal activity in response to peer pressure. It is extremely difficult for most adolescents to separate from the values of the peer group with which they identify.

Acceptance of peer values, such as positive regard for sexual activity with resulting pregnancy, abortion, sexually transmitted diseases or AIDS can, for example, be the source of considerable conflict between adolescents and parents. The nurse can be caught between the anger and duties of the parents and the defensiveness and vulnerability of the adolescent. Each believes that his or her choice is the right one. Each expects that the nurse will advocate and actively support his or her position. For example, the 13-year-old seeking an abortion without parental knowledge expects unconditional support from the abortion unit as patient advocate. This adolescent insists on carrying the burden of guilt or regret regarding the abortion decision and of her fear of the procedure without the parental support she might otherwise receive. The nurse tries to help the young person identify and analyze her perceptions of her family in the hope that parents will be viewed in a positive light. The adolescent's negative reasons may be substantive, including abuse and incest. The pregnant adolescent may fear both punishment and rejection from a family that has forbidden premarital sexual activity. The nurse as patient advocate and in accordance with the *Code for Nurses* supports such a patient's self-determination while giving information relevant to making an informed judgment. Such information includes the possible helpfulness of parental support and participation in the decision, the alternatives of full-term delivery, adoption, or abortion, the steps and effects of the procedure, and the patient's right to receive or to refuse treatment. Relevant information also includes referrals to family planning for counseling and information regarding contraception. Supportive nursing care includes concern and interest for the tragic choice faced by the young adolescent. Anticipatory guidance is directed toward prevention of future unintended pregnancies, along with adolescent evaluation of personal values expressed in behavior and in relationships.

The second level of advocacy is for a nurse to refer a sexually active adolescent to a family planning unit or physician for contraceptives or individual counseling. Such agencies aim to counsel, educate, and guide the adolescent toward control of pregnancies and of matters of general health. Care is usually low-cost or free.

A third level of advocacy is appeal to the courts. Department of Health and Human Resources regulations require that all family planning projects receiving federal funds make "services . . . available without regard for religion, creed, age, sex, parity, or marital status."[33] A 15-year-old whose family was receiving Aid to Families with Dependent Children sued the Planned Parenthood Association of Utah for denying her contraceptives without parental permission. A three-judge federal court in Utah held that the parental consent requirement was in conflict with federal requirements. To deprive the adolescent of contraceptives from agencies receiving federal assistance was therefore unconstitutional. The court further ruled that the requirement for parental consent was a violation of the minor's right of privacy. Therefore, the federal regulations were to be enforced.[34]

The controversy between parental authority and adolescent autonomy continues. At times, the nurse's role may be much like that of a broker, trying to reconcile the adolescent's insistence on rights to sexual activity, contraception, and abortion with parental authority, parental concern for the adolescent's welfare, and such consequences as unintended pregnancies. The parent may argue justifiably that the adolescent's rights are limited by her inability to care for a child and her dependence on parental support, or that sexual freedom, contraceptives, abortion are wrong and therefore undesirable. The nurse may suggest to parents the unrealistic expectations for adolescent sexual abstinence. The nurse may then be in the position of advocating the adolescent's right to contraception as a lesser evil than unintended pregnancies, abortion, and sexually transmitted diseases, including AIDS.

The dilemma of adolescent sexual activity, contraceptive use, abortion, and child-bearing outside of marriage is a serious and persistent problem. The birthrate for unwed mothers increased by 70% from 1983 to 1993 to 6.3 million children.[35] The adolescent may be asserting her right to sexual freedom, but the exercise of a right requires a correlative duty of someone to provide for that right. According to this argument, it is the duty of a parent to provide decent conditions for a fulfilling life for the child produced, because most adolescents cannot do so.

Births out of wedlock have "been cited as a factor in a host of social problems, including increased crime, drug abuse, welfare dependency, and poor educational attainment."[36] The issue for the nurse then becomes one of presenting rational alternatives to adversarial parents and adolescents, if possible. Moral and social consequences of behavior are elicited and analyzed together by parents, adolescents, and the nurse. Assumptions of parental support by providing the necessary goods and services to the adolescent regardless of lifestyle and choices need examination and evaluation by both parents and adolescents.

Adolescents, too, can engage in the process of morally justifying their major decisions. Little recognition is given to adolescent responsibilities for analyzing and evaluating the moral dimensions and consequences of behavior. In the public media, particularly, the adolescent is regarded as glamorous and exciting when experimenting with drugs, alcohol, sexual activity, music, dress, and unconventional lifestyles. The central issue for the nurse becomes one of supporting those adolescent rights that facilitate a decent, fulfilling life or, as in the case of Karen, the right to die as a release from excessive or pointless suffering. This is the role of the patient advocate in support of the individual's moral right to rational decision making or autonomy. As illustrated by the problems of adolescent sexual activity in the form of pregnancy, abortion, AIDS and other sexually transmitted diseases, child-bearing, child abuse, and substance abuse, there are morally justifiable limits to adolescent rights. The boundaries to adolescent rights may come from several sources. For example, in some states, compulsory driver education has made a significant statistical difference in the accident rates of adolescents. In family relationships, the development of responsibilities and trust goes with the exercise of rights. This shows the relation of rights and virtues. To paraphrase Kant, rights without virtues are empty; virtues without rights are blind. One without the other is incomplete. Thus, the adolescent learns to be both a provider and a recipient of goods and services rather than a mere right holder in a world of rapidly increasing rights and shrinking resources.

ETHICAL CONSIDERATIONS IN THE ADOLESCENT-NURSE-PARENT RELATIONSHIP

The fact that one shares social life with others has an important bearing on adolescent development. A socially worthwhile life calls for an adolescent to recognize not only rights but also responsibilities commensurate with the growing physical power to do good or harm to the self and others. The moral education of an adolescent includes the point that social life is shared and people depend on one another. Human relationships call for reciprocal give-and-take, the mutual recognition of rights and responsibilities.

Consequently, one may argue that the moral-correlativity thesis of rights may well apply to adolescents. This means that in order for them to have rights, they must demonstrate the capacity to live up to corresponding responsibilities. Driving a car calls for an adolescent's ability to drive safely. It may call for the adolescent to pay for part or all of the cost of driving. The adolescent may also be expected to refrain from drinking alcohol while driving. Similar constraints govern the use of drugs. These are constraints imposed equally on adult members of society who are expected to fulfill social and economic responsibilities. Thus, the new rights adolescents gain, such as driving, may be said to be "earned rights," which depend on appropriate assumption of responsibilities. Similar constraints may well govern sexual activities. Adolescents of school and college age who are not yet ready to assume adult responsibilities in bearing and rearing children are not free to engage in sexual activities without appropriate constraints, such as the proper use of condoms.

The governing principle in determining the rights and responsibilities of adolescents is to decide whether such rights and responsibilities are conducive to leading a socially worthwhile life. This ideal rules out socially destructive behavior such as unsafe sex, unsafe driving, drug experimentation, vandalism, violence, and lack of concern for others. The point is that one does not want adolescents to become veritable savages, like those portrayed in William Golding's *Lord of the Flies* (1954).[37] Such behavior is unacceptable in our society.

The role of the nurse, as well as other health professionals, is to be a health educator and therapist in reinforcing positive social values. The nurse supports values that help an individual adolescent become a responsible, upstanding member of society. The nurse helps the adolescent learn both to contribute and to allocate, and facilitates adolescents' functioning together. In this connection, the concept of physical, social, psychological, and economic well-being becomes a decidedly important nursing model. In a recent position statement on adolescent care, the American Nurses Association (ANA) views the role of the nurse to function as advocate, spokesperson, care provider, administrative case manager, and volunteer with an interdisciplinary approach and a multicultural, socioeconomic, and multiracial perspective.[38]

A socially worthwhile life also calls for appropriate recognition of and training in standards and skills of sustained intellectual judgment. Such judgment requires a common understanding of the methods and results of cognitive disciplines with appropriate regard for and familiarity with rules of evidence in the sciences. The relevance to ethics is that enormous good or evil comes by either considering or ignoring rules of evidence.

THE BIOLOGICAL/BIOGRAPHICAL/SOCIAL/COGNITIVE DISTINCTION APPLIED TO ADOLESCENTS

The biological/biographical/social/cognitive distinction discussed herein raises questions about the quality of some adolescents' lives as persons if they have been comatose for a long time. Such questions are raised on the grounds that they lack a biographical life, a life with conscious activities. These distinctions also raise questions as to what kinds of persons they are if they have extreme physical, intellectual, social, or psychological handicaps, such as substance addiction or criminal or antisocial behavior. These biographical and social distinctions also support an adolescent's right to terminate her fifth pregnancy on grounds that she is unlikely to provide a worthwhile human life for yet another child. The biographical/social/cognitive distinction also rules against a biology major's refusal to dissect animals in the course of study. The social/cognitive distinction rationally counts against a nurse's refusal to participate in surgical repair of a boy's cleft palate or in an abortion indicated by social and cognitive considerations. By implication, the cognitive requirement (respect for and familiarity with scientific methods and results) gives a reason against a nurse's recommending laetrile or faith healing as a rational alternative to scientifically verifiable health care measures.

The biological/biographical/social/cognitive distinction also rules against the behavior of sociopaths and bigots who kill and maim other people or who believe that the Holocaust never occurred. These adolescents rule themselves out of the pale of moral discourse. Such adolescents (as well as adults) may even be regarded as persons, but not as very good persons.

Some people ask: "Who decides?" or "Who shall have the justifiable authority to decide whether an adolescent's life is no longer worth sustaining?" One move in philosophy consists in rephrasing the question to ask: "What criteria do a rational person appeal to in deciding nurse adolescent-parent issues?" or "What counts as a good reason or as evidence?" In some cases, such as the faith-healing issue, appeal to scientific evidence is appropriate because it works; and the reason it works is that it has a truth value that appeal to faith healing lacks. The reason for believing in the truth value of cleft-palate surgery over faith healing is that the verifiable evidence favors the results—a clear victory for utilitarianism.

In other kinds of cases, such as saving the life of a Jehovah's Witness by giving a necessary blood transfusion, one effective and wise appeal is to conventional or "common morality."[39] While it is true that a common morality is not the whole of morality, it does address itself to the common moral sentiments and virtues, such as honesty, affection, generosity, wisdom, courage, and happiness, and to the survival and well-being of people.

One aspect of nursing ethics is the use of a checklist among major ethical theories and their principles. These include duty-based ethics, with its principle of autonomy, fidelity, and truth-telling; love-based ethics with its golden rule principle;

utilitarianism, and the majority happiness principle; and the Rawlsian justice as fairness principle. These ethical theories all espouse beneficence and the duty to refrain from harm.[40] (Other ethical theories are cited in Chapters 3 through 7.)

To practice nursing ethics is to reflect on these principles and to use formal, inductive, and dialectic reasoning. Along with this process, one uses moral intuitions to select principles and practices over competing principles. From the case of Kenneth Darling, an adolescent who injured his leg in a football game and whose leg had to be amputated (the hospital, the physician, and a nurse were found guilty of negligence), one learns that a nurse is valued for her trained intelligence, caring, and skilled observation. This type of case, along with the "faith healing" cases and the Chad Green case, adds moral strength to the Platonic principle that "knowledge is a virtue."

Whereas knowledge of ethical theories and their principles and practices produce no certainty, the continuous use of reasoned argument on behalf of some ethical theories and against their rivals brings a powerful moral force to nursing practice.

A distinction made earlier between various models of health care (see Chapter 2) by Emmanuel and Emmanuel applies to the issue of restraints versus the freedom of infants, children, and adolescents. As children grow into adolescence, some form of the guidance-cooperation model increasingly applies. Young adolescents are expected to learn how to develop increasing degrees of independence and self-sufficiency. The adult, including the nurse, will be analogous to the driver's education teacher who sits next to the student and guides the student's driving activities. These models correspond to our ownership, club membership, and partnership models.

The third model, mutual participation, as with partnership (the goal sought for in a democratic society), is a society of approximate equals. This goal guides and orients adolescents on their way to and through adulthood.

SUMMARY

The main moral problem in each developmental span—infancy, childhood, and adolescence—are different in some aspects and similar in others. Adolescents are similar in concerns to other human beings throughout all phases of growth. They are self-respecting persons; they learn to respect others; and they live by sharing social life. As such, young people are brought up to be not only dependent or independent, but to be interdependent human beings. The adult, and the nurse as health educator, who brings up a child only to think of himself or herself is overlooking a crucial reality consideration that governs social life. For example, adolescents who drive at high speeds with their friends threaten their friends' safety. The role of the nurse as health educator is to teach children and adolescents appropriate health behavior. There are other rules of social life under which the development of a person is aimed not only at independence but at interdependence.

These rules admonish a child to eat a nutritious breakfast, to have wholesome physical, intellectual, cultural, and emotional activities, and to avoid drug and alcohol abuse, premature and unsafe sexual activity, crime, and violence.

The development of persons with rights and reciprocal responsibilities constitutes goals that apply from birth to death and do not vary from infancy to childhood and adolescence. As Harry Stack Sullivan, the eminent American psychiatrist, said, "Everyone is much more simply human than otherwise."[41]

The moral differences in the three phases of growth are many, but they center on dependence in infancy, development of independence in childhood, and developing interdependence in adolescence. Each phase brings moral problems, some of which have no completely satisfactory answers, as in the attempt to decide whether to save an infant, child, or adolescent with few or marginal prospects of living a full life. Moral problems are thorniest at the fringes. The core of morality is fairly well-settled. Phillip Becker's foster parents were morally right to insist on his cardiac surgery. Karen was not wrong to choose to die. Martin Sieferth's father is clearly wrong. On what grounds do we say this? On the grounds that Martin has rights, as does Phillip. But do these grounds justify the conclusion? That is a further question.

In the nurse's role as health educator, patient advocate, agent of reality, and therapist, the nurse is not alone. Because of the common morality, one that generally aims at the well-being of everyone, the nurse has many allies and resources to call on for help while coping with the admittedly real hindrances and obstacles of adolescence.

Discussion Questions

1. On what grounds did Karen, the adolescent kidney patient in Case 13.1, have a right to refuse dialysis and thus end her life? Give reasons for and against your position.

2. What reasons might one give both for and against Martin Sieferth's father refusing surgical repair of his son's cleft palate (Case 13.3)? Which reasons outweigh which others?

3. What health care rights and responsibilities does an adolescent have? May adolescents refuse to drink milk and eat the nutritious foods their parents serve them at home?

4. Which doctrine, if any, best applies toward guiding adolescent decision making in health care, the "substitute judgment" doctrine (put yourself in another's shoes) or the "best interest" doctrine (doing or not doing X in your child's best interests)? Critically evaluate the application of either of these doctrines. From a caring perspective, what are the strengths and weaknesses of the substitute judgment and the best interest doctrines?

5. How do substitute judgment and best interest standards apply to the tragic plight of an adolescent AIDS case?

REFERENCES

1. Muscari ME. When to worry about adolescent angst. *Am J Nursing* 1998;98(3):22–23.
2. ibid.
3. ibid.
4. ibid.
5. ibid.
6. Young R. In the interests of children and adolescents. In: Aiken W, LaFollette H (eds). *Whose child? Children's rights, parental authority and state power.* Totowa, NJ: Littlefield, Adams. 1980;179.
7. ibid, p. 180.
8. Hoffman ND. The health of american adoescents: Current issues and service gaps. In: Bluestein J, Levin C, Dubler NN (eds). *The adolescent alone.* Cambridge: Cambridge University Press. 1999;50–77.
9. ibid.
10. ibid.
11. ibid.
12. ibid.
13. ibid.
14. ibid.
15. Will G. Condoms don't belong in schools. *Daily Hampshire Gazette.* January 10, 1994;16.
16. ibid.
17. ibid.
18. ibid.
19. ibid.
20. ibid.
21. ibid.
22. Schowalter JE et al. The adolescent patient's decision to die. *Pediatrics* 1973;51(1):97–103.
23. ibid, p. 98.
24. ibid.
25. Bandman E, Bandman B. The nurse's role in protecting the patient's right to live or die. *Advances Nursing Sci* 1979;1(3):21–35.
26. Will G. The case of Phillip Becker. *Newsweek.* April 14, 1980;112.
27. ibid.
28. Ruddick W. In the matter of Sieferth. In: O'Neill O, Ruddick W (eds). *Having children.* New York: Oxford University Press. 1979;139.
29. Holder A. *Legal issues in pediatrics and adolescent medicine.* (2nd ed) New Haven, Conn: Yale University Press. 1985;240.
30. ibid, p. 239.
31. ibid.
32. Aiken W, LaFollette H. *Whose child? Children's rights, parental authority and state power.* Totowa, NJ: Littlefield, Adams. 1980.
33. Holder A. *Legal issues in pediatrics and adolescent medicine.* (2nd ed).
34. ibid.
35. Holmes SA. Birthrate for unwed women up 70 percent since 1983 study shows. *The New York Times.* July 20, 1994;1.
36. ibid.
37. Golding W. *Lord of the flies.* New York: Putnam;1954.

38. Adolescent Health Task Force Position Statement on Adolescent Health. American Nurses Association: Washington, DC; 1998.
39. Donnegan A. *The theory of morality.* Chicago: University of Chicago Press. 1977;6,7, 28–31,102,172,210–243.
40. Hamblet J. Ethics and the pediatric preoperative nurse. *Today's OR Nurse* 1994; 16(2):16.
41. Sullivan HS. *The interpersonal theory of psychiatry.* New York: Norton. 1953;32.

14

Ethical Issues in the Nursing Care of Adults

Study of this chapter enables the learner to:

1. Understand adult development in relation to the moral issues significant to this phase of human development.
2. Apply ethical principles of the prevention of harm, truth-telling, informed consent, the right to receive and to refuse treatment, and the right to privacy and confidentiality in practice with adult clients.
3. Utilize the AHA's *Patient's Bill of Rights* in development of the nursing role as patient advocate.
4. Facilitate the patient's right to self-determination and well-being through shared decision making in relation to the client's life goals, rational plans, and values.

OVERVIEW

A person's passage from childhood and adolescence to youth or early adulthood is one of the most exciting times of life. Romantic love and attachment to another person marks this period as a peak experience in life. Vigorous health is the norm for youth and young adults. Therefore, serious or chronic illness is devastating to lifestyles, educational and social goals, careers, family planning, and the realization of hopes.

ADULT DEVELOPMENT

Adulthood is the longest and most productive phase of human development. The process is one of continuing change characterized by growth, development, and slow decline. The rate of change differs considerably among individuals. Consequently, all divisions of the adult life span are somewhat arbitrary and apply only generally to a particular individual.

Young Adulthood

Young adulthood is regarded as the years up to age 35. In this period, persons are establishing themselves in occupations and in situations of interpersonal intimacy, including marriage.

Customary developmental tasks of young adults include gradual independence from parents with progressive involvement in the world of education and work. The young adult is concerned with a role in the community and in selected groups. Marriage, childbearing, and child rearing are characteristic of this phase of development.

Young people are expected to provide for the health, education, and care of their children and for their own welfare and future. Serious illness at this age is unexpected and catastrophic to all members of the family system. Chronic illness in a spouse can be disruptive to the marital relationship and to the security of the children. Ethical decisions regarding life prolonging measures of comatose spouses can be especially difficult at this age, because they involve a healthy spouse and children in need of social, emotional, and financial resources. If, however, the young family enjoys good health and good fortune, then the couple gradually moves into the developmental tasks of middle age.

Youth. In contrast to this traditional path of development, there are those young adults who are unable to accept the traditional values they were taught without reexamination and anguish. Keniston has defined an emerging developmental phase called "youth," which he describes as an "optional stage, not a universal one. . . . Most young Americans who enter this stage of life tend to be between the ages of 18 and 30."[1]

The term describes a new generation born in the nuclear age and usually of college and graduate-school age. They refuse to settle down in traditional ways and "often vehemently challenge the existing social order."[2]

A central concern is the issue of individual autonomy that is expressed in a variety of ways. One expression is that of living and working arrangements that seek independence from the money economy of the larger society. Protests against the use of nuclear power and the use and disposal of toxic substances is another expression of autonomy.

This group assumes moral responsibility for the dwindling resources of the planet by conservation measures. Consequently, nutritional patterns are often vegetarian. Another issue is concern for the second-rate status of women, racial and ethnic minorities, and other disadvantaged groups. The attempt is to bring about fundamental change in society's distribution of goods and services on the basis of fairness and need. If such youth were successful in their efforts to create basic change in social institutions, a system free of war-making machines and ideology and of greed and corruption, society would be vastly different in its goals and processes. This may mean more support for holistic health approaches and for health care as a right enjoyed equally by everyone. These new ways of youth include home deliveries and natural methods of healing. These young people will question the reasons for care provided. They expect to participate fully in the decisions affecting them and to reserve the privilege of deciding the ethical issues for themselves.

Middle Age

The years of middle age, from age 35 to age 65, are regarded as the most productive. In these years, individuals consolidate and expand their financial and occupa-
tional security. These are years of focus on the rearing, education, and enjoyment
of children. There may be additional responsibilities for aged parents. In these
years, nursing plays a role in ongoing health education. There is less obstetric care
and more care for growing children, in emergencies and in crises. The nurse can
be a significant influence in facilitating the processes of moral deliberation in
health care that guide the family in its choices of action.

Middle-aged women and men recognize that theirs is the most powerful age
group, that it is they who make most decisions and carry forward social norms. Although our society is youth-oriented, it is under the control of the middle-aged population.[3] The middle-aged have most to lose from ill health, incapacitation, and death.
This phase of life is the period of maximum competence in self-assessment and cognitive problem-solving abilities. The middle-aged person has developed a wide range
of coping strategies. New appreciations come from in-between relationships with
younger and older generations. Middle-aged persons find themselves in control and
in the driver's seat, in contrast to their youth or to their expectations of old age.

Middle age can also be seen as a period of losses and crises. Some women see
menopause and the departure of grown children as tragic. Other women celebrate
the launching of children into adult independence. Members of both sexes may
regard with bitterness the inevitable decline in youthful good looks, strength, energy, and sexual drive. Other individuals see these as turning points toward serenity and deeper expressions of love and affection.

The occurrence of unexpected events such as sudden serious illness, forced
retirement or unemployment, or death of the spouse or of a child out of the natural sequence is highly traumatic for both young or middle-aged individuals and
families. Nurses can play a supportive role by helping the family in anticipatory
grieving when there is time, or by encouraging appropriate grief after an unanticipated loss. Nurses can be helpful to clients in working through feelings of unrealistic self-blame. It is the unanticipated event that is likely to cause major
stresses, ". . . events that upset the sequence and rhythm of the expected life
cycle."[4] Consequently, serious illness, impending death of self or actual death of
spouse or child, accidents, and loss of job or income are severe stresses, particularly to the middle-aged adult. The nurse can help alleviate this stress through
helping the family identify its strengths and values.

Widespread social change in the form of increasing longevity for both sexes
along with the inclusion of nearly half of all women in the work force emphasizes
values of personhood and self-actualization for the middle-aged individual. Values
of respect for self and others are expressed in demands for accessible health care
oriented to the needs and rights of the adult. Women, particularly, are seeking
health care that respects their sensitivities and special needs of combining a career, parenthood, marriage, homemaking, and possible further education. Women
are not only living longer than men, but are expressing a new sense of freedom in
their increased status, reproductive control, economic independence, and the assumption of new career and civic roles.[5]

THE APPLICATION OF ETHICAL PRINCIPLES TO SELECTED CASES

Selected cases illustrate the major ethical issues that affect the adult developmental phase. Major issues are the enforcement of patients' rights.

Prevention of Harm

CASE 14.1.   Herbert, age 28, a depressed, suicidal patient, tells Nurse M that he has a right to end his life in the hospital and that she has no right to restrain him.[6] The issue here is the patient's autonomy and self-determination versus the principles of "do no harm" and "do good," which the Nurse M may invoke as guides to action.

The Allocation of Scarce Resources

CASE 14.2.   Phillip, age 57, an alcoholic, derelict patient, claims a right to unlimited medical care, including three dialysis treatments per week costing more than $200 per treatment, or more than $31,000 per year. Phillip has now applied for a kidney transplant and is on the waiting list. Should a good match occur, is it fair to give Phillip the scarce and precious organ while others go without? Phillip is not a young person making useful social and economic contributions to society. The issue here is whether or not any person who is noncontributing with a self-destructive lifestyle has unlimited rights to health care and to the community's scarce resources.

CASE 14.3.   Allan, a 29-year-old college student, rode his motorcycle without wearing a helmet. One Saturday night Allan was hit by an uninsured drunken driver and sustained severe head and spinal injuries. Although Allan was employed part-time, health care costs were so high that he qualified as a medical indigent eligible for public aid. Allan is one of 105 injured motorcyclists in Washington state whose medical care was 63% subsidized by public money, state and federal, mostly Medicaid.[7] The ethical issue concerns the conflict between the freedom not to wear helmets and the heavy cost to the public of medical care for injured riders. What moral reasons, if any, are there for motorcyclists to be legally forced to wear helmets and carry insurance? What moral reasons are there for the public to be forced to subsidize Allan's very costly treatment and care for the remainder of his life?

Truth-Telling and Deception

CASE 14.4.   Robert, age 27, is a handsome, successful Wall Street account executive. He proposed marriage to a beautiful, 21-year-old recent graduate of an ivy league university nursing program. His application to an exclusive health club required a comprehensive health examination. Tests and retests of his blood show him to be unmistakenly positive for the human immunodeficiency virus (HIV). Nevertheless, Robert sees advantages in marrying and not telling his nurse friend the truth. He believes that she will care for him devotedly as her husband when the disease becomes symptomatic. She has useful scientific, medical, and nursing knowledge of the treatment of disease that may prolong his life. Once infected, she will have less reason to abandon him. The examining physician and the nurse practitioner reflect on the morality of notifying the girlfriend and other possible contacts of the facts of Robert's health status. Should they tell? Is not informing the girlfriend, although not a falsehood, a deception?

CASE 14.5. In a case adapted from Brock,[8] Edward, a high-anxiety cardiac patient with several previous near-fatal heart attacks, refuses tranquilizers. The head nurse, in consultation with the attending physician, gives Edward tranquilizers, but without Edward's knowledge or permission. The nurse does this for life-saving reasons, thus setting aside the patient's right to know what is being done to his body.[9] The other nurses, Ms. C and Ms. G, are instructed to lie about the real content and effects of the drug given. Ms. C believes the head nurse, the authority figure, knows best. Ms. G thinks the patient has the right to decide what is done to his body. Who is right, and why?

CASE 14.6. Another example of the patient's right to know the truth about diagnosis, prognosis, proposed treatment, alternatives, risks, and benefits is a case adapted from Brody.[10] A 54-year-old mother of four grown children, Ms. Jones is admitted complaining of severe abdominal pain. She fears cancer. Surgery reveals advanced cervical cancer and distant metastases. The 5-year survival rate is less than 20%. The chief resident avoids the word "cancer." He believes that a diagnosis of incurable cancer will prompt the patient to harm herself. The resident later tells the patient that the malignant process has been removed. The patient then confronts the nurse with the statement, "I really have cancer, don't I? And they don't want to tell me the truth." The nurse evaluates the patient's situation and her need to prepare her children, husband, and herself for dying and death. The nurse considers the possible but unlikely event that the patient will react to the news in a self-destructive fashion, and ponders the assignment of guilt and responsibility for such an act. The nurse then analyzes his own responsibility and loyalty to the chief resident as a member of the team in need of support in a difficult situation, and a nurse's vulnerable status in contradicting a physician's word to a patient. The nurse weighs the use of meaningful silence and verbal reflection of the patient's concern for her diagnosis and prognosis. Finally, the nurse is able to separate the issue of whether to tell the truth or not from the issues of what truth shall be told by whom and in what words and circumstances. The ethical issue has priority, the ways and means are secondary.

The Principle of Informed Consent

Another major issue is the patient's right to informed consent regarding proposed medical, diagnostic, or surgical procedures. This right is implied by the right of respect. Informed consent includes diagnosis, prognosis, and the risks, benefits, and alternatives to the proposed measures conveyed in words the patient can understand. Few patients know or are told that a second opinion before consenting to surgery is not only a precaution against unnecessary surgery but is paid for by health insurance plans.

Glaring examples of the failure to seek informed consent include the coercive consent of parents of mentally retarded children in the Willowbrook hepatitis experiments, and the use of 600 US Army servicemen for an LSD experiment without their knowledge.[11]

The Right to Receive and to Refuse Treatment

A further significant ethical issue in the adult development phase is the right to receive and to refuse treatment.

CASE 14.7. An example is the case of John, age 32, married with two children. His wife is unable to tolerate oral contraceptives or intrauterine devices, and the couple finds condoms unsatisfactory. On the recommendation of the family nurse practitioner, the couple considers a vasectomy among their contraceptive alternatives. John and his wife conclude that a vasectomy best fits their situation because their family is the ideal size. John's request for a vasectomy is refused by the urologist who feels that John is too young, he might change his mind or remarry, and that the operation is irreversible.[12] The urologist may argue that the right to life includes the right to reproduce. This right is inalienable, which means John may not renounce the right to reproduce through vasectomy.

The family nurse practitioner is in a dilemma concerning her relationship with the family and the urologist. As patient advocate, the nurse's loyalty is to the family's autonomy and self-determination. In that case, she would support John's decision and furnish him with the names of other urologists. The nurse considers the possibility that in the future, after a vasectomy, the patient may remarry and bitterly resent the irreversibility of the procedure and the nurse's advice. The nurse also considers the refusal of the urologist to perform the vasectomy as an infringement of the patient's right to receive treatment. Because this urologist is the only available one in the surrounding community, the patient will have difficulty and incur financial cost in securing the services of a urologist in a distant large city. The nurse's dilemma is that of upholding the patient's right to treatment or agreeing with the urologist's right to refuse treatment on grounds of the patient's best interests.

CASE 14.8. Despite the best-intentioned and well-planned strategies, psychiatric nurses are still confronted with young, deeply disturbed psychiatric patients who refuse neuroleptic medications. For example, Jane, a 22-year-old, unmarried, graduate student, does not want to risk repulsive adverse effects such as tardive dyskinesia in the form of uncontrollable grimaces, which appear in some patients, and also regards drugs as a form of intrusion and control. She may also refuse drugs on the basis of their effects on mental acuity, the "snowed under" or "zombie" effect. If Jane is a voluntary patient, the refusal is honored. Jane may be discharged, however, if she continues to refuse treatment and fails to improve. In extreme cases, the patient's status is converted to involuntary admission and the patient is declared incompetent and forced to take prescribed medication.

The nurse, in possession of all of the facts surrounding the use and misuse of medication and adverse effects of tardive dyskinesia and dystonias, may be in a genuine dilemma in relation to Jane's refusal. The nurse may deplore the sleepiness and sealing over of acute anxiety that comes from the use of medication. On the other hand, the nurse may, out of loyalty to fellow nurses and workers who prefer quiet patients, feel strongly motivated to influence or coerce Jane to take the strong tranquilizers. Another dimension of the nurse's dilemma is that of the community's desire for conformity to social norms and laws. Community pressure on nurses and the mental health establishment to tranquilize troubled or troublesome patients raises questions concerning the nurse's role. The psychiatric nurse is placed in the role of double agent—for the community's good versus the patient's good. In this example, what began as simple truth-telling about the intended effects of drugs to facilitate a patient's compliance with the drug regimen became a genuine dilemma when the psychiatric patient refused medication on reasonable grounds.

CASE 14.9. Virginia, age 26, a Jehovah's Witness and mother of three, is wheeled into an emergency room department unconscious and hemorrhaging as a result of a car accident. Her husband refuses blood transfusions on religious grounds. Again, two nurses, along with the interns, are faced with the problem of what is to be done to either save or not save Virginia's life. What is the right thing to do, and how would you reason to a conclusion?

The Right to Privacy and Confidentiality

CASE 14.10. Jim, 26 years old, is brought into the emergency department following a seizure in a movie theater. Jim is known to the emergency department nursing staff because he has previously been treated for seizures due to failure to take prescribed anticonvulsive drugs. Meanwhile, Jim drives his fellow workers in a car pool 1 week out of 4 and drives twice monthly to a neighboring town to visit his mother. Under the licensing requirements of that state, an individual with uncontrolled seizures is ineligible for a driver's license. The patient begs that the nurses not report him, because he depends on his driver's license and jobs are very scarce.[13] The nurses debate the patient's right to confidentiality and privacy versus the right of others to expect a safe driver on the road who will not endanger innocent human life.

CASE 14.11. George is a 25-year-old homosexual patient hospitalized in a large medical center on the East Coast. He is seriously ill with an AIDS-related disease and wishes to see his parents before he dies. When George left his home on a sheep ranch in Montana at the age of 18, his parents had no knowledge of his lifestyle, nor have they seen him since. George does not want his parents to know the cause or the seriousness of his illness or the nature of his lifestyle. He asks the staff to respond to his parents' questions regarding his illness as some form of leukemia or other exotic disease of which they have no knowledge. After 3 days of visiting their obviously dying son, the parents ask the nurse, "Does he have

AIDS?" Should the patient's right to privacy and confidentiality take priority over the parents' right to the truth?

MORAL-PHILOSOPHICAL CONSIDERATIONS

To examine these cases and issues effectively, one must consider several moral-philosophical theories, concepts, and principles.

Informed Consent, Openness, and Self-Corrective Feedback

To the extent that information is available to health professionals and is communicable and understandable, the principle of *informed consent* applies. Informed consent means that both patients and subjects are entitled to updated information on which to base their consent or dissent to a proposed health care procedure. The publicness test once proposed by Rawls is relevant. According to Rawls, a procedure of justice is fair if, among other conditions, it conforms to the test of publicity.[14] This means that procedures used are openly aired. We may call this the "fishbowl" view of health care, in which procedures and processes such as x-rays are subject to public scrutiny. The growth of health care procedures performed in doctors' offices may be a trend away from openness and publicity of procedures. The publicness principle or fishbowl metaphor point to the advantages of the teaching hospital, in which mistakes are used as a source of health care learning in the form of self-corrective feedback.

The Right to the Prevention of Harm

In a world filled with dangers and vicissitudes, one cannot possibly guarantee the right to prevent harm. Natural catastrophes, as well as human misjudgments and foibles, make the world unsafe from chance and fatality. However, one has the right to live in a society that seeks to practice the prevention, or rather minimization, of harm. The concept of doing no harm figured prominently in Plato's concept of justice, which emphasizes not doing harm to anyone. To fail was to countenance injustice, an intolerable obstacle to being civilized. Thus, a standard was set, however woeful or deficient in practice. The prevention of harm in health care also includes the alleviation of suffering. This brings us to the case of Herbert (Case 14.1), who believes he has a right to jump out of the 22nd-story hospital window. Nurse M, sensing that there is a viable life in Herbert, attempts to restrain him, and succeeds. One may wonder if Nurse M is right or wrong.

A central issue of nurse-patient relationships concerns the role of negative and positive rights. Negative rights are those rights to be left alone, to choose regardless of consequences to oneself. If a person is helpless, too bad for him or her. On this view, no one has a right to be given help.

This view has recently been called the "will" or "choice" view of rights,[15] an unduly stout form of anti-paternalism. That view seems morally impoverished, for it fails to account for a person's incapacity to express option or autonomy rights if a person is too poor, too sick, too unenlightened, and too powerless to express those autonomy or self-determination rights. There are cases in which a person does not know best and in which he or she needs help to make the wisest decision.[16] This provides a counterexample against a client's right to do whatever the client wants to do at the moment. The example of restraining Herbert shows that to identify one's autonomy right with one's choice of the moment is a faulty moral practice in nursing. Nurse M was justified in interfering. There are limits to one's self-determination. Identifying one's rights with one's will and desire exclusively is not the only way to determine one's most vital rights. One may also connect one's rights to one's rational best interests. There are grounds of justified interference with one's liberty both for one's interest and for the good of others. One may be restrained from unknowingly harming oneself, as by taking medically inadvisable forms of treatment. One may also be counseled to take appropriate measures to prolong one's life where the evidence on behalf of the viability of life warrants doing so.

MacCormick developed a distinction between a "will" based view of rights, which emphasizes values associated with freedom, and an interest-based view, which emphasizes benefits conferred equally on all persons, regardless of the capacity to exercise one's will.[17] In the United Nations *Declaration of Human Rights*, Articles 1 to 21 are oriented by a will-based view, whereas Articles 22 to 27, which include the right to a decent standard of living and the right to health care for everyone, are oriented by an interest-based view. These newer positive rights to be cared for are rights of another kind. Such rights are not recognized by those who believe that rights are only negative rights to be free from interference by others. These newer rights include the right to food, clothing, shelter, education, and health care.

The Right to Truth-Telling and the Avoidance of Deception

To show how rights to be cared for may have priority over liberty rights in certain cases, some examples given earlier will be considered. In Case 14.4, Robert is about to be married and does not tell his fiancée about his HIV-positive status. Edward, the high-anxiety cardiac patient in Case 14.5, is given a tranquilizer without his consent, and Ms. Jones, the woman in Case 14.6 with cervical cancer, is not told the truth because her physician fears she will end her life. The right to truthful information and avoidance of deception is ordinarily an important part of the right to be treated as a rational person. The truth enables a person to decide for himself or herself what course to follow. Ordinarily, a person's will-based negative rights are a vital feature of one's complement of human rights. Paternalism, too often practiced, undermines an essential aspect of one's complement of human rights. Having rights to decide shows respect for a person as a rationally autonomous being. These rights to decide include the right to be told the truth and not be brainwashed, told falsehoods, or deceived by having information withheld. For health care team members to withhold information from Robert's intended bride is a gross violation of her right to know the truth about his condition as the basis for informed consent to the marriage. Withholding the fact that he is HIV-positive interferes with his future and that of his intended bride. Does the fiancée's right to the prevention of harm override Robert's right to confidentiality?

According to Brock, "medical advisability" does not override a patient's precious autonomy rights by "withholding relevant information from the patient. . . ."[18] Brock appeals to "our right to control what is done to our body" to justify being given "relevant available information."[19] Brock also appeals to the metaphor of ownership of one's body as the basis for the right to truthful relevant available information. The right to truthful information then serves as a moral standard for criticizing lies, deception, and withholding of information. One cannot be morally free without access to truth about one's body. The case of Ms. Jones, who has cervical cancer and was told, "We got it all," is an example of a lie and a violation of her right to know the truth about her body. In the absence of demonstrable morally compelling reasons for overriding her right, such a lie is reprehensible.

In a pinch, however, showing how rights to be cared for may have priority over liberty (autonomy) rights leads one to consider the case of Edward, the high-anxiety cardiac patient. If one believes in the moral priority of the right to prevent harm, even over truth-telling, a case may be made showing that the health team respects the fundamental interest-based rights of the patient by withholding information. The concept of medical advisability, cited in *A Patient's Bill of Rights*, may in some cases give grounds for overriding a patient's autonomy rights. Therefore, Brock rather than *A Patient's Bill of Rights* may be mistaken. The right to live and not be seriously harmed, on an interest-based view of rights, is in a pinch prior to the right to self-determination. The health care team members may know in some selected types of cases, such as the case of Edward, that the only way to save a patient's life is to not tell him that he is being given tranquilizers. If a wise nurse believes that there is still a viable and enjoyable life to be lived in which the patient who is prevented from harm or death could retrospectively say after a time, "Thank you for not listening to me when I wanted to refuse help," then we do not think such a nurse wrongs the patient. Such a patient may become grateful for his life.

On the self-determination view, the nurse will be apt to perceive himself or herself as the servant and instrument of the patient, willing to assist the patient and to take the client at his or her word. It may be better, however, for the nurse to perceive himself or herself as a friend of the client in Aristotle's sense—one who cares with intelligence and wise judgment. One could set aside a patient's will-based rights in such cases by considering a person's more fundamental, deep, interest-based rights that are preemptive and compelling and that shine over all else. Truth-telling is precious, but in certain situations, prevention of harm overrides truth-telling. This does not mean, however, that truth-telling is canceled, only that truth-telling has a few justifiable classes of exceptions. The Biblical injunction, "The truth shall make you free," is not vacated by a small number of morally certifiable exceptions.

Informed Consent

Truth-telling and the right to informed consent are closely related. Nevertheless, there are differences. One difference is that truth-telling, which is more generic than informed consent, covers accurate information governing all health care states, processes, and procedures. Informed consent enables patients to have the right to decide whether to undergo medical procedures before they occur. Informed consent implies the patient's permission for surgery and stipulates the extent of morally permissible procedures.

Informed consent is an example of a patient's special right to adequate relevant information prior to medically invasive procedures or interventions. The infamous Tuskeegee syphilis experiment and the shameful Nazi Holocaust experiments are examples of violations of the right to informed consent. Similar violations occur when prisoners are offered early parole or other bribes in exchange for their willingness to be subjects of medical experimentation with untested drugs. Such consent may be termed consent by coercion.

But even on the principle of informed consent, there are marginal cases that give rise to legal and moral issues. One such case is *Canterbury v. Spence* (464F.2D 772 (1977):785–89) in which an unexpected and unwanted result of surgery occurred of which the victim claimed to be uninformed. In response, Judge S. Robinson reiterated the powerful moral appeal to the right to self-determination in this way:

> The root premise, fundamental in American jurisprudence [is] that "every human being of adult years and sound mind has a right to determine what shall be done with his own body." True consent is held in this case to be contingent upon the informed exercise of a choice and thus the physician's disclosure must provide the patient an opportunity to assess available options and attendant risks. As to sufficiency of information, the court holds, "The patient's right of self-decision shapes the boundaries of the duty to reveal. The right can be effectively exercised only if the patient possesses enough information to enable an intelligent choice."[20]

Thus, the right to informed consent cannot easily be overridden, according to principles of our common morality.

The Right to Respect and the Right to Receive and to Refuse Treatment

The rights to prevention of harm, truth-telling, and informed consent imply a trilogy of patients' rights: the right to respect, the right to receive treatment, and the right to refuse treatment. The right to respect is manifested in giving kind, considerate, quality care, and in honoring every patient's right to receive and to refuse treatment.

A patient's right to respect means that one applies Kant's principle of treating all patients as ends in themselves, not as "means only" of securing a higher income or gaining some other advantage. Respect means treating the other in the highest rational regard that one would accord to oneself when one is rational. According to Kant, respect consists in treating each human being as a member of the "kingdom of ends."[21] Respect is the treatment of oneself and others as intrinsically, rather than instrumentally, worthwhile. In the vasectomy case (Case 14.7), the urologist violated John's right to decide whether to reproduce or not. Again, it is John's body, and thus his right to seek this procedure.

In the case of Phillip (Case 14.2), the 57-year-old alcoholic who demands too much, the right to receive treatment must be weighed against the rights of others and thus cannot be an absolute, unchallengeable right because the concept of rights involves the equal rights of all. Because rights are limited by resources, no one individual can have rights to unlimited medical resources.

The case of Jane, 22-year-old graduate student (Case 14.8), presents a no-win situation, an unsolvable dilemma from the point of view of knowing what is best. Although the behavior-modifying drugs are indicated, the adverse effects are unwanted. However, because no compelling moral reason, (i.e., prevention of harm) clearly presents itself and Jane is competent, her right to refuse cannot be overridden. To do so is to violate her autonomy rights. If Jane's symptoms worsen, resulting in danger to herself or others, then her autonomous rights to refuse might be overridden in favor of her interest-based rights.

On just such grounds as the interest-based rights, one may consider the case of Virginia, the Jehovah's Witness in Case 14.9 who is unconscious in the emergency department. Her husband refuses blood transfusions on her behalf. Is he her advocate, however? In a life-and-death situation, Virginia, were she able to speak, might prefer to have a blood transfusion and live rather than die without one.

To respect a patient's right is to know when to honor the patient's right to refuse treatment and when to override that right. A precedent for overriding the husband's substitute decision in Case 14.9 is given by the apostle of liberty rights, J. S. Mill, who wrote:

> If either a public officer or anyone else saw a person attempting to cross a bridge, which had been ascertained to be unsafe, and there was no time to warn him of his danger, they might seize him and turn him back with out any real infringement on his liberty; for liberty consists in doing what one desires, and he does not desire to fall into the river.[22]

Mill continues that people may act to prevent a crime before it is committed and if the only function of poison were murder, then "it would be right to prohibit [its] manufacture and sale."[23] There is a tacit presumption in society that life is precious. Therefore, the right to seek prevention of harm overrides the right of personal choice. Thus, by a parity of reasoning, one might similarly safeguard a Jehovah's Witness's real desire to live. If, however, Virginia were conscious and in need of blood transfusions, but refused based on her religious beliefs, then the nurse must consider whether Virginia really prefers no transfusion and resulting death, or if she prefers to have her life saved at the expense of her religious belief. Virginia's autonomy rights cannot be discounted. They may have to give way in the face of the stronger rights invested in protecting life, endorsed by the common morality. People and subcultures, as Plato long ago observed, are not islands isolated from human relationships with other people. Neither the right to receive nor to refuse treatment is sacrosanct. These are important rights, however, and cannot be ignored or sidestepped. Weighty moral reasons must be given for overriding either the patient's right to receive or to refuse treatment. Such reasons will involve every person's equal right to respect on behalf of everyone's freedom and well-being.

The Right to Privacy and Confidentiality

Our last example is that of Jim, who drives fellow workers to work in a car pool (Case 14.10). Jim experiences seizures because he does not take his prescribed medications. He begs the emergency department nurses not to report him to the motor vehicles department and promises to take his medication from now on. This type of case is in some ways like *Tarasoff v. Regents of University of California* (1976) in which a patient reportedly told his therapist that he would murder a young woman, Ms. Tarasoff, who spurned him. The patient did murder her; the psychiatrist failed to warn her on grounds of patient-therapist confidentiality. The psychiatrist might have prevented this murder.[24] Joseph Fletcher recounts a similar case to that of Jim involving an English doctor's patient.

> A railway signalman suffers with [such] severe asthmatic attacks that he blacks out altogether. . . . The man works alone in a signal box, regulating fast, express passenger trains. At any time, he may lose consciousness and let a train be wrecked. The doctor would like to warn the company but his patient threatens to sue him for libel.[25]

The rights to confidentiality and privacy, again being crucial autonomy rights, merit high moral consideration. But there are extenuating circumstances in which the paramount right to the prevention of harm overrides even the right of confidentiality and privacy. Therefore, in the Tarasoff and Jim examples, the right to confidentiality and privacy may be overridden. This does not mean due regard is not given to these important autonomy rights. As with the rights to receive and to refuse treatment, they can in rare classes of justifiable exceptions be overridden, and only by demonstrably compelling reasons in which the equal freedom to live well is a central factor.

ETHICAL AND PHILOSOPHICAL CONSIDERATIONS OF PERSONHOOD

Reason and Freedom as Marks of Personhood

Several philosophical concepts help to clarify the cases and HIV-AIDS problems presented. In the adult years, a human being is preeminently a person who has rights and responsibilities.

Personhood.   To be a person, as distinct from being human, derives from the Latin *persona,* meaning a mask from which an actor spoke.[26] In subsequent Roman law, a person was identified as a bearer of rights and responsibilities. A person is a human being who is in a position to perform social roles, like being a nurse, physician, engineer, teacher, waiter, spouse, father, or mother. Human characteristics, such as laughing, crying, eating, drinking, eliminating, and being hungry, thirsty, and afraid, are biological features. These answer the question: What is a human being? To have social roles and acquire recognition as a member of a community means, for example, that one can write and read, work, take a vacation, vote, treat patients, reconcile conflicts, develop friendships, and show sympathy for others. To be able to do so is to live not only as a human being, but as a person, a high-order achievement. As humanhood is biological, personhood is biographical. Personhood calls for respect and recognition of individual rights and responsibilities. Such rights provide individuals with freedoms, powers, entitlements, responsibilities, and boundaries that others may not trespass without a rightholder's permission.

According to Feinberg, a person is said to have consciousness, a self-concept, self-awareness, the capacity to experience emotions, to reason and to acquire understanding, to plan ahead, to act on plans, and to feel pleasure and pain.[27] One could add other features of personhood, such as the capacity to form significant human relationships evident in long-term, harmonious marriage and parent-child relationships and friendships. In addition to Feinberg's conditions, Engelhardt adds a further characteristic of a person: the capacity to develop moral relationships.[28] For Engelhardt and for Kant before him, a person is also a moral individual. A moral person is one who lives in freedom in the sense that he or she has an internalized sense of freedom, is a rational being, and is not constrained or coerced into his or her actions, because reason, rather than compulsion or coercion, governs a rational person's actions

Pivotal to a person as a rightholder is the right to informed consent, a point well made by Ramsey, who writes that "a human being or person is more than a patient or experimental subject, he is a personal subject. . . ."[29] According to Ramsey, consent establishes and sustains a relation of fidelity between persons. Singer endorses the *Oxford English Dictionary* definition of a person as "a self-conscious or rational being."[30] Although Fletcher refers to humans, the criteria he uses aptly identify persons. Fletcher's criteria of personhood include neocortical activity; an effective intelligence quotient (IQ) of at least 20–40 exemplified in a sense of the past and future, self-awareness, consciousness of others; the capacity to communicate with others; and the ability to form and sustain significant human relationships with others.[31] One who has hopes, plans, projects, history, a sense of the present, joys, frustration, the capacity to regret, and a sense of a future with expectations and prospects, all of which presuppose consciousness, is said to have a life as a person.[32] If one can plan a vacation, drive a car, play a musical instrument, or have some similar project, then one is living a biographical life and is said to be a person. To live as a person is more than just breathing and eliminating.

A reason for distinguishing a human from a person is that additional restrictions can be agreed upon and imposed on those who qualify as worthy of receiving scarce health care resources. This distinction facilitates ethical decision making in regard to those who have priority for being helped to live and those who are valued as being less important.

A related reason is that one invests scarce health care resources and medical attention on persons, treating them as ends, never as means only, in accordance with Kant's substantive ethical principle. One form this principle takes is the right to informed consent and respect for a person as a rightholder, one who has some control of what happens in and to his or her life and body. This is sometimes referred to as the right to autonomy. As a rightholder, a person has a veto power, a moral barrier over what others may morally do to him or her.

A further reason for distinguishing a human from a person is to restrict the attribute of being a person to beings who meet the personhood criteria. Becoming human happens over time. Potentiality is a term that applies to biological processes rather than to social roles. To speak of a potential or unborn person or child is a contradiction, because personhood is a conferred role that depends on social role achievements.

A disadvantage in distinguishing humans from persons is that one is apt to decide quite arbitrarily who counts as a person and consequently rule out those whom one dislikes or deems unworthy. The application of flat deductive rules, such as deciding who lives or dies on the grounds of personhood without reference to a case-by-case approach, commits an ethnocentric fallacy of simply preferring one's own kind. This practice leaves the resolution of who lives or dies to those with the most power. Making "person" synonymous with being a member of an elite club or of the powerful is an obvious misuse of language.

Nevertheless, there are advantages in distinguishing humans from persons, as long as such a distinction is not excessively restrictive, for one needs some criteria for deciding who lives or dies. Those with severe mental, social, or emotional incompetence may not qualify as persons. When there is only so much room at the table, hard choices must be made. The softest of these is a reasonably restrictive set of criteria for personhood, such as a minimum IQ and the capacity to form and sustain beneficial interpersonal relationships.

RIGHTS IN AND TO HEALTH CARE

HIV/AIDS

A test case for these moral-philosophical theories, concepts, and principles in adult health care ethics is to consider the HIV/AIDS crisis, which is perhaps the most difficult health care issue of our time.

The HIV epidemic has changed dramatically from one originally identified with homosexual men to one that affects men, women, infants, children, and adolescents of all ethnic and socioeconomic groups and sexual orientation.[33] The World Health Organization (WHO) predicted that 30 to 40 million people worldwide will be infected by the year 2000[34]; others predict 110 million infected persons.[35] WHO projects that AIDS will be the third leading cause of death in the United States by the turn of the century.[36]

Even though AIDS is a fatal disease, there is an asymptomatic period which, for the fortunate few, may last a decade or more. During this period, there are medical, nursing, psychological, and social interventions that can improve the patient's quality of life. Early intervention is regarded as most effective in maintaining the patient's good health and in delaying the advance of symptoms and disease. Lack of access to services and to promising new drugs can delay the necessary testing, assessment, and early intervention. "Enrollment in clinical trials has been slow in reaching women, adolescents, and minority groups, in particular. Continued efforts are needed to remove the obstacles that hinder participation of these patients in trials such as lack of support services, outreach, and education in existing programs. Linking clinical trials to the primary care setting is essential. Providers are responsible for sharing . . . current information on these trials and treatments and facilitating access to them."[37] These interventions call for the nurse to endorse Plato's rational paternalistic principle that knowledge is virtue.

For the patient, the decision whether to disclose his or her illness to family, significant others, employers, associates, friends, or support groups is a moral issue of truth-telling. On the grounds of the Kantian principle of truth-telling and the principle of "do no harm," the patient is morally obligated to disclose his or her HIV status to significant others, especially sexual and needle-sharing partners, in order to prevent the transmission of the disease to others.[38]

The whole family is affected by HIV and AIDS, moving from one crisis to another: hospitalization of a member; the continuing lack of needed services, and the expenditure of the short supply of energy, time, and money spent seeking care; the pain of rejection; stigmatization and discrimination throughout this long process; the death of a child, parent, or spouse; and the need for present or future placement of an orphaned, possibly infected, child or children.[39] All of this is painful, tragic, and very expensive to both the family and the community.

Is the AIDS epidemic getting more or less than its share of health care resources?

AIDS advocacy groups charge that society is not attempting to cope with the widening epidemic. Advocates charge that there is too little research and too few drugs being tested and approved by the US Food and Drug Administration (FDA). Most important, the nation is spending too little money to do what needs to be done.[40]

Critics charge that the tactics of the AIDS advocacy groups resulted in the public's distorted response that may have damaged the whole of the health care system by allocating more money to the AIDS program than to cancer (which kills 12 times more people) or to the heart disease program (the leading cause of death in the United States).[41] The critics view this allocation as a gross injustice.[42] Moreover, they point to the traditional methods of controlling epidemics by placing the focus on the uninfected population and measures to protect it in contrast to the emphasis on developing effective treatments for those already infected.[43] Thus, twice as much money has been spent on treatment than on prevention—a poor strategy from a utilitarian view of the greatest happiness for the greatest number. Critics say that lack of prevention has left vulnerable populations—intravenous drug users and their partners and poor, inner-city minorities—without necessary information and help. These groups are the disadvantaged deprived of justice in the form of a fair chance at prevention and treatment.[44]

Critics also charge that AIDS advocacy groups forced change in the federal drug approval system, a self-serving act that resulted in the approval of an experimental drug that killed several people before it was banned.[45] The most severe criticism of the AIDS advocacy groups is that they have secured support for themselves in self-serving ways far beyond what advocates for diseases that kill many more people have been able to do—a gross injustice.[46]

Ethical analysis of HIV/AIDS patients' claims to health care.

Two significant moral issues arise from the HIV/AIDS epidemic. The first issue involves HIV/AIDS patients' rights to and in health care in relation to all other ill people.

The second issue is how they shall be treated by society in relation to their contagion, their freedom, and their personhood.

There are many unanswered moral and philosophical questions about HIV/AIDS. Do infected individuals have a right to unlimited health care, welfare, and social and financial support? Do employers, friends, family, significant others, relatives, co-workers, and others have a right to know the person's seropositive status?

Moral-philosophical responses to HIV/AIDS. People embrace a spectrum of values and attitudes about HIV/AIDS patients, ranging from "Treat them as evil" to "Treat them as good." There are several moral-philosophical positions on HIV/AIDS. These include categories that are candidates for social policies that engage health care and nursing ethics. We can map out six types of responses to the ethical issues raised by the HIV/AIDS epidemic. One is to reject such patients as outcasts to be shunned, vilified, or ignored. Some proponents of legal moralism claim that these diseases are a just retribution for the lifestyle of those people who engage in drug abuse, homosexuality, or sexual promiscuity. A difficulty with this argument is that innocent people—adults transfused with infected blood and infants born of infected mothers—contract, suffer, and die of the disease. Moreover, punishing such patients does not minimize the disease or its tragic consequences. This position denies their humanity.

A second type of response to AIDS patients is to quarantine them; isolate them from the public as health hazards to society. (HIV/AIDS patients are currently quarantined in Cuba, for example.) Other victims of dreaded diseases such as typhoid fever, cholera, and measles have been quarantined with the aim of preventing transmission to others. By placing HIV/AIDS patients in quarantine, their liberty rights, and their rights of informed consent, of confidentiality and of privacy are violated. Yet the very difficult question remains of what to do with known infected persons who are sexually active.

A third policy option is to treat HIV/AIDS patients like criminals who deserve to be punished for wrongdoing. According to the criminal view, by and large, they have themselves to blame. Innocent victims of HIV/AIDS (on a utilitarian perspective) are also regarded as criminals, because to do so on the grounds of overall social consequences supplies the greatest happiness for the greatest number for those who are not afflicted. Thus, both innocent and noninnocent HIV/AIDS patients receive minimal health care benefits on this option.

A fourth option is to treat HIV/AIDS patients as public nuisances who, if carefully observed and controlled, are not detrimental to a healthy society, as the mentally ill are regarded. They are not criminals and do not deserve to be punished unless they willfully infect others. They may, however, be morally neglected for there is the moral option of not wasting health care resources on treating their disease or doing much research on it. They are like people "lost at sea." This may be regarded as the "benign neglect" policy option.

A fifth perspective and policy option is that HIV/AIDS victims have a right to live as well as possible. Their rights imply everyone's obligation to assimilate, integrate, and help them to the best of our ability. To do less is to fall below the standard of being minimally decent samaritans (see Chapter 8 for a discussion of minimally decent samaritanism).

A sixth response is to intervene, treat, and interact with the victims and carriers of HIV/AIDS. Although health professionals incur a very slight risk of infection by treating infected patients, active intervention is the course leading to the control and cure of this disease. Active intervention also poses risk for infection to those of general public who work and socialize with unidentified AIDS and HIV-positive individuals. Public education through mass media, educational institutions, and individual counseling appear to be the only alternatives to mandatory blood testing for HIV/AIDS, public exposure, and the unnecessary but certain stigma that attaches to these diseases.

Intervention has the advantage that one takes care of problems by dealing with them, not by evading them. Treating AIDS patients, who require enormous amounts of highly skilled nursing care, requires demonstrations of nurses' commitment to the ethical principles of care, compassion, and altruism. Therefore, the nurse has an obligation to interact with the dying son and parents mentioned in Case 14.11 in a compassionate manner that facilitates their communication.

Lastly, the "Good Samaritan" view of the HIV/AIDS policy option says: Do everything to help those among us who are "least advantaged." This option says to give priority to HIV/AIDS research above heart disease and cancer.

From the Rawlsian veil of ignorance concept, one could ask, "If I had HIV/AIDS, what would I want done?" "As much as society can afford, but not everything." Why? "Because, on the veil of ignorance, I might have heart disease, cancer, or tuberculosis instead and I would want research and treatment in these areas as well." On love-based, rational paternalist, and duty-based and rights-based ethical theories, "a common morality" would reject the first three options as anti-human and irrational, and regard the fourth option, benign neglect, as morally less justifiable than the minimally decent samaritan position.

The sixth position would favor HIV/AIDS research at the expense of other morally justifiable programs. These reasons favor the fifth position (of minimally decent samaritan) over the first four and over the sixth.

THE NURSE'S ROLE

The American Hospital Association's statement of *A Patient's Bill of Rights* may be one response to public criticism of the lack of active meaningful patient participation in hospital care. The various professional codes, such as the American Nurses Association's *Code for Nurses,* are another answer to the patient's need for an advocate who will defend the patient's autonomy. Malpractice and negligence suits against physicians, hospitals, and sometimes nurses are another patient response to perceived neglect, errors, or omissions of care. Another response is the hiring of a patient advocate by community health boards; this advocate functions independently of administrative control in hospitals. Other hospitals have employed persons (usually nurses) called patient relations coordinators, who respond to patient complaints and problems. The most effective hope for patient advocates, however, is in nurses who are intelligently involved in patient care. Although they are participants in hospital technology and bureaucracy, nurses are the main source of personal, intimate, and continuous contact with patients. More than any other health professionals, nurses have frequent opportunities to facilitate and manifest respect for patients' rights. Modern hospital care and medical technology have largely developed into a team effort of highly specialized members. Nurses are the part of the team that implements the delivery of that care to a particular individual. This provides the nurse with frequent opportunities to inform and to educate the patient, and to tell patients the truth about the procedure that the nurse or another professional is about to perform in terms the patient can understand. The nurse has many opportunities to inform patients about special diets and the indications for those diets. The nurse who gives medications can inform patients about drugs given, dosages, and expected effects and side effects. The nurse can convey accurate information concerning the patient's body temperature, blood pressure level, and laboratory results.

These nursing practices of health teaching and counseling function to convey truthful information to patients and to facilitate the individual's responsibility for his or her own health.[47] The patient's possession of information regarding health status enhances the patient's independence and self-determination in decisions of health care. Accurate information contributes to the possibility of the patient's choice of the best option from among the alternatives.

The nurse's respect for people extends beyond self and patient to include others who share in care, such as physicians, social workers, and family. Ideally, therefore, nurses and fellow care providers jointly resolve such major issues as telling a young or middle-aged adult the truth about a diagnosis of a fatal condition. One goal is to seek consensus among team members concerning how the truth will be communicated to the patient, who will be the bearer of bad news, and what hope can realistically and honestly be given to the patient. In this way, each member of the team is prepared to support the patient's exploration of what it means to receive a diagnosis of a serious, life-threatening, or fatal disease. Because nurses have the most intimate and continuous contact with patients receiving such news, nurses are in the forefront of those who show respect for the patient and for the patient's right to receive and to refuse treatment. Nurses respect the patient's right to information by answering all of the patient's questions, explicit as well as implicit, in a relevant, accurate, sympathetic, and understandable way, as friends of the patient. This means that the patient is not burdened with technical or anatomical details in which he or she has no interest. When, for example, the patient asks how irradiation or chemotherapy will affect him or her, this indicates a knowledge deficit about the side effects, which the nurse fills with relevant facts only.

If the patient inquires about life after a colostomy or similar radical surgery, the nurse again shows respect for patients by sharing relevant information and experiences that are helpful to educating the patient. The nurse is sensitive to feelings and to what are perceived as unstated questions, such as "Can I have sex after a colostomy?" A nurse who lacks up-to-date knowledge has the obligation to tell the patient that he or she doesn't know but will find out or communicate with others who do know. The nurse's duty then is to return to the patient with the latest information or to refer the question to someone more capable of response.

Respect for people implies patients' rights to know as well as not to know diagnosis, prognosis, treatment alternatives, risks, and benefits. An individual may simply say, "I don't want to know what I have. Just do what you think is best. You're the experts." But does the right to know imply the right to decide not to know? There are two possible responses the nurse might give to such an individual. One is to offer unconditional support for the patient's right not to know; for example, a statement such as, "It is your right not to know, since this is your body, after all, and you'll decide when you want to know what is happening and being done to your body." This statement supports the patient's right not to know, while clearly indicating that the choice to receive or to refuse treatment is almost always up to the patient. In this way, the nurse indicates the patient's strong right to seek knowledge when, where, and from whom the patient wishes. The nurse's statement defines and supports the patient's autonomy. As time passes, the patients' defense-mechanism processes of denial lessen. The patient then becomes concerned about what is happening in and to his or her body and seeks to regain control on the basis of relevant information.

A different nursing response is that given by Mary Kohnke, who recommends confronting the client with the consequences of not knowing. Kohnke's experience is that the client agrees to know certain things and not others; the nurse then records what the client has and has not been told and why.[48] The patient's family is often the first to know of the presence of cancer, for example, from the surgeon, while the patient is still in the intensive care unit or recovery room. Some families specifically request that the patient not be told of the cancer, or of the extent of its life-threatening properties. In such cases, there are several objections that nurses in contact with the family can offer. One argument is that not all cancers are fatal; some may be cured. Only a few cancers are immediately fatal; other cancers may be treated with good life expectancy for the patient. The second argument is that the patient will naturally want to know the outcome of the surgery and the reason for such treatments as irradiation or chemotherapy. It is the patient's right to know. A third argument is that the nurses' and physicians' primary relationship is with the patient, and this relationship is based on trust and honesty. The patient has the right to a truthful answer to the question of "Did you find cancer?"

Educating and informing the patient of the diagnosis, prognosis, proposed treatments, risks, benefits, and alternatives tend to raise questions in the patient's mind, such as "Do I want to suffer the adverse effects of chemotherapy for the small and remote possibility of a short remission of my leukemia?"

Another moral issue for the nurse is the question of supporting the patient's right to receive and to refuse treatment. The example of the young father who sought a vasectomy as the best method of contraception (Case 14.7) is a case in point of the importance of the nurse's role in supporting patients' rights. Despite the nurse's own misgivings regarding the possibility that the client might change his mind about having more children and the urologist's denial of that right, the *Code for Nurses* supports the client's moral right to determine what will be done with his or her person; to be given the information necessary for making informed judgments; to be told the possible effects of care; and to accept, refuse or terminate treatment.[49]

In accordance with the *Code,* once the nurse is satisfied that the patient has a complete understanding of the procedure, including the fact that it is generally irreversible, and that the wife concurs, the nurse is obligated to refer the patient to another physician or facility for a vasectomy in as helpful a way as referring a patient for non-elective surgery, such as a herniorrhaphy. It is the patient's right to receive treatment of his choice.

The right of psychiatric patients to refuse treatment is more complex because exercise of this right may delay the patient's recovery and return to the community. The use of neuroleptic drugs carry the probability of undesirable adverse effects, some of which are irreversible. As in Case 14.8, the possibility that a young woman may develop unsightly muscular movements of her lips, mouth, face, or extremities is an unhappy one. The possibility that the same young woman will languish in a mental institution without treatment and become progressively disturbed over a long period of time is also an unhappy one. The situation becomes one of trade-off—the drugs versus prolonged illness. In such cases, the nurse depends on an accurate store of knowledge of the particular drugs prescribed, the possible adverse effects, and the effectiveness of the measures used to control such effects. The nurse supports the patient's participation in regulating the dose, the timing of administration, and the possibility of drug holidays in conjunction with the physician's recommendations and the goals of the treatment plan.

The alternative is for the nurse to support the patient's refusal of drugs, with disclosure of the full range of consequences to the patient and possibly to the nurse. Kohnke recommends that the advocate support the patient's decision without "falling into a defending or rescuing position, in which responsibility for decision making belongs to the advocate and not the client. . . . Supporting a client's right to make a decision does not mean giving approval for the decision."[50]

One could disagree with Kohnke's position on the grounds that the patient's perception of the nurse's support of refusal of surgery, of neuroleptic drugs, or of electroconvulsive therapy is one of approval. Colleagues may share the same perception. Some nurses view their role as one of rescuing patients who are victims of the excesses of medical technology in the form of radical surgery and radical drug therapy. In such instances, patients tend to react globally to the physician as omnipotent and lifesaving or to the nurse as one who really knows the qualifications of the physician and the merits of the case.

The effective nurse tries to avoid the position of broker or intermediary between physician and patient. Instead, the nurse informs and educates the patient regarding measures designed to restore health and prevent illness. The nurse recognizes the physician as a valuable ally in attempting to reach the patient's health goals. The nurse seeks to involve the physician in the process of the patient's deliberations in every possible way.

One way of supporting the patient's right to receive and to refuse treatment is to inform the physician that the patient has questions and doubts about prescribed treatment. Another way to involve physicians in patients' deliberative processes is to suggest that the patient formulate and write down relevant questions for discussion over the phone or during an office visit. The patient's right to a consultation or second opinion is part of what it means to have the right to know.

The nurse who informs patients of the content and therapeutic purpose of nursing actions as their right to know effectively helps to demystify medical and hospital infallibility. The nurse is an approachable person who shares expertise and encourages the patient to ask questions of nurses, physicians, and technicians that are relevant to the patient's illness and recovery.

Unlike the nurse's advocate role in protecting infants and children from harm, the nurse who works with adults promotes the autonomy and self-determination of his or her patients. Through nursing activities aimed at case finding, educating, and counseling the patient, the nurse consciously seeks to facilitate the patient's exercise of rights to information concerning diagnosis, prognosis, treatment, risks, benefits, costs, and alternatives as the basis for informed consent and the right to receive or refuse treatment. In this respect, a nurse functions as a health educator, which is a valuable form for expressing nurse advocacy.

AMERICAN HOSPITAL ASSOCIATION: *A PATIENT'S BILL OF RIGHTS*

The revised version (1992) of *A Patient's Bill of Rights* developed by the American Hospital Association is found in the Appendix of this textbook. It supports all of the ethical principles and practices identified in this chapter. The *Bill* is a detailed and comprehensive identification and provision for safeguarding the patient's rights in hospitals.[51]

The *Bill* begins with the right to considerate and respectful care that ensures the role of patients in decision making with sensitivity to cultural, racial, religious, linguistic, age, sex, and other differences. It covers the patient's right to know and to be informed of their diagnoses, treatments, prognoses, risks and benefits, identity of care providers, and other circumstances necessary to the patient's informed consent. Moreover, patients have a right to refuse treatment, to have advance directives, to considerations of privacy and confidentiality, to review medical records, to appropriate medical care and services including referrals or transfers to other facilities, to continuity of care, and to the nature of relationships between care providers and institutions.

Of major importance are patients' rights to be informed of hospital policies and practices that are related to care, such as ethics committees, patient representatives, or other institutional mechanisms for resolving conflicts, disputes, and grievances. These rights are related to patients being enabled to look after their own best interest. Patients, in turn, are expected to be responsible for providing medical, hospitalization, and health histories, advance directives, and necessary information for health insurance claims, for these rights are in a reciprocal relation to patient responsibilities. Patients are obliged to make reasonable adjustments to the needs of other patients, such as not blasting the volume of their television sets or abusing staff members. Patients are responsible for communicating anticipated problems in following prescribed treatments.

This document is significant because it recognizes the patient as a person with human rights to know and to make decisions about his or her care. It also recognizes that these rights can be exercised on the patient's behalf by designated surrogates or proxy decision makers if the patient lacks decision-making capacities or is legally incompetent, or is a minor. This *Bill* is an advance over previous paternalistic practices and has been adopted in various versions by most states and most care providing institutions, with a pending federal version that will deal with health maintenance organization (HMO) provisions and problems, such as the denial of care. The enforcement of this *Bill* is of paramount importance to patients as a characteristic of a just and humane health care system.

SUMMARY

Adults are more independent and also more interdependent than other persons, including children and the elderly. Consequently, nursing care is more verbal and interactive with adults than with younger and older age groups. Adulthood is the longest, most significant aspect of personhood and the standard for judging qualities and degrees of personhood. Cases were cited illustrating the centrality of ethical issues. These were discussed under several principles: prevention of harm, truth-telling, informed consent, the right to receive and to refuse treatment, and privacy and confidentiality. These cases dovetailed with key provisions of *A Patient's Bill of Rights* and the *Code for Nurses*.

The ethical issues considered in these topics and cases centered on the values of freedom and autonomy, rationality, well-being, and optimum health care. These ideals are buffeted by world social and economic reality: a growing population with more demands than resources. There are also conflicts within these goals. Prevention of harm, for example, may collide with freedom of expression of a Jehovah's Witness. There are other moral conflicts such as those presented by the HIV/AIDS crisis. New, difficult cases sometimes refute entrenched principles, as our AIDS example helped illustrate.

The relation of principle to practice shows that, to paraphrase Kant, principles without nursing practices are empty; but nursing practices without principles are blind. For moral principles are like the stars or beacons that guide the nurse and health care navigators through the shoals of ethical and clinical challenges. Such principles are part of the common morality that function as moral standards and a steady rebuttal that all values are solely relative to time and place. It is frustrating that there is no single principle, but rather a plurality of them requiring thought and choice without certainty. That, however, is the price one pays for being human and working in the ethics of adult health care without surrendering to dogma.

Nursing implications show how the principles of the common morality are implemented in daily health care practices. These nursing practices, in turn, show how the principles are strengthened or weakened in accord with Kant's principle that he who agrees with the ends also agrees with the means.[52]

Discussion Questions

1. What moral reasons, if any, are there for persons in high-risk groups to be subject to mandatory testing for HIV? What happens to confidentiality?
2. Are insurance companies or employers entitled to test applicants for HIV? Why or why not?
3. What moral reasons are there for arguing that helmetless motorcycling is morally permissible or impermissible?

REFERENCES

1. Keniston K. Youth and its ideology. In: Arieti S (ed). *American handbook of psychiatry.* Vol. 1 (2nd ed) New York: Basic Books. 1974;422.
2. ibid, p. 403.
3. Neugarten BL, Datan N. The middle years. In: Arieti S (ed). *American hand-book of psychiatry.* Vol 1 (2nd ed) New York: Basic Books. 1974;596.
4. ibid, p. 606.
5. ibid, p. 593.
6. Bandman E. The dilemma of life and death: Shall we let them die? *Nursing Forum* 1978;17(2):118–132.
7. Study cites public expense of injuries to motorcyclists. *The New York Times.* July 14, 1988;B7.
8. Brock D. The nurse-patient relation: Some rights and duties. In: Beauchamp T, Walters L (eds). *Contemporary issues in bioethics.* (2nd ed) Belmont, Calif: Wadsworth. 1982;144.
9. Bandman B, Bandman EL. The nurse's role in an interest-based view of patients' rights. In: Spicker S, Gadow S (eds). *Nursing—Images and ideals.* New York: Springer. 1980;135.
10. Brody H. *Ethical decisions in medicine.* (2nd ed) Boston: Little, Brown. 1981;46–47.
11. Bandman EL, Bandman B. Rights are not automatic. *Am J Nurs.* 1977;77(5):867.
12. Brody H. *Ethical decisions in medicine.* (2nd ed) Boston: Little, Brown. 1981;46–47.
13. ibid, p. 53.
14. Rawls J. *A theory of justice.* Cambridge, Mass: Harvard University Press. 1971;133.
15. Hart HLA. Bentham on legal rights. In: Simpson AWB (ed). *Jurisprudence.* New York: Oxford University Press. 1973;170–201.
16. Bandman E. The dilemma of life and death: Shall we let them die? *Nursing Forum* 1978;17(2):118–132.
17. MacCormick DN. Rights in legislation. In: Hacker P, Raz J (eds). *Law, morality and society: Essays in honor of H.L.A. Hart.* New York: Oxford University Press. 1977; 188–209.
18. Brock D. The nurse-patient relation: Some rights and duties. In: Beauchamp T, Walters L (eds). *Contemporary issues in bioethics.* (2nd ed) Belmont, Calif: Wadsworth. 1982;145.
19. ibid.
20. Beauchamp T. The disclosure of information. In: Beauchamp T, Walters L (eds). *Contemporary issues in bioethics.* (2nd ed) Belmont, Calif: Wadsworth. 1982;172.

21. Kant I. *Fundamental principles of the metaphysics of morals* (1748). New York: Liberal Arts. 1949;38.

22. Mill JS. *Utilitarianism, liberty and representative government.* London: Dent. 1948;151.

23. ibid.

24. California Supreme Court. *Tarasoff v. Regents of the University of California,* 131 California Reporter. In: Beauchamp T, Walter L (eds). *Contemporary issues in bioethics.* (2nd ed) Belmont, Calif: Wadsworth. 1982;204–210.

25. Fletcher J. *Morals and medicine.* Boston: Beacon. 1954;58.

26. Downie RS. *Roles and values.* London: Methuen. 1971;131.

27. Feinberg J. The problem of personhood. In: Beauchamp T, Walter L (eds). *Contemporary issues in bioethics.* (2nd ed) Belmont, Calif: Wadsworth. 1982;108–116.

28. Engelhardt HT. Medicine and the concept of person. In: Beauchamp T, Walter L (eds). *Contemporary issues in bioethics.* (2nd ed) Belmont, Calif: Wadsworth. 1982;95.

29. Ramsey P. *The patient as person.* New Haven: Yale University Press. 1970;5.

30. Singer P. Value of life. In: Reich W (ed) *Encyclopedia of bioethics.* New York: Macmillan, 1978.

31. Fletcher J. Four indicators of humanhood: The enquiry matures. *Hastings Center Report* 1974;4(6):51.

32. Ruddick W. Parents, children and medical decisions. In: *Bioethics and human rights: A reader for health professionals.* Lanham, Md: University Press of America. 1986, 165–170.

33. Agency for Health Care Policy and Research. *Evaluation and management of early HIV infection: Clinical practice guideline.* US Department of Health and Human Services, Public Health Service. 1994;7. Publication no. 7.

34. ibid.

35. ibid.

36. ibid.

37. ibid, p. 8.

38. ibid, p. 2.

39. ibid, p. 9.

40. Munson R. *Intervention and reflection: Basic issues in medical ethics.* (4th ed) Belmont, Calif: Wadsworth. 1992;226.

41. ibid, p. 227.

42. ibid.

43. ibid.

44. ibid.

45. ibid.

46. ibid.

47. American Nurses Association. *Nursing: A social policy statement.* Kansas City, Mo; 1980;18.

48. Kohnke MF. *Advocacy: Risk and reality.* St. Louis: Mosby. 1982;18.

49. American Nurses Association. *Code for nurses with interpretive statements.* Kansas City, Mo; 1976;4.

50. Kohnke. *Advocacy: Risk and reality.* St. Louis: Mosby. 1982;5.

51. American Hospital Association. *A Patient's Bill of Rights.* Chicago; 1992.

52. Kant I. *Fundamental principles of the metaphysics of morals.* Indianapolis: Bobbs-Merrill. 1949;34.

15

Ethical Issues in the Nursing
Care of the Elderly

Study of this chapter will enable the learner to:

1. Understand the developmental tasks of the elderly in relation to ethical problems of health care.
2. Identify ethical issues of special relevance to the elderly population such as the macrolevel and microlevel of allocation of scarce resources, rights, competence, and quality of life.
3. Formulate the role of the nurse as patient advocate in facilitating the elderly person's participation in shared decision making based on goals, values, and rational life plans.
4. Use utilitarian and Kantian principles to analyze lifeboat, triage, cost-benefit, and lottery methods of allocating health care.

● OVERVIEW

According to one viewpoint, growing old is and ought to be a special time to anyone fortunate enough to have reached old age. Old age is a time for savoring and evaluating life's myriad experiences of people, places, and events shared with intimates and with strangers. One's older years provide an opportunity to reflect on the time left, rather than regret the time of life spent. Life goals and processes take on special significance, like the last brilliant colors of autumn.

● DEVELOPMENTAL HIGHLIGHTS: RETIREMENT, ADVANCED OLD AGE, THE FRAIL ELDERLY, DEMENTIA

Since the passage of federal Social Security legislation, the age of 65 has become a developmental landmark; it marks the entry point into old age. Time has, however, different meanings for the elderly. Some predominantly grieve the death of a spouse, relations, and friends, and feel saddened and nostalgic about the passing of happier years. Others mainly look forward to the years ahead with optimistic anticipation. All fervently hope for health and independence.

Some persons at the age of 65 are little changed from the middle years. If they have been fortunate enough to escape disease, they look upon themselves as competent, complete, and capable of independence and self-care. Physical changes such as decreasing sexual drive occur without diminishing desires for intimacy and affection. As men lose some muscularity and women lose their rounded contours, both sexes look more alike. Likewise, men "become less aggressive and women more assertive as they enter old age and both tend to diminish their activities and become less involved with people."[1] Old friends, relatives, and family become more important, because new friends tend to be less involved. Spousal relationships become more interdependent as the need for help increases. Sexual activity may continue into advanced old age. The wife may regard the growing number of widows with alarm and guard her husband's health jealously.

Retirement

According to the US Bureau of Labor statistics for 1990, the majority of both men and women are retired from the labor force by age 65.[2] Women in the 55 to 64 age bracket, however, joined the work force in large numbers and largely remain in the work force after age 65 owing to several reasons; for example, older women face a longer life span—about 7 years longer than men—with lower income expectations.[3] Many single or widowed women live in poverty in old age. Working women, along with workers needing a second job to maintain their standard of living, are sometimes described as "the overworked American."[4]

Moody defines retirement as "an expansion of leisure time in the last stage of life."[5] Leisure can be regarded positively as providing opportunities for relaxation, recreation, personal development, and service to the family or community.[6] Negatively, leisure can be regarded as freedom from work in conflict with the ethical ideal of work as desirable, meaningful, healthful, virtuous, and productive. The work ethic "holds that it is ennobling to be exerting oneself in the world."[7] Therefore, some retired and unengaged patients are depressed and bitter. They adjust poorly to what they now perceive as their roleless status. They tend to be difficult and unhappy patients. On the other hand, some members of the retired group are delighted to be free of work, responsibility, and obligation. However, most retired persons pursue what Ekerdt calls "the busy ethic," the offspring of the work ethic, which "like any ethic is a set of beliefs and values that identifies what is good and affirms ideals of conduct. It provides criteria for the evaluation of behavior and action."[8] The work ethic is not abandoned but transformed by those retirees who pursue the busy ethic. This transformation allows a moral continuity between work and retirement by: 1) conducting daily life according to the busy ethic, and 2) regarding pensions as earned entitlements for former productivity. The status of these retirees is thereby thought to justify pension income without working, maintains the self-respect of retirees, and "keeps retirement consistent with the dominant social prestige system which regards members primarily to the extent that they are economically productive."[9]

The social status of the formerly productive worker practicing the busy ethic is in stark contrast to the status of aging welfare recipients, homeless people, the mentally ill, and substance abusers, who are regarded as outsiders to the productive process.[10] Their states of idleness incur moral censure, and they are grudgingly given financial support. As patients, the nonproductive aged person may be regarded as not worthwhile, and denied the respect and attention due a sick person. Ill health, based on indolent and unkempt conditions, is still regarded by many as evidence of moral failure.[11]

Advanced Old Age

Advanced old age is viewed as beginning at age 75. Persons of this age hope "to live out their lives with dignity, to remain capable of caring for themselves and their spouses, to continue managing things between themselves."[12] These elderly people hope to be useful, if not significant, to others. They also hope not to become burdens through illness or senility. Some are serene and content, despite the ever present fear of needing nursing home or mental hospital care.

The Frail Elderly

Eventually, the elderly become frail and must depend on others, including nurses. Such dependencies can provoke family conflict and apprehension in the elderly individual in need of help.

The nurse caring for elderly patients in the community or in health care facilities can play a significant role in maintaining respect for each person by the time, attention, and quality of nursing care provided. Medical technology, such as improved cataract operations with implanted contact lenses, electronic hearing aids, and motorized wheelchairs, can be of great assistance to the elderly with such needs.

Hospitalization may be a threat that becomes actualized for the elderly person fearing separation, mutilation, pain, and incapacitation. The hospital may be seen as a last resort from which the individual is transferred to a nursing home because of the inability to care for himself or herself. Here, home care nursing has a role.

Dementia

For the elderly person living in the community with assistance, the hospital and surgery experience may necessitate transfer to a nursing home. A radical prostatectomy for a man of 80 to 90 years of age who is confused and forgetful may emphasize his growing dependence on others for what was formerly part of self-care. It may then become obvious to everyone that the critical integrative functions of memory, judgment, and problem solving are seriously impaired. That individual is ideally given full-time nursing care and supervision. On the other hand, all elderly persons may be completely but temporarily disoriented by such factors as the toxic effects of drugs, anesthesia, dehydration, anoxia, diabetes, and urine retention. As soon as the illness is resolved, the individual becomes oriented and rational and is discharged with community nursing supervision. It follows, then, that each elderly person, no matter what the diagnosis, requires respect and attention. A prejudgment of dementia may be premature or inaccurate.

The most characteristic feature of dementia is memory failure regarding recent events, with only memories of childhood remaining. Thus, people with dementia live and act as if in the past, and are unable to care for themselves. Such persons are disoriented as to time and place and need monitoring.[13] There is some loss of control of emotions, and impulses, suspicion, and anger are freely expressed. Loss of inhibitions and judgment may occur, followed by unacceptable behavior. The onset of dementia may be gradual or suddenly precipitated by circulatory deficits, drug toxicity, trauma, death of a spouse, or a move to a new and complex environment.

The quality of health care and human services given in nursing homes is a direct reflection of the respect for the rights of the elderly person to a decent, fulfilling life. A society that rejects its elderly and consigns them to brutalized care in virtual warehouses suffers from ethical insensitivity and moral callousness. However, no previous society has been faced with the numbers of elderly people now living and the responsibility for providing for them.

A sad story that reflects some societal attitudes against the elderly is told about a prison physician who amputates a prisoner's mutilated finger and, as he throws it into the garbage can, says to the prisoner, "You won't be needing that anymore." Such a remark captures the way that elderly people feel about themselves, that they are symbolized by the amputated finger, fit only for waste disposal. Some elderly people feel acutely that they will not be needed any more, and that they no longer rate having their needs satisfied. A dilemma for society is either meeting the needs of the elderly, with all the utilization of health care resources this implies, or limiting the utilization of these resources on grounds of fairness to other age groups.

PROBLEMS AND PROSPECTS FOR THE ELDERLY

Erikson views old age as the ripening period for the fruits of earlier stages. It is the result of taking care of things and people, of bearing and rearing children, or generating products and ideas, and of adjusting to the inevitable triumphs and disappointments of life. He calls this ripening process "ego integrity. It is the acceptance of one's one and only life cycle as something that had to be and that . . . permitted of no substitutions. . . ."[14] Lidz characterizes Erikson's "integrity" as the phase that "requires the wisdom to realize that there are no 'ifs' in life; that one was born with certain capacities, a set of parents, . . . the past cannot be altered. . . . It is too late to start out on a new life."[15] Integrity means one recognizes that one has fewer "ifs," fewer options. In later life, one rounds out one's goals and way of life, but does not start anew. To Erikson, even for the poorest of human beings who understands that birth into a particular culture at a particular time is an historical accident, but who has lived by its precepts with the awareness of integrity, death has no sting. The one and only life cycle is accepted as final and death is not feared. For those persons living with integrity, old age can be a harvest of contentment and pleasure. Lidz points to the relief from striving and struggle that comes from the lessening of the passions and of unfulfilled ambitions. Leisure can be rewarding, as can be the achievements of grandchildren or the societies and organizations one helped develop. It can be, in Lidz's words, "a time of relaxed closure of life that still contains much to experience and enjoy."[16]

In comparison, Butler and Lewis view this picture of the tranquility and serenity of old age enjoying the fruits of labor as mythical. It does not square with the values of the general public and its disdain and neglect of the elderly. They see ageism as a national prejudice based on a systematic stereotyping and discrimination against older people. Older people tend to be classified as ugly, rigid, senile, garrulous, and as less than full human beings. As with any form of prejudice, the aged victims believe this negative definition to be true, place a negative value on themselves, and expect and accept the discriminatory treatment given them. Other negative societal attitudes stem from the high values placed on productivity, with contempt given the nonproducer. Significantly, this society places positive values on youth and negative values on the elderly. Prejudice against the elderly may be a manifestation of the inability to face the inevitabilities of one's own aging process and death.[17]

Siegel notes the social and economic implications for health services related to the elderly in this society. An obvious finding is that the elderly are the largest users of health resources.[18] Demand and need rise with age. It follows, therefore, that an increasing amount of health care resources will be utilized for an increasing number of elderly persons. "The elderly, while representing only 12 percent of the population, consume 29 percent of the national budget, and fully 51 percent of all government expenditures for social services."[19] Furthermore, "Minority elders and the 'oldest old' aged 85 and above have extremely high rates of poverty and are the fastest growing segment of the population."[20]

This raises ethical issues of the allocation of limited resources. Moreover, as health care and medical technology improves, such as drugs, organ transplants, surgery, and dialysis, the elderly will increase their utilization. Additionally, the availability of insurance plans, such as Medicaid and Medicare, support more equal and thereby increased utilization of health care resources by all income groups. However, the scarce distribution of health care resources remains problematic to the elderly in inner cities and in nonurban areas.[21]

Another problem is the need to gear health services toward elderly women because of their much higher proportion among the elderly population. With declining birth rates, the elderly person will have fewer siblings or relatives and a diminished family support system. This raises ethical issues of enabling elderly persons to die if they choose, rather than requiring them to prolong their lives. The plight of these elderly persons also raises issues regarding the obligations of their offspring, who may be supporting their own children. The proportion of smaller kinship networks also raises issues concerning a greater role for government in providing health and human services to the elderly and raises problems of the allocation of limited resources. Some writers such as Daniels, advocate a lifelong rationing scheme into which one contributes, analogous to Social Security.[22] Another aspect of the allocation of limited resources concerns the quality of care given to the 5% of the elderly who reside in nursing homes and other group-care facilities. These persons may be institutionalized to provide needed care for their incapacities or for social convenience. The moral issue is the provision of care that enhances the human dignity and health status of the elderly. Some elderly persons in nursing homes have been neglected or abused, exist on substandard food and live in unsafe environmental conditions. The provision of adequate and appropriate nursing services could make a significant difference in the care of the elderly.

Moral problems of distributive justice are acutely felt by the frail elderly and by those who are terminally ill. Do they have a right to decide to live with dignity and to choose when to terminate life support systems? Or are they required to live as long as they breathe?

SELECTED CASES AND PRINCIPLES

We will consider eight fairly typical cases that involve moral issues in the health care of the elderly.

CASE 15.1: Allocation of Scarce Resources.   Mr. H, a 23-year-old motorcycle accident victim, is seriously injured and requires a life-support system in the intensive care unit. There are no empty beds. Ms. K, age 66, in a coma following a major stroke and on a life-support system, is the oldest patient in the intensive care unit. The nurse must recommend which of these two patients will be given the cardiopulmonary support unit.

CASE 15.2: Assisting the Patient with Suicide.   "Suicide rates for males are higher after age 65 than in younger men. That is because male suicide rates increase from age 15 to 85 in a straight line."[23] There is a substantial increase in suicides of both sexes in the age category of 75 and above.[24]

Nurse A covers the night shift for a member of the regular staff whose is ill. One of her patients is Dr. D, age 75, a well-known neurosurgeon and a retired member of the medical school faculty. He has recently been admitted for severe, intractable back pain with increasing difficulty in walking. His wife is dead and his three children are successful medical practitioners. Dr. D lives alone with domestic help in the same large family home in the suburbs, and he attends medical meetings. Since his radical prostatectomy for a malignancy, his medical practice ceased. There is every reason to believe that examinations performed on this admission will reveal extensive metastatic cancer to the spine. Dr. D may suspect his true prognosis despite the professionally cheerful and respectful manner staff members accord to him.

Nurse A is about to leave his room to prepare the prescribed injection of narcotics in response to his request. Before she leaves, Dr. D asks the nurse to increase his dose of morphine sufficiently to cause his death. He tells her that his son, a resident physician who visits his father every night, is on call and will immediately write the order for the increased dose. Nurse A is very fond of Dr. D and wonders if it is not his right to determine what shall be done with his disease-ridden, pain-wracked body. She also thinks about the sanctity of every life and the irreversibility of this act. What reasons are there for the nurse either to follow or not follow the request?

CASE 15.3: A Patient's Right to Decide.   Mr. M was an unmarried 82-year-old resident of a nursing home, independent in self-care but needing assistance in dressing and able to ambulate with a walker. Despite occasional episodes of memory loss and confusion, he continued to care for himself. His loss of hearing interfered with social activities, but he resisted the use of a hearing aid. The development of dysuria led to the diagnosis of benign prostatic hypertrophy and the recommendation of a transurethral prostatectomy operation. When informed of the necessity for surgery, Mr. M readily consented. His nephew and only relative, however, refused to consent to surgery on the grounds that owing to the uncle's mental status, his life was without dignity and should not be sustained by extraordinary means. The nephew believed that the uncle had already lived a long life anyway. The nurse appealed for consent for surgery, but to no avail. Without the surgery, Mr. M's condition rapidly declined, and he died of uremic complications within 6 weeks. What of the patient's right to decide to accept or to refuse treatment and the nurse's role as patient advocate?

CASE 15.4: Competence and the Patient's Right to Refuse.   Annas relates the case of a 60-year-old woman, Ms. Yetter, who had been involuntarily committed to a mental hospital with a diagnosis of schizophrenia.[25] A lump in her breast was discovered and a biopsy ordered, to be followed by a mastectomy if the biopsy showed malignant tissue. Ms. Yetter refused permission for the procedure on the grounds that she was afraid of the operation because her aunt had died following a similar procedure. Moreover, she believed the surgery would interfere with her genital system and prevent her from having babies and a career in the movies. The judge decided that although she was delusional, she consistently refused the surgery even in lucid periods. Therefore, the court found Ms. Yetter competent to refuse the biopsy and surgery. What reasons would justify continuing attempts to persuade Ms. Yetter to consent to the surgery or to refrain from attempting to persuade her on the grounds that the patient is "competent"?

CASE 15.5: A Conflict of Rights.   Annas reports a related case involving a 77-year-old woman who suffered from gangrene and refused to undergo a recommended amputation. Although the court found that the patient was combative . . . that her train of thought wandered and her conception of time was distorted, it also found that she demonstrated a high degree of awareness and acuity. The patient made clear that she did not wish to have the operation, even though she knew that decision would probably lead shortly to her death.[26]

The woman made a choice fully aware of the consequences and was therefore "found to be competent."[27] The court said, "The law protects her right to make her own decision to accept or reject treatment, whether this decision is wise or unwise."[28] The moral issue is whether the nurse is to educate the patient regarding the nature of gangrene and the importance of amputation as a condition for the patient's survival or simply supports the patient's decision as an act of self determination?

CASE 15.6: A Case of Truth-Telling. Ms. G, an active, independent, cheerful, 68-year-old grandmother who smokes heavily, is admitted to the hospital for an acute bout of pneumonia requiring intensive care. Her diagnostic tests reveal a widespread, metastatic, inoperable cancer of the lungs. She is expected to live only a few months. Her devoted children and husband are told the diagnosis while the patient is in intensive care. The family insists that the patient not be told the truth so that the patient's remaining time at home will be as happy as possible. When her nurse comes into the room to prepare her for discharge, Ms. G says to the nurse, "I know that I've had a lot of special tests and x-rays of my lungs. I have the feeling that something important is being kept from me. I believe that I have the right to know what's wrong with me." The issue is the patient's right to know the truth.

What are the possible responses the nurse may make and what are the ethical justifications? After one evaluates both the utilitarian and Kantian arguments for what a morally sensitive and knowledgeable nurse might say in response, it seems that the Kantian emphasis on truth-telling and integrity prevails.

CASE 15.7: The Nurse as Patient Advocate. This example, adapted from Barry,[29] involves Ms. R, a 78-year-old, independent, nearly deaf convalescent-home patient. The patient had suffered a cerebrovascular accident (stroke) and her prognosis was uncertain. She was a difficult patient to please. Her family was devoted and concerned. Ms. R contracted a case of influenza and the family demanded reasons of the nurse as to why Ms. R seemed to be getting worse and why she had not been seen by her physician. On admission, the physician reportedly told the family that with rest and physical therapy, Ms. R would soon be her old self. The nurse knew, however, that when the head nurse called the doctor for medication and treatment, "he instructed her simply to have us make 'R' as comfortable as possible because she wasn't going to last very long anyway."[30] The nurse concluded, "I knew, of course, that professionally I should keep my mouth shut and not make anybody look bad. But I felt sorry for R, and I thought the daughter-in-law was getting the runaround."[31]

Barry then asks what if the reader were the nurse, what would she or he do? Barry then cites some alternatives, one of which is to tell what the nurse knows. Another alternative for the nurse is to put on the professional hat and "stonewall" the daughter-in-law. A third alternative is to refer the daughter-in-law to one's superiors, again the professionally approved route. There is also the problem of not saying anything derogatory about a doctor, fellow nurse, or hospital. There is also the moral issue of the nurse, as patient advocate, informing the daughter-in-law that the physician has not seen the patient for 2 months despite being notified of the patient's illness and decline. What is the nurse justified in doing? The Kantian principle of truth-telling seems to prevail in this case, if one believes in a patient's right to respect, autonomy, and being treated rationally. But the important question here is: What do you think is the morally right thing for the nurse to do or say?

CASE 15.8: Allocation of Nursing Resources. Barry reports an essentially true case of Professor A, age 84, who was considered to be a "brilliant jurist and legal scholar." He was a giant of a man, and he had an admirable "sense of independence," which even "bordered on conceit."[32] He was married to Kate for over 50 years. They were childless but proud of their independence. At age 82, he was diagnosed with diabetes, and by age 84 he lost his sight and hearing. He then suffered a total heart block and needed a pacemaker. His independence vanished by painful degrees. He was diapered and put on a waterbed mattress. Professor A's self-esteem suffered, in addition to the pain of his physical losses.

In an adaptation of Barry's account, the scenario continues. The hospital physician concluded that Professor A no longer needed the facilities of an acute care setting. Much against his wife's wishes, he was transferred to a facility giving highly skilled nursing care. His wife visited him every day. She was at his bedside from early morning to early evening. Although she participated in and observed the high level of skilled nursing care he was given, she respectfully but continually interrupted the nurses' work with other patients because of her extreme solicitude for her husband. She held his hand, watched his face, and rang for the nurse every time he moved or made a sound. Some nurses on the unit felt that Professor A was receiving more than his fair share of the available nursing care on that unit and gave reasons for curtailing the time and resources spent on him. These nurses argued for the utilitarian concept of the greatest happiness of the greatest number. Other nurses on the unit argued that this patient and his wife needed and deserved that care, as should every other patient on that unit. These nurses argued for the Kantian principle of treating every patient as an end and not solely as a means. The problem was to determine what was a fair distribution of limited nursing services. What is a fair share of nursing resources when all the health care needs cannot be met?

ETHICAL-PHILOSOPHICAL CONSIDERATIONS IN THE NURSING CARE OF THE ELDERLY: FIVE METHODS OF ALLOCATING HEALTH CARE

There are five alternative methods of distributing health care: 1) the Holmes lifeboat method (egoist); 2) the triage or some cost-benefit calculation of worth (utilitarian); 3) the lottery method of treatment; 4) equal shares; and 5) equal consideration.

The Lifeboat Method

The Holmes method stems from an 1846 shipwreck in which Mr. Holmes, the officer in charge of a lifeboat, ordered the "unfit" thrown overboard. Rescue followed shortly, and the moral question remains to this day whether Holmes should have been charged with the murder for which he was found legally guilty. The lifeboat method is the egoist solution, sometimes called "survival of the fittest." The lifeboat method does not, however, save or serve a maximum number of persons. Nor does it work in the long run by helping a large-scale, complex culture to flourish. Among those thrown overboard, for example, may be some who are physically unfit but intellectually more fit to help the whole group survive. On this ground, the nurse's decision in Case 15.1 is to allocate the bed and life-support system in the intensive care unit to the younger person and, in effect, throw Ms. K overboard.

The idea that elderly people belong on the scrap heap, illustrated in examples of neglect and ignoring the needs of the elderly in need of a prostatectomy and of medical care (Cases 15.3 and 15.7), is morally callous. One argument against lifeboat morality is the classic "is-ought" fallacy: what is, such as existing power, does not by itself justify what ought to be. In effect, the is-ought fallacy exposes the invalidity of the claim that "might makes right." (See Chapters 3 and 6). There are additional powerful positive moral arguments on behalf of allocating limited health care resources to the elderly. One argument is the appeal to Rawls's "veil of ignorance,"[33] in which one agrees to rules without knowing one's life circumstances.

The Utilitarian Method

A second method of allocation to the elderly is addressed in ethics by utilitarianism. The utilitarian emphasis is on providing the greatest happiness for the majority. Because the elderly constitute only a minority of the population, one might argue that they do not, on that ground alone, have much claim to limited social and economic resources. If one adds another utilitarian argument to the previous one, that the elderly are less likely to grow to be as productive and creative as children, adolescents, and young adults, one may conclude that the elderly deserve less than younger people. A rejoinder to this point is that the elderly as a group helped the young and adults to achieve; therefore, the elderly now merit the allocation of health care resources that they helped make available. The elderly also collectively contribute to the quality of human life through their experience and their wisdom. A variation of this view holds that society owes the elderly for what they contributed in the past.

Readers of Mill's version of utilitarianism will appreciate his conception of the quality of human life as more than the quantity of pleasure. The quality of human life for Mill means that it is better to be "a human being dissatisfied than a pig satisfied; better to be Socrates dissatisfied than a fool satisfied."[34] A patient who wishes not to be kept alive under all conditions appeals to the "quality of life" argument. A refined form of utilitarianism recognizes the equal right of each individual to happiness regardless of age, sex, race, color, or creed. This view is expressed in Bentham's famous rule, cited by Mill, that "everyone is to count for one, nobody for more than one."[35] The emphasis on equality, on the equal right of everyone to count, implies a restraint on crude utilitarianism, which either rules by a hypothetical majority that old people do not deserve ample resources, or that it is enough to repay old people for what they have done. For if everyone counts equally, no persons, young or old, are likely to pursue happiness by voting against their interests.

A similar principle is expressed by Kant's substantive principle "to treat humanity, whether in thine own person or in that of any other, in every case as an end, never as means only."[36] Kant's principle—to treat people as ends—as well as his categorical imperative to act so that one's action is at the same time a universal moral law, calls for equal treatment of all people, regardless of their intellectual, cultural, or economic contributions or age.

A practical utilitarianistic health care goal calls for a maximum number of persons, but not everyone, to be helped. The "optimum number" and "everyone" may make a telling difference, especially in crunch cases in which the only practical moral solution is to apply triage. Triage serves the maximum number. Triage in health care emergencies means that one sorts people out into three groups: the worst off, those who will die anyway; the best off, those who are most likely to recover on their own or with little help; and the median group, those to whom maximum medical and health care attention will most likely make the most difference. Because health care resources are limited, one serves the largest number by distinguishing them into these three groups and singling out the median group on whom to confer benefits. Triage implies the general utilitarian formula called cost-benefit analysis and cost-efficient analysis; in other words, serve the largest number most effectively.

This utilitarian formula is identified with "diagnostically related groupings" (DRGs) and similar methods of federally funded reimbursement programs for the elderly. According to DRGs, patients are allocated hospitalization according to their diseases, rather than their individual hospital needs. Triage provides more widespread distributive benefits for the cost expanded, and also is more cost-efficient than any other method of distributing health care under limited conditions.

The Lottery Method

The lottery method allocates health care on the basis of equal chance for treatment. The lottery method has a serious difficulty: The losers receive no care. One can appreciate the general unserviceability of the lottery in deciding, for example, which of 30 emergency patients to care for first or whether to help Mr. H or Ms. K (Case 15.1) with the pulmonary lifesaving unit, for one of them will be untreated. A key premise in having a life-choosing lottery is that of scarcity. This premise may rest on a fallacious moral assumption that allocating adequate health care for the elderly is not worthwhile in relation to other social values. Like musical chairs, the lottery may begin by allocating too few resources, thus compelling small numbers of winners and large numbers of losers. The method may seem fair, but not if the initial allocations are unfairly limited. If a member of the best-off or worst-off group picks the lucky straw, health care resources will have been wasted. The lottery method is based on luck. Yet in some kinds of cases, the lottery method is regarded as the fairest when resources are limited and there is near equality of conditions among candidates.[37] The lottery treats individuals equally in some situations, providing that resources are also limited. For example, the shortage of vaccines and drugs in experimental cancer and AIDS research shows the difficulty of achieving distributive justice by using the lottery method. A practice may seem fair, but not be wise. When deciding whether to use a lottery or triage in some nonacute resource-limited situations, the utilitarian triage method is the wisest choice. In other types of cases, such as deciding to save the most intelligent person, a form of elitism or egoism or paternalism may be the best solution. In a battle, one helps the general officer before helping a soldier.

The lottery leaves to chance what may be unwise. Some shortages are genuine, whereas others are artificial. One alternative to the lottery—lining up on a first come first served basis—may seem to eliminate the difficulty of having losers; but those who line up too late suffer health care deprivations similar to those who do not pick the lucky straw.

The Principle of Equality

The principle of equality can be interpreted to mean either equal chance, equal shares, or equal consideration. Equal chance was discussed as the lottery method, and its serious deficiencies were identified. The principle of equal shares means that everyone gets the same amount of health care resources. For the person in robust health, this method of distribution may be eminently satisfactory. For the person born with serious congenital malformations, or for the person with chronic disabling illness, or for the person with HIV, this method may be tragic. The share of health care resources for such people is grossly inadequate. The advantages are that people are given equal shares, but their needs are different. This method works only if people are all equal. But people's value in society is not equal; therefore, the method does not work.

The equal shares argument has as the right to health care several serious objections. One objection is that those who have not worked as diligently, as long, or as effectively as others would rate equally in having their health needs met. This is the objection expressed by supporters of individual merit, and it cannot be discounted. For example, people who save for sickness in old age and who go without better homes, vacations, and entertainment believe that it is not right that those who spent their earnings receive equal shares. One version of this argument is that if health care resources are distributed equally, then the nonsmokers, nondrinkers, and weight watchers may have to pay the bills for the smokers, alcoholics, and the obese. This anti-equality argument is sometimes referred to as the "anti-freeloader" argument.

A second serious objection to the equal shares argument is that people's value to society is unequal. The idea that all people are equal, if it is unqualified by some such phrase as "in the eyes of the law," is a myth. In some societies the oldest people are the least economically valuable. As proponents of the is-ought fallacy point out, however, that fact is not a justifiable basis for a moral policy that deprives aging persons of needed health care.

A third difficulty with the equal shares argument is that all health care cannot be satisfied with available limited resources. Veatch has pointed out that those most in need, "the incurably ill . . . would end up with all the medical resources. This is . . . inefficient. Furthermore, if they do not benefit from the commitment of resources, it is hard to see why it is just that they get those resources."[38]

To say "X has a need due to old age" does not translate into "X has a right due to old age." Needs, unlike rights, are refusable without contradiction. If one were to say, however, that X has a right due to old age, X's right would not be refusable without a reason. The needs argument, therefore, does not have many teeth in it. All people have many health care needs, but needs are not a sufficient ground for distributing limited health care resources.

Appeals to love, charity, and one's obligations to others, even appeals to decency, are morally refusable in a way that appeals to the survival of the race or to a well-established right are not. One has to reach for stronger reasons to cancel the application of a right. One can refuse a beggar without being morally blamed for doing so. For however great the beggar's need, to be given anything is not the beggar's right. In contrast, if patients have a right to health care compensation or if nurses have a right to be paid their due, to refuse to give the patient compensation or to refuse to pay nurses their due is morally and also legally blameworthy as a violation of their rights. The appeal to the moral sentiment that elderly people have needs will not by itself carry the day. Their needs are also morally refusable.

Another problem is that health care resources may be inadequate. The health care everyone receives may be too little to be effective, like dividing a slice of bread into 25 parts. Distributing equal shares in health care practice means that if health care resources are distributed equally, health care resources are distributed too thinly.

The Principle of Equal Consideration

If the aim of distribution is social justice, then everyone must receive equal consideration, rather than equal shares. For example, nurses give more care to acutely ill patients than to ambulatory patients. This does not imply that the ambulatory patient is neglected or abandoned. It is just that she or he needs less care.

A presupposition of equal consideration is that there are ample health care resources, including personnel of intelligence, experience, and merit. The problem is that, in health care situations, there are not sufficient resources to give everyone with a health care need equal consideration. Equal consideration does not work if hospitals have too few nurses and too many seriously ill patients. Currently, this society is unwilling to allocate the necessary resources to provide equal consideration to everyone.

Equal consideration depends upon ample resources, both human and material. The quality and often the quantity of these resources depend on human intelligence and talent, including persons of merit.

The problem of providing distributive justice in health care is to combine the principle of equal consideration, with appropriate development and recognition of merit. What Jesus ostensibly did in multiplying the loaves and fishes and what Edison did by inventing the electric light bulb combine equality and merit. Appropriately rewarding persons of merit, such as expert nurses, developing trained intelligence, and supporting medical technology can provide enough intensive care units so that young and old patients do not have to compete for a life-support system. The combination of equality and merit has already been achieved in the production and distribution of antibiotics, making them no longer scarce. One can then give effective equal consideration to each elderly patient who has a need for antibiotics.

In giving equal consideration to everyone's health care, one appeals to the reciprocity of everyone's needs, like living under a large-scale insurance plan called the social contract. According to the golden rule argument, one is to treat others as one wants to be treated. This means that one lives by giving and taking on a roughly reciprocal basis. One practical solution then is to have health care insurance plans into which subscribers pay a fair share throughout their lives. This response means that the beneficiaries share the burdens, in accordance with Rawls's principle that benefits and burdens be shared equally. On this view, the health care right Professor A has in Case 15.8 is limited. He cannot have unlimited health care resources, and he may have to stand in line like everyone else, literally and figuratively, as when he must wait his turn for a rare but highly desirable drug and a nurse's attention.

In geriatric nursing practice, scarcity of personnel, facilities, or resources may not justify inadequate and negligent treatment of patients who need help. This is illustrated in the case of Ms. R (Case 15.7) who suffered from lack of medical attention and negligence. The use of Kantian ethics supports the principle of equal consideration. A strength of Kantian ethics is to remind us of ideals, principles, and rights that ought to govern human conduct. This strength is illustrated in Case 15.3 when the nurse advocates Mr. M's right to a prostatectomy, despite the nephew's refusal to sign a consent form.

Truth-telling provides a further example of the strength of the Kantian orientation. Truth-telling is a vital obligation nurses have to elderly patients, as well as to other patients. Treating a patient with respect, which is the patient's right, rather than as a mere symptom bearer to be diagnosed and treated, is another example of applying a Kantian principle to geriatric nursing. To paraphrase Kant, a health care policy of benefits to the elderly without appraisal of costs is empty; a health care policy without widespread decent benefits is blind.

Appeal to either equality or merit alone is inadequate. Yet each, in pointing to the weaknesses of the other, reveals moral considerations worth taking seriously. For example, a society cannot function or flourish without merit. But a society that fails to make large-scale provision for legitimate human needs would be heartless and inhumane and, in a very important sense, immoral. To adapt a statement attributed to Dostoevsky, one can judge a civilization by how it takes care of its prisoners; thus, one may judge a society by how it takes care of its elderly. The problem remains to reconcile the moral relation between the appeals to needs and merit in a world of limited resources.

A TRILOGY OF ELDERLY PATIENTS' RIGHTS

Despite controversies over the meaning of elderly people's rights, three important rights emerge on the basis of the general human rights of all persons. These provide a basis for hope, love, justice and wisdom in considering the allocation of health care resources to the elderly. These rights are the client's 1) right to respect, 2) right to receive treatment, and 3) the right to refuse treatment. Each of these rights has an impact on nurse-client relations and issues in the care of the elderly. The elderly patient's right to respect includes the right to dignity and regard as a rational person, and as an end, not as a means or instrument of someone else's will only. An elderly person's right to respect implies the right to be treated on the basis of informed consent. The right to informed consent is the client's right to know what treatment is proposed, what its procedures and processes are, and what its expected results are, as well as the alternatives including no treatment. The right to respect also implies the right to privacy and confidentiality.

The right to receive appropriate treatment implements the right to respect. The right to receive treatment is the right to effective diagnosis and treatment by qualified health care persons, including nurses. A social, political, and economic issue that occurs with the right to receive treatment is that of receiving treatment at no individual cost versus treatment given on an individually payable basis. Because this issue is controversial, one may refer to the right to receive treatment in either of two senses: the right to receive treatment on an individually payable basis, and the right to receive nationally paid-for treatment from a national health care system, as in Canada and western European countries.

The third in the trilogy of health care rights is the client's right to terminate or refuse treatment. There are several views on whether to override an elderly patient's right to refuse. One position is the libertarian one, which says to respect a patient at face value and comply, as long as risks of failing to act are carefully explained. "It's his or her life, after all." Another view is the paternalistic view, which holds that patients' rights may be overridden in their own best interests or in the best interests of the state. A third position, a utilitarian view, holds that a patient's right may be overridden on the grounds of cost-benefit analysis, which may include the patient's good or the good of society.

COMPETENCE AND THE RIGHTS OF ELDERLY PATIENTS

A difficulty arises if a patient refuses treatment that will aid him or her to achieve the autonomy that a rational patient would prefer. Macklin gives a compelling reason for overriding a psychiatric patient's right to refuse: a patient's rational powers and autonomy would be increased as a result of treatment when the patient's consenting organ is affected.[39]

According to Annas, to be mentally ill (a psychiatric concept) is not necessarily to be incompetent (a legal concept) Annas cites an example of a 60-year-old woman, Ms. Yetter (Case 15.4), who refused a breast biopsy and was found competent to refuse surgery because she consistently opposed it in lucid periods.[40] The court was assured that she understood that she might die as a result of having refused.[41]

A moral and philosophical issue raised by the case of Ms. Yetter is to consider under what conditions to override an elderly patient as incompetent. In Plato's *Republic,* Socrates uses the example of whether to deprive a patient of the right to be given back a weapon the patient has lent someone. Socrates points out that if a person lends one a weapon and then goes mad and demands the weapon back, one would be quite justified in not returning the weapon out of concern for preventing harm.[42] Thus, one ground for overriding elderly patients' rights to refuse treatment is to prevent harm, either to themselves or to others. Socrates quite formidably presented the obvious paradigm for the morally right action in that type of instance and identified one meaning of "incompetence" as doing harm.

There are, however, other borderline ambiguities that make judgments of competence unclear. In this connection, one may consider several distinctions Feinberg has recently proposed that may help clarify the concept of competence.[43] Feinberg cites three scenarios, the first two of which show that a patient is incompetent, while the third shows the patient to be quite competent. In the first scenario, the patient, a layperson, disagrees with a physician about the properties of drug X, which the physician refuses to prescribe. The patient is *factually* incompetent. In the second scenario, the patient is told that drug X, which the patient wishes the physician to prescribe, will be harmful. The patient says that is exactly what he or she wants. In this scenario, the patient is *normatively* incompetent. In the third scenario, the patient wants drug X, realizes the harm, but says that X will give enough pleasure to make it worthwhile running the risk for physical harm. In this scenario, according to Feinberg, the patient is competent. For the patient shows recognition of risk and, in doing so, reveals an awareness of making value judgments in the real world.

Unnecessary drug use, alcohol dependency, smoking, driving too fast, overeating, and eating the wrong foods are examples of the third scenario. This scenario shows that one can disagree morally without being incompetent.

The question is to determine which of these three scenarios, if any, appropriately applies to Ms. Yetter's refusal of a biopsy. Ms. Yetter is delusional about a Hollywood career and having children at age 60. If there is adequate evidence that her biopsy would lead to effective lifesaving treatment, then one would have a rational consideration for overriding her right to refuse. If a form of treatment a patient refuses leads to worthy health values that the patient wants, then in that case, one would have reason to override the patient's right to refuse. The appeal to a patient's own best interests might also be used to override the 77-year-old woman in Case 15.5 who refused to have her gangrenous foot amputated. The patient's own good might again be cited as a reason for Nurse A's morally justifiable action in refusing Dr. D, who requested a lethal dose of narcotics (Case 15.2). However, in the case of a woman who requests not to be resuscitated so that her kidneys may be donated to a suitable recipient, the nurse may be justified in supporting the patient's wish. The reasoning here is libertarian. One's liberty rights offer an initial presumption of a person's rights as a person. One's prima facie liberty rights are usually honored, unless there is a morally better reason to override one's liberty rights by other moral considerations, such as prevention of harm to oneself or others. The reasonable moral grounds for honoring this woman's wishes when her life no longer seems viable to her or anyone else seems to place a moral stop sign on all overriding reasons. Even to override an elderly patient's right to refuse treatment does not mean one refuses the patient's right to respect. The reason for overriding, as a nurse might do in a case like Ms. Yetter's if her chances for living longer would rationally be improved by surgery, shows more rather than less respect. Even if one overrides an elderly patient's right to refuse treatment, this does not overrule the right to respect. For within the trilogy, the right to respect is accorded priority or is preemptive. This means that an elderly patient's right to treatment or the right to refuse may be overridden by the right to respect. To again appeal to a counterfactual conditional judgment, the right to respect means one would do for the patient what the client would, if rational, retrospectively want to have done. The right to respect gives one moral grounds for overriding or preempting Ms. Yetter's right to refuse a breast biopsy, providing a breast biopsy is medically indicated and that she will be helped by it.

JUSTICE BETWEEN GENERATIONS

Questions arise as to what adults owe their elderly patients. The answer to this question has a bearing on what obligation a society has to care for the elderly, and the role of nurses in carrying out this obligation. Six main ethical theories address this question. First is the traditional Chinese view, in which an unbreakable filial bond places the parent first, even if it means forfeiting the grown child's life. Second, the European-American view places elderly parents second to one's spouse and children. One treats one's parents like one treats good friends, on a third view. A fourth attitude is the bookkeeping reciprocal view that requires children to give back roughly the good they were given. On a fifth view, grown children treat their elderly parents like one treats beggars or strangers. On a sixth view, adults perceive their parents as one sees undesirable aliens, or as opponents or enemies. Such adults view their parents with hatred, hostility, abuse, and even violence.

Of these six views, the most flexible and helpful seems to be the third view, whereby one treats one's parents with care, hope, love, and shared wisdom in the spirit of Erik Erikson's concept of "mutuality and reciprocity." Friendships and partnerships seem to be appropriate forms of intergenerational relationships that enable justice to be practiced between generations. According to Moody, when we turn from professional relationships to family relationships, we find a need for an "ethics of filial responsibility."[44] To Moody, another alternative to the dominant ethics is phenomenological (or existentialist) ethics, with its emphasis on an individual patient's consciousness involving a person's "lived experience, intimacy, moral complexity, conflict, and tragedy."[45] Moody endorses this spectrum of alternatives, which include aspects of Marxism, feminist theory, and Habermas's critical theory.[46] Moody assembles the tragic decline of Alzheimer's patients in his partial critique of the dominant model, and attempts to supplement the dominant ethics with alternative ethical perspectives.

The view one might take regarding both the dominant ethical theories and the alternative ethical theories is to draw from J. R. Oppenheimer's analogy of the thruways and the side roads. We benefit by having and using both. The thruway gives us the big view. The side roads give us the detail of villages we would miss on the thruway. Analogously, the dominant ethics helps one to appreciate the abstract principles and general issues, such as truth-telling. The alternative ethical theories help us with the concrete, tragic event; in the day-to-day struggles of patients such as those with heart disease, cancer, AIDS, and Alzheimer's disease.

But our effort to supplement Moody's account rests on an adaptation of a Kantian aphorism: "Concepts without percepts are empty; and percepts without concepts are blind."[47] Adapting Kant's remark to the two kinds of ethics, the presence of the dominant ethics without alternative ethical theories is empty;

and alternative ethical theories without the dominant ethics (e.g., goal-based, duty-based, rights-based ethics) is blind and purposeless.

NURSING IMPLICATIONS

Freedom Versus Control and Prevention of Harm

As identified in Chapter 1, these two important principles may be in conflict. This is especially evident in caring for the elderly who are in need of restraints.

CASE 15.9: A Case of Restraint. Ms. Gardener, an 88-year-old dementia patient, is hospitalized with pneumonia. She attempts to free herself from her gastronomy tube and get out of bed. To prevent the patient from falling and pulling out the tube, the nurse applies wrist and body restraints. Even though she has an order for restraints, the nurse is uneasy with her decision.[48] Why? Research has shown the negative effects of restraints on patients: Two-fold increase in hospital stay; eight-fold increase in mortality; increased removal of tubes; increased falls with more serious injuries; and increased mortality due to asphyxiation.[49]

Despite the promulgation of national standards and government regulations recommending restraint-free care and the use of alternatives, the practice of restraints continued in three nursing homes surveyed with restraint reduction programs.[50] Restraint alternatives begin with the development of preventive strategies based on preserving patients' rights, dignity, and well-being during use.[51] Qualified physicians and registered nurses assess the least restrictive method of patient care in accordance with physicians' and nurses' responsibilities for monitoring patient's safety, conditions for renewing orders, and written documentation.[52] Nurses are in key positions to identify and correct underlying problems, such as adverse effects of drugs that alter mental status, and irritating tubes and catheters.[53]

In the case of Ms. Gardner, the nurse returned to try something different. She removed the wrist restraints and wrapped an abdominal binder around the patient's waist without impeding the flow of the tube feeding. The nurse then seated the patient in a reclining chair near the nurse's station, with obvious relief to the patient.[54]

Abuse of the Elderly Patient

CASE 15.10: A Case of Probable Abuse. Ms. Cox, a 75-year-old widow, walks into the emergency department with her 52-year-old son, with whom she resides. The patient has a broken arm from a spiral fracture related to twisting motions, and numerous bruises at different stages of healing. The patient explains her injuries as the result of falling down the stairs. The son stays close to his mother and answers all the questions for her.

Lynch states physical, psychological, or financial abusers to be usually family members with a history of psychological or financial dependence on the parent.[55] Therefore, victims are usually widowed, elderly, mentally or physically impaired, and socially isolated. There are protective services for the elderly in every state and usually a "hotline" to report abuse that requires prompt response and investigation. The situation in Case 15.10 is a red flag for the nurse to be a patient advocate.

Elder abuse in nursing homes falls largely on impaired patients who are incapable of the activities of daily living and are vulnerable to abuse, neglect, or maltreatment. Victims of abuse or neglect are likely to be residents with few or no visitors and limited resources for asserting their rights. Abuse, neglect, and maltreatment occur frequently in nursing homes lacking adequate staff, positive feedback to employees, and scheduled staff meetings focused on patient care.[56] Abuse is frequently identified with job stress, low job status, low regard for patients, belief in patients' need for discipline, conflicts among staff members, burnout, and personal stress. The prediction of an increase in the incidence of abuse, neglect, and maltreatment of nursing home residents is attributed to the rise in the elderly population, the negligence of administration, financial interests, and the lack of professional interest in nursing programs that focus on nursing home care. Again, as in home or hospital care, the law requires the nurse and others to report instances of suspected or actual abuse, neglect or maltreatment to the appropriate state office. Every state has elder abuse reporting laws that protect the whistle-blower from reprisal.

Among the kinds of abuse—physical, psychological, financial, or neglect—the most obvious is physical abuse. In abuse cases, nurses provide privacy for patients, avoid confrontation, perform assessments based on physical examinations and medical histories of their patients. Patients may be admitted for their protection. After victims are removed from danger, abusers are relieved of responsibilities and stresses, are directed toward counseling and education services as well as rehabilitation for any drug and alcohol abuse. Adult Protective Services, in accordance with the law for incompetent patients, can provide for guardianships, financial assistance, foster care, case workers, counselors, and legal aid.[57] A competent patient may refuse intervention; consequently, the nurse informs the patient of available services, written emergency numbers, and the possibility that the frequency and severity of abuse may continue. Nurses must still contact Adult Protective Services for the sake of patient safety.

Self-neglect or caregiver neglect occurs when the demands of the required care exceed the ability or the commitment of the responsible individuals. Depression, addiction, personality problems, or ignorance of available community services contribute to neglect. If educational services are ineffective, legal intervention by means of adult protective services, the police, and abuse hotlines are necessary.

> More than 2 million elderly persons, especially those over 75 years of age, are abused by family members, neighbors, or informal caregivers who reside with the victim. Although abuse crosses racial, social, and religious lines, most victims are isolated, caucasian, poor women who experience temporary or permanent physical, cognitive or emotional impairments . . . who lose self-esteem, are shamed and humiliated and unable . . . to convey their abuse experiences to designated authorities in the community.[58]

Role of Patient Advocate

Nurses play pivotal and, in some cases, indispensable roles in providing health care for the elderly. The elderly are in the majority in most nursing units of a general hospital. They are in need of daily dressing, medications, getting out of bed, and various therapies. The elderly in surgical and intensive care units are a particular source of concern for the nurse, because every aspect of their care over a 24-hour period is provided by nurses.

Nursing care plans and goals are set by nurses. The success or failure of these plans is the outcome both of the wisdom of the plans and goals and the quality and quantity of nursing care given in support of those goals. Homebound elderly persons for whom nursing services are the main source of health care are also dependent on the appropriateness, frequency, and effectiveness of that care for survival. The nurse is not only indispensable to the delivery of nursing services, but also for coordinating other health and human services on behalf of the patient. Therefore, nurses identify and secure whatever other health services the patient needs. It is the nurse who identifies shortness of breath, irregular pulse, untoward effects of medication, and signs and symptoms of pain, and then secures medical help both in the home and hospital setting. The nurse identifies deficits in the delivery of effective care, and safeguards the patient from an unsafe environment. The nurse then contacts those health care and social services responsible for correcting personnel or environmental hazards.

This view of nursing care as a total responsibility for the elderly patients' health care by coordination of nursing services with medical care and with diagnostic and therapeutic services presumes the role of the nurse as patient advocate. In no other client group except children are patients so vulnerable to outside influences, neglect, and abuse.

Several definitions of the role of patient advocate may clarify this concept and its application to the nursing care of the elderly. Kohnke defines the role of the nurse advocate working with conscious patients who are able to speak or act as two-fold. The advocate's first function is to inform the patient by providing information "in a way that is meaningful to the client."[59] The nurse informs the patient of essential knowledge regarding the client's health and welfare or regarding the patient's rights, or provides answers to the patient's questions. The second function Kohnke views as the nurses' support of whatever decision the client makes. "The role of advocate comprises only two functions: to inform and to support."[60] A common example of nurse-patient interaction that provides the nurse with an easy, natural opportunity to be a patient advocate is "Must I have this surgery?"

The patient advocate's function in Case 15.4, according to Kohnke, would be to inform. Because this patient requested information, she deserved an honest, direct answer informing her that she had both a moral and legal right to refuse surgery. If the patient then refused surgery, the nurse as patient advocate is bound to support that decision, in Kohnke's definition of the role. Evidently, Ms. Yetter's nurse assumed that others, such as the physician, would not want Ms. Yetter to be informed regarding her right to refuse treatment. However, because many states, hospitals, and nursing homes have adopted variations of the American Hospital Association's *A Patient's Bill of Rights,* first proposed in 1973, the nurse may have been incorrect in that assumption. Nurses may well be supported by institutions in informing patients of their right to refuse treatment. Some nurses are unduly intimidated by the presumed authority of physicians over nursing practice. As a consequence, such nurses misperceive the situation as one in which their continued employment is threatened when the facts indicate otherwise.

Kohnke recommends that the nurse learn how to support the client's decision without either defending the decision or rescuing the patient. Her reasoning is that clients are responsible for their decisions, which the nurse supports without necessarily approving. Nor, in Kohnke's view, is the advocate obligated "to fight [patients'] battles for them."[61] Such behavior may be regarded as disloyal to colleagues and family members, who also claim to give priority to the patient's best interests.

The nurse who seeks to be effective as patient advocate becomes familiar with the policies and goals of the institution, the supervisory and administrative practices of the staff, and the provisions of the law. This kind of knowledge enables nursing staff members to develop and test strategies for developing the role of patient advocate and for coping with the risks that may come with implementation. Some groups of nurses have become enormously creative in advocating for patients' rights by pointing out the legal pitfalls of less-than-informed patient consent or unsafe conditions of patient care. Utilizing the provisions and protection of a nursing contract with the facility in which the patient-nurse ratio is specified, or specifying the American Nurses Association code of ethics as a guideline to practice may be useful to the nursing staff striving to develop the role of patient advocate. The ethical orientation examined in this book may serve as the basis for principles stated in the plan of nursing governance and the body of ethical principle in support of that governance. If, for example, support of patients' rights is considered to be an essential feature of nursing care, then the role of patient advocate follows naturally. Hopefully, it results in dialogue and resolution without coercing the patient to consent to or to refuse treatment.

The American Nurses Association develops the concept of the patient advocate as that of guardian of patients' care and safety. In this role, the nurse is expected to "take appropriate action regarding any instances of incompetent, unethical or illegal practice(s) by any member of the health care team or the health care system itself, or any action on the part of others that is prejudicial to the client's best interests."[62]

Informed Consent
The patient's problems become the nurses' problems, as patients turn to nurses as the persons most involved in their care and closest to them in socioeconomic status and the level of language used. As patient advocate, the autonomous nurse has the duty to remedy the patient's knowledge gap, preferably before the surgery or treatment so that there is time for discussion. The nurse notifies the physician and surgeon of the patient's questions so that the information gap will be closed in ways most useful to patients and families. This may prevent lawsuits.

A further ethical problem for nurses is to respect the patient's right to decide in giving nursing care that involves drug studies, electroconvulsive therapy, or surgery for elderly and possibly brain-damaged patients. One example of this problem was that of Mr. M in Case 15.3. He needed surgery, but his nephew refused to consent. The patient's life could have been saved. Yet, this and similar decisions of whether or not to operate, or to resuscitate, are made for the patient by the family and physician. The rationalization is that the family, not the patient, will sue if dissatisfied with care provided, so that it is their wishes that are honored, not the patient's rights. Advocacy groups for the elderly are formed to prevent just such abuses. The American Nurses Association clearly states that "each client has the moral right to determine what will be done with his or her person."[63]

The issue of whose consent is to be respected and whose passed over is a significant problem that requires vigilance by nurses individually and collectively, so that prompt action may be taken through the appropriate nursing, medical, and legal channels of the health care facility. One example of the failure of vigilance was in the case of elderly residents of a nursing home in Brooklyn, New York. They were asked to participate in research and they agreed. These elderly patients were then injected with live cancer virus. At the time of the injection, the effects of these live viruses were unknown. Clearly, informed consent means more than the act of a nurse witnessing the patient's signature, which is the extent of the nurse's legal commitment. As advocate, informed consent means the nurse's moral commitment to the patient's clear understanding of the proposed procedure, surgery, medication, or research. This can best be done by the nurse's presence and participation in the physician's explanation to the patient. The nurse can then ask in the presence of the physician, as in Case 15.5, "Do you understand what the word 'amputation' means?" If no response is forthcoming, the nurse may say, "Dr. Smith is talking about cutting off your leg to save your life. Your leg is not healing because there's no circulation. The gangrene will spread and threaten your life. But you can learn to walk again using an artificial leg. We'll all help you." Thus, the nurse actively facilitates dialogue between the patient, the nurse, and the physician. In this way, the nurse can be a patient's advocate and health educator who willingly witnesses the signature of the patient secure in the knowledge that the patient understands what procedure will be done and the consequences, and consents on that basis. Then the nurse is free to do all of the patient teaching helpful to that situation. If the nurse works in the community, a phone call or a visit to the physician's office may facilitate a clear understanding of the procedure and the need for patient education. The easily remediable problem is that not all elderly patients are allowed the necessary respect, time, and effort needed to give them an understanding of the proposed treatment. Elderly persons easily accept and expect the lack of interest shown in their welfare as a necessary part of being old; they view themselves as discards. The caring nurse expects that her elderly clients will be given sufficient information, help, and time to consider consequences and alternatives as the basis for informed consent.

THE SANCTITY OF LIFE VERSUS THE QUALITY OF LIFE

One of the most difficult dilemmas for the nurse to face is between advocating courses of action that favor as primary considerations the sanctity of life and those that favor as primary considerations the quality of life of the elderly person. Nurses working in intensive care units must sometimes rank patients in terms of prognosis, so that a new admission may be given a bed, as in Case 15.1. Age and prognosis are factors to be considered. The dilemma is in assigning weights to the variables as the basis for decisions that are fair. This poses ethical problems for the nursing staff of the intensive care unit having to decide or to recommend a transfer of an elderly patient out of the unit to give a younger person a chance. The question is whether it is fair, if the younger person was injured as a result of drunken driving, to condemn the older person to certain death. If, however, the elderly person's time is short anyway, the question is whether her life is less precious than the younger man's. There is no easy answer to these questions. They call for careful consideration of ethical principles and all of the relevant data as the bases for a decision.

The dilemma of the sanctity of life versus the quality of life also arises in deciding whether to resuscitate. Some elderly patients with pain and a fatal prognosis specifically request that they not be resuscitated. If that patient's family wants "everything done for the patient," as might be the case with Professor A in Case 15.8, and the hospital has no policy, the question is to determine the moral basis on which the nurse makes the decision. A patient advocate would press for respect and consideration of the patient's wishes. Before the particular event, it is easier to work with colleagues to arrive at a clear and unequivocal policy on resuscitation, which calls for written "no code" orders. It is morally indefensible to accept tacit and sly orders such as "Make haste slowly" in cardiac arrest or pencil-written orders not to resuscitate, to be erased on the patient's death for the purpose of defense against malpractice suits. The opposite situation, which also presents a dilemma, prevails on some intensive care units in which a patient is repeatedly resuscitated by an exhausted, frustrated, and perplexed staff. Annas cites one example of a 70-year-old woman who was resuscitated over 70 times within the span of a few days.[64]

Truth-Telling

The question "Am I going to die?" raises an important issue of truth-telling. Aged persons long in touch with their body functions and feeling states are sometimes knowledgeable about their terminal conditions. Such individuals gain great comfort in discussing the disposition of their property, their funeral arrangements, and the living arrangements for a surviving spouse. Visits from family members and friends are cherished and eye contact is maintained even when the patient is unable to speak. The nurse's confirmation of the patient's knowledge of impending death may be simple assent to the patient's question. Some patients, however, steadfastly deny the obvious decline of their bodies and neither ask nor wish to hear information regarding their condition. Perhaps all patients, even the most curious and determined individuals, need time and preparation, assuming one can prepare for death, before hearing the most profound truth, "You will soon die." Therefore, even the nurse advocate who supports truth-telling may, out of consideration, surround this final truth regarding dying with sufficient focus on the "here and now" of reality to enable individuals to reach their own conclusions. Harsh, naked truth can be destructive to the aging person's capacity to face this last test of ego mastery and control in the face of the "unthinkable" loss of one's life. The decision to tell the truth is aided by the seasoning of compassion and wisdom.

SUMMARY

To grow old is also to grow in "integrity," in Erikson's term. Advanced age sharpens one's awareness of where one has been and who one is, even though one may become vague and unsteady around the edges. Old age can be an ironic time. One may be both sharper and more aware and yet more forgetful and slower. There are reasons to value and also to disvalue old age. Wisdom, long associated with old age, goes side by side with infantile regression.

Attitudes toward the elderly are also paradoxical. The elderly are castigated, reviled, and regarded with contempt by some, yet others see and appreciate successful elderly people as exemplars and models for others to follow. Great elderly women and men are cited and looked up to with admiration. These opposing attitudes are reflected in allocating health care to the elderly, and in dealing with the tough problems of deciding who gets what and how much. Like a seesaw, striking a balance between what a society can provide for its elderly and how much to allocate to the young, to adults, and for other human goals, such as environmental concerns and education, leaves deep questions and moral uncertainty.

Geriatric training for nurses implies a common set of moral principles, culled from various ethical views. One principle implicit in geriatric nursing is the prevention of harm. Another principle is truth-telling. Other moral values include respect for equality and fairness, autonomy, regard for merit, and recognition of individual rights. These common values have an initial presumption of soundness. On this view, nurses ought, for example, to prevent harm, tell the truth, and respect the elderly patient's autonomy. Nurses are also obligated to treat patients fairly and equally. Compelling reasons need to be given for overriding these values. The purpose of this chapter has been to clarify some of the ethical considerations that arise in deciding on the amount and quality of nursing care for the elderly.

Discussion Questions

1. In Case 15.6 what reasons could the nurse give for telling the patient the truth or for withholding the truth?
2. What reasons are there for a nurse to assist or refuse to assist an elderly suicidal patient?

3. As science and technology make more health care possible, the elderly want more and more, with never enough to go around. What just rationing scheme provides the maximal health care needs for the elderly without bankrupting the rest of society?
4. What do you think it feels like to be an elderly person? How does your sympathy help or hinder your responses to your elderly patients?
5. What is the relation between individual freedom and the conditions for forming and maintaining attachments among the elderly?

REFERENCES

1. Lidz T. *The person.* (rev. ed) New York: Basic Books. 1976;512.
2. Bureau of Labor Statistics: Labor Force Participation of Older Men. In: Moody HR (ed). *Aging: Concepts and controversies.* Thousand Oaks, Calif: Pine Forge Press. 1994;298–300.
3. ibid.
4. ibid, p. 303.
5. Moody HR (ed). *Aging: Concepts and controversies.* Thousand Oaks, Calif: Pine Forge Press. 1994;300.
6. ibid.
7. Ekerdt DJ. The busy ethic: Moral continuity between work and retirement. In: Moody HR (ed). *Aging: Concepts and controversies.* Thousand Oaks, Calif: Pine Forge Press. 1994;334.
8. ibid, p. 329.
9. ibid, p. 330.
10. ibid.
11. ibid, p. 334.
12. Lidz T. *The person.* (rev. ed) New York: Basic Books. 1976;521.
13. ibid, p. 525.
14. Erikson EH. *Childhood and society.* (2nd ed) New York: Norton. 1963;268.
15. Lidz T. *The person.* (rev. ed) New York: Basic Books. 1976;512.
16. ibid, p. 514.
17. Butler RN, Lewis MI. *Aging and mental health.* (2nd ed) St. Louis: Mosby. 1977;ix.
18. Siegel JS. Recent and prospective demographic trends for the elderly population and some implications for health care. In: *Second conference on the epidemiology of aging.* Washington, DC: US Department of Health and Human Services. 1980;309.
19. Minkler M. Generational equity and the new victim blaming: Critical perspectives on aging. In: Minkler M, Esters C (eds). *The political and moral economy of aging.* Amityville, NY: Baywood Publishing Company. 1991;67–79.
20. ibid.
21. Siegel JS. Recent and prospective demographic trends for the elderly population and some implications for health care. In: *Second conference on the epidemiology of aging.* Washington, DC: US Department of Health and Human Services. 1980;309.
22. Daniels N. *Just health care.* Cambridge, Mass: Cambridge University Press. 1985; 14–15, 90–96.
23. Atchley RC. Aging and suicide: Reflection on the quality of life? In: *Second conference on the epidemiology of aging.* Washington, DC: US Department of Health and Human Services. 1980;141.

24. ibid, p. 143.
25. Annas G et al. *The rights of doctors, nurses and allied health professionals.* New York: Avon. 1981;80.
26. ibid, p. 81.
27. ibid.
28. ibid.
29. Barry V. *Moral aspects of health care.* Belmont, Calif: Wadsworth. 1982;3.
30. ibid.
31. ibid.
32. ibid, p. 266–267.
33. Rawls J. *A theory of justice.* Cambridge, Mass: Harvard University Press. 1971.
34. Mill JS. *Utilitarianism.* Indianapolis: The Liberal Arts Press. 1957;14.
35. ibid, p. 76.
36. Kant I. *Fundamental principles of the metaphysics of morals.* Indianapolis: Liberal Arts Press. 1949;46.
37. Childress J. Who shall live when all cannot live? *Soundings* 1970;53:339–355.
38. Veatch R. What is a "just" health care delivery? In: Veatch R, Branson R (eds). *Ethics and health policy.* Cambridge, Mass: Ballinger. 1976;134.
39. Macklin R. *Man, mind, and morality: The ethics of behavior control.* Englewood Cliffs, NJ: Prentice-Hall. 1982;90, 91–95.
40. Annas G et al. *The rights of doctors, nurses and allied health professionals.* New York: Avon. 1981;80–81.
41. ibid.
42. Plato. *Republic.* (GMA Grube, trans.) Indianapolis: Hackett. 1974;5–6.
43. Feinberg J. *Social philosophy.* Englewood Cliffs, NJ: Prentice-Hall. 1973;50–51.
44. Moody HR. *Ethics in an aging society.* Baltimore: Johns Hopkins University Press. 1992;34.
45. ibid, p. 34–35.
46. ibid, p. 34–38.
47. Kant I. *Fundamental principles of the metaphysics of morals.* Indianapolis: Liberal Arts Press. 1949;46.
48. Rogers PD, Bocchino NL. Restraint-free care: Is it possible? *Am J Nurs* 1999;99(10): 27–33.
49. ibid.
50. ibid.
51. ibid.
52. ibid.
53. ibid.
54. ibid.
55. Lynch SH. Elder abuse: What to look for, how to intervene. *Am J Nurs* 1977;97(1): 27–30.
56. New York State Nurses Association. Position Statement: Patient abuse, neglect, and maltreatment in nursing homes. 1993.
57. Lynch SH. Elder abuse: What to look for, how to intervene. *Am J Nurs* 1977;97(1): 27–30.
58. New York State Nurses Association. Position Statement: Patient abuse, neglect, and maltreatment, 1993.
59. Kohnke M. *Advocacy: Risk and reality.* St. Louis: Mosby. 1982;5.
60. ibid, p. 2.

61. ibid, p. 5.
62. American Nurses Association. *Code for nurses with interpretive statements.* Kansas City, Mo; 1976;8.
63. ibid, p. 4.
64. Annas G. Remarks on the law-medicine relation: A philosophical critique. Presented at: Trans-Disciplinary Symposium on Philosophy and Medicine. Farmington, Conn: University of Connecticut Health Center. November 11, 1978.

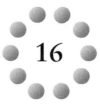

16

Ethical Issues in the Nursing Care of the Dying

Study of this chapter enables the learner to:

1. Apply ethical principles of respect for the dignity and worth of the dying person.
2. Advocate for the individual's right to accept, refuse, or terminate treatment.
3. Evaluate ethical principles for the relief of suffering versus the principle of double effect, ordinary versus extraordinary treatment, the active versus passive distinction, voluntary versus involuntary euthanasia, and suicide.
4. Counsel clients in the provisions of the living will and organ donation.
5. Distinguish between definitions of circulatory and respiratory death.
6. Respect the religious values and practices of the patient and family.
7. Implement supportive physical and psychological care to the dying patient.

OVERVIEW

Although nurses are intimately involved with the care of the dying, to be a nurse in every important sense of that term is to be on the side of a good quality of life. The profession and the activities of nursing support the most fundamental value beliefs of human beings. These values are two-fold:

1. We want to live well as persons.
2. We want nurses and physicians to help us live a long, healthy, and happy life.

This simple means-ends belief was a reasonable goal throughout nursing and medical history. Until recent times, intense and continuous skilled nursing care was the only hope of saving lives. There were no miracle drugs, radical surgery, or life-sustaining machines. Beyond using heat, cold, food, fluid, rest, and a sanitary environment, nurses and physicians relied on the natural healing powers of the body. If the body failed to heal and the patient died despite the efforts of nurses and physicians, the conditions of the professional means-ends value statement had been met. Nurses and physicians fulfilled their moral obligations on the side of life. Their power was simply not equal to the strength of the disease, and their sense of moral obligation was reinforced by the nature of the struggle against death.

The leading causes of death in the United States are now heart disease, cancer, and cerebrovascular disease. These diseases are progressive and occur in later life. The affected individual is usually receiving health care and medical interventions. With the advent of "miracle" drugs, radical surgery, and life-sustaining technologies available in hospitals, persons with heretofore life-threatening prognoses are now seeking continuation of life and improved functioning.

The capacity to prolong life and to ease the plight of dying patients has improved to the extent that almost all acutely ill and seriously ill persons are hospitalized. As a consequence, most deaths now occur in institutions.[1]

MEANINGS AND DEFINITIONS OF DEATH

Increasingly, death comes quietly in the presence of the blinking lights of the monitors, pumps, drips, and suctions of critical care units. Under such conditions, death is impersonal. It appears to be merely a separation of body from tubes and machines. Death may be due to someone's decision, rather than the failure of the heart to pump blood. There is only a deteriorating organ system present. In some cases, the essence of the patient has long been absent. The family has exhausted its grief during the prolonged period when the patient was neither responsive nor dying, seemingly neither dead nor alive. The family aches for resolution of an ambiguous situation in which neither grief nor hope is appropriate. The family longs to resume normal feelings, responses, and living.

Nurses are central characters in these dramas intimately and continuously involved with the dying patient and significant others. This care involves the coordination of nursing with health care services of other disciplines, medicine particularly, on behalf of the patient. Care of the dying may require prolonged close contact with the dying person's family and friends. Those who are concerned may look to the nurse for guidance or information that will be helpful in reaching decisions of life-and-death proportions. Thus, one function of the nurse is to facilitate communication and the dissemination of information among all the participants involved in the care of the dying person. Another function is to be an advocate for dying patients, who quite often are unable to talk or to fend for themselves.

Definitions of Death
Deciding what death is depends on one of two definitions: irreversible cessation of respiration and circulation, or "irreversible cessation of all functions of the brain."[2] A brain-death definition is appealed to for deciding vegetative cases, in which "cerebral silence" is a basis for donating organs for transplant.

The concept of death masks an ambiguity between the heart and brain definitions. The brain-death definition affords more latitude for bodily experimentation and transplant uses than the heart-death definition. Because "there is no possibility that a person fitting the brain-death criteria "will return to useful life,"[3] by identifying such beings as dead, one is then morally free to treat the remains as one treats other objects. If such a moral policy is generally adopted, it provides a ringing tribute to a 17th century philosopher, René Descartes (1596–1650), who said that for a human being to exist is to think, and that for a human being not to think is not to exist.

A practical difficulty is that by ruling that if one organ is dead then the organism is dead, one is free to use the "dead" as means for other ends on the assumption that cerebral activity defines the person. The question is: Can one be a non-thinking person? If the answer is "No," then the brain-death definition is morally acceptable, with all of its social and economic consequences, including elitism. If, however, the answer is "Yes," then the world will soon be overpopulated with mindless or brainless beings who may morally not be tampered with because they are not yet regarded as dead. However, they are cared for by others and receive the benefit of resources.

The growing appeal of the brain-death definition is not only a tribute to Descartes, it is also a way of showing the role of the mind-body problem in relation to health care ethics. Although people now speak of the brain in place of the mind, the two are equivalent, at least on the identity theory, which holds that the mind is nothing more than a brain state. Second, the mind-body problem of showing how the body and the brain or mind are related is also a basic presupposition of teaching right from wrong and of practicing health care ethics. For if our brains and bodies were different, then our ethics would be also. If we had the brains of bats, we might have no ethics. We could expect either more or less responsibility from one another if we had either greater or fewer mental capacities. We are defined by our minds and by our being recognized as persons.

SELECTED CASES AND PRINCIPLES INVOLVING NURSING JUDGMENTS AND ACTIONS

We cite the following cases to illustrate moral issues in the care of dying persons.

CASE 16.1: A Case of Active-Passive Euthanasia.   A baby with Down syndrome "was born with an intestinal obstruction at Johns Hopkins Hospital. The parents . . . refused to give consent to surgical repair of the duodenal obstruction. The infant could not be fed and died within 15 days."[4]

Two issues arise in this case. First, if Nurse A believes in the infant's right to life, and Nurse B believes that the parents have a right to decide, what argument is there for either side? Second, in this case, is passive euthanasia morally equivalent to active euthanasia?

CASE 16.2: A Case of Active Euthanasia.   Sandy, age 5, had a malignant brain tumor, and underwent three major operations. The scars on her head looked like zippers. Her condition worsened and she slipped into a coma. Her mother, distraught, attempted suicide. The nurse said, "One night, Sandy stopped breathing . . . and some nut jumped on her chest and her heart started beating again." She was put on a respirator. When infection developed, the doctors gave her antibiotics. Nurse A said the child's arm looked "like a pincushion. She was black and blue. Nothing worked. She smelled like decaying flesh. She had been such a pretty little girl. . . . I went into her room to bathe her. This time, I closed the door, took her off the respirator, bathed her and powdered her. I hooked her up again, but her heart had stopped. I felt relief."[5]

In this case, Nurse A committed active euthanasia. What if you were Nurse B and learned about Nurse A, what would your response be?

CASE 16.3: Should the Plug Be Pulled?   Jack, age 14, was injured in a football accident and was comatose for 2 months. Jack's mother asks the nurse to "just un-plug the respirator. . . ." The physician, who has not discussed this case with the parents, . . . has adopted a "wait and see" attitude because he knows of a similar case where a patient on a respirator is now back in school.[6]

This case illustrates a conflict between the mother and the physician. Nurse A believes her role is to inform the mother that she has a right to know the patient's diagnosis, prognosis, treatment, risks, and alternatives as the basis for accepting, terminating, or refusing care. The physician is the best source for this information. Nurse B believes that she should not comply with the mother's wishes.

CASE 16.4: A Patient's Right to Know the Truth.   Carolyn, age 21, is dying of leukemia. She wants to know what is happening to her. However, her devoted mother believes in shielding Carolyn from this prognosis. Nurse A believes her client, who repeatedly asks about her worsening signs and symptoms, has a right to know the truth. Carolyn's mother, a wealthy, influential woman, threatens to sue the hospital if her daughter finds out that she's dying. Nurse A wishes to support the pa-tient's right to know the truth. Nurse B wishes to acquiesce to the mother's wishes.

CASE 16.5: The Right to Suicide.   Tom, age 26, is a brilliant and handsome young man who has contracted AIDS and is dying. His family, friends, and lover have abandoned him because of fear of contagion. Nurse Smith, a community health nurse, finds a lethal supply of barbiturates in the drawer of his bedside table in the course of her nursing care. Should the nurse confiscate the pills or confront the patient?

This case illustrates a conflict for both patient and the nurse. If Nurse Smith believes in the self-determination rights of patients, she may perceive her role as letting the patient take the barbiturates at will. If, however, she sees herself as pro-tecting the best interest of the patient, then she may see her role as removing the drugs. Using a counterfactual conditional judgment, if you were the nurse, what do you think would be the right thing to do, and what reasons would you give to support your position?

CASE 16.6: An Adult's Right to Die.   Mr. C, age 40, is blind and has end-stage renal failure due to diabetes. He wants to die. When Mr. C has a cardiac arrest, he is resuscitated in accordance with hospital policy. Despite his protests, Mr. C is re-suscitated several more times. The hospital authorities contend that life must be preserved and this is their policies. Mr. C's family then sues the hospital on behalf of his right to die. By this time, Mr. C has become comatose. The hospital is finally required by the court to comply with Mr. C's wishes.[7]

Three nurses discuss Mr. C's right to die versus the hospital's moral and legal duty to preserve life. Nurse A takes the position that Mr. C's right to die is his alone and must be honored. Nurse B maintains that hospital staff members have no right to commit murder. Nurse C says that the physician ought to decide. In this case, which nurse is right, and on what moral grounds?

CASE 16.7: Who Decides Not to Resuscitate?

Mrs. W, age 50, has burns over 50% of her body. She has been alert, cheerful, happy, and positive. When Nurse A returned to her room after an hour, Mrs. W was not breathing. "I decided not to call a code. . . . I remembered the doctor saying 'Her spirits are good, but I still don't think she'll make it, but . . .' There would have been so much pain, and there was practically no chance that she would have survived the burns."[8] Nurse A told Dr. C and he decided not to resuscitate, because he did not know how much time had elapsed since Mrs. W had stopped breathing.

Unlike Mr. C in Case 16.6, Mrs. W had not expressed a wish to die. Would an additional lifesaving effort have been morally justified in this case? Nurse B believes so, but not Nurse A, who knew Mrs. W better and found her not breathing. Who is right ethically and why?

CASE 16.8: Honoring the Patient's Wishes for a "Do Not Resuscitate" Directive.

Ms. M is a 52-year-old woman who faces surgery for a possible malignancy of the brain. She has asked not to be resuscitated. The order was written on her chart. When she suffered a cardiac arrest following surgery in which an inoperable cancer was found, the nurse resuscitated her. The result was that after 3 days, the kidneys she wished to donate were unusable.[9]

This case, unlike the case of Mr. C, could have resulted in a kidney transplant, which might have aided some other person. Was the nurse wrong to resuscitate the patient? On what grounds do you base your decision?

CASE 16.9: Paternalism versus Libertarianism.

Mr. W, age 75, was admitted to a community hospital with pneumonia, advanced pulmonary edema, urinary tract infection, and anemia. He did not respond well to treatment, but his wife asked that everything be done for him. On the fourteenth day, he stopped breathing. Nurse A, on finding him, reported that "vital signs were absent." She summoned Dr. B, who immediately gave a "do not resuscitate" order. The cause of death was recorded as ventricular fibrillation. Mr. W had not been sent to the intensive care unit "due to a shortage of beds." Dr. B said afterwards, "I saw no sense calling Code Blue with a 75-year-old who has no future to look forward to. That's doing him a disservice with increasing hospital costs."[10] Nurse B disagrees with Nurse A and Dr. B.

In this case, should Nurse A have called Code Blue instead of calling Dr. B? Was Dr. B "playing God" or responding to medical reality? But then why did Dr. B make a gratuitous observation about Mr. W having no future? And why wasn't Mr. W put in the intensive care unit where he might have had a better chance to be resuscitated? What role is there for a nurse advocate in aiding Mr. W's best interests?

RELATED ETHICAL ISSUES

Trilogy of Rights of Dying Patients

To respect a person consists in recognizing the dignity and inherent worth of that individual as being uncompromisable. Respect for persons is in some religiously oriented traditions defined as reverence for persons. Mother Theresa expressed this tradition when she said that her mission was to convert the lepers, the homeless, the poor and abandoned children, and the dying persons of Indian cities into angels. An example of respect is to treat patients in the order in which they arrive, but on the principle of treating the sickest person first. This replaces preferential treatment or unfavorable treatment based on prestige or social or economic standing. A patient's right to respect means that the patient is treated as an end, not as a means only, in Kant's sense. In that sense, the patient's right to respect includes the right to know the truth and to be told the truth insofar as it is known. A conscious patient's right to respect implies the right to informed consent prior to treatment or nontreatment. Based on a patient's right to respect, Carolyn (Case 16.4) has a right to know the truth about her diagnosis of leukemia and her imminent death. In another example, Mr. C. (Case 16.6) has a right to have his wish to die respected, as does Ms. M in Case 16.8, who does not wish to be resuscitated.

A second right, the right to receive treatment, means that a patient has the right to be given the best available treatment. The right to treatment stems from the right to respect and is a special health care right. The patient's right to treatment means that the patient is not ignored or given custodial or palliative care if more aggressive measures are needed. For example, Mr. W's right to treatment (Case 16.7) includes the right to the intensive care unit, where he would in all likelihood have been resuscitated.

The patient's right to refuse and even to terminate all treatment is an especially important right of competent patients. Such a right assumes that hospital personnel are willing to take on the legal and moral responsibility associated with the death of patients who wish to discontinue treatment. This decision implies that health professionals will accept corresponding duties, such as providing competent, compassionate care while the patient is dying. The patient's right to terminate treatment also applies to Mr. C in Case 16.6. He too has the right to have his wishes honored. So does Ms. M, the woman with a brain tumor who refused resuscitation because she wanted to donate her kidneys.

Finally, the third right of a dying patient means he or she is treated with care and comfort and not left alone. For to show respect for a dying person is to provide maximum well-being for that person as long as life is present.

ETHICAL PRINCIPLES IN THE CARE OF THE DYING

Quality Versus Length of Life

Some of the cases cited illustrate the moral issue between the principle of saving all life versus the principle of preserving only a life of quality. Those who say that all of life is a gift aim to protect all life, regardless of its quality. Others defend the idea that control of one's life and body are fundamental rights. Other individuals are likely to evaluate the quality of life and would discontinue the respirator for brain-dead patients in particular. On the other hand, deciding who shall live or die can present a serious moral dilemma. The physician in the case of Mr. W (Case 16.7) arbitrarily decided that the patient's quality of life did not warrant his admission to an intensive care unit. Those who invoke a quality-of-life argument are, in effect, playing God. Thus, a safeguard to a quality of life argument is to obtain freely given first-person consents for health professionals' interventions.

Relief of Individual Suffering versus the Principle of Double Effect

Another issue that concerns a dying patient is whether to relieve suffering in the presence of competing goals, expressed through the doctrine of *double effect* (see Chapter 3). This doctrine recommends doing the least of several evils when evil cannot be avoided. One example of double effect is that of giving a suffering terminal patient increasing doses of morphine, which relieves pain but also inhibits respiration. Pope Pius XII addressed this topic specifically in 1957. He said, "If. . .the actual administration of drugs brings about two distinct effects, one the relief of pain and the other the shortening of life, the action is lawful."[11] According to the President's Commission for the Study of Ethical Problems in Medicine and Biomedical and Behavioral Research, "health care professionals may provide treatment to relieve the symptoms of dying patients even when that treatment entails substantial risks of causing an earlier death."[12] The American Nurses Association supports this principle.

Ordinary versus Extraordinary Treatment

Treatment which at one time is extraordinary, scarce, and expensive later becomes ordinary. Antibiotics, dialysis, open-heart surgery, organ transplants, and cardiopulmonary resuscitation are examples of formerly extraordinary treatments and procedures that have become ordinary. In an important papal statement in 1957, Pope Pius XII said, "One is held to use only ordinary means—according to circumstances of persons, places, times and culture—means that do not involve any grave burden for oneself or another."[13] The Pope's statement seems to say that deciding who lives and dies, especially among elderly patients, is relative to the degree of available technology in one's time and place.

In any event, the words "ordinary" and "extraordinary" are fraught with vagueness and ambiguity. The President's Commission identifies several often confusing and conflicting meanings of terms, such as "usualness," "complexity," "invasiveness," "artificiality," "expense," or "availability."[14] The Commission prefers "useful" and "burdensome to an individual patient" as having an important advantage over other distinctions, such as "common/usual."[15] A difficulty with the useful/burdensome distinction is that despite the reference "to an individual patient," this distinction overlooks other problems. What about the burden to the physician, nurses, family members, other hospital personnel, the patient, society in general? A further question is: Who decides whether a treatment or procedure is useful or burdensome to the patient if the patient cannot speak for himself or herself?

In one standard sense of the "ordinary" and "extraordinary" distinction, the extraordinary is associated with doing for a patient something exceptional, extra, heroic, or supererogatory. On this view, "ordinary" means applying conventional procedures and treatments, which are routine. However, to associate "ordinary" medicine with "useful" medicine and "extraordinary" with "burdensome to an individual" may do a disservice to the advancement of health care. The efforts made for the recipient of the first artificial heart show that advances in health care depend occasionally on extraordinary rather than ordinary efforts. Unknown patients who selected burdensome, extraordinary means for themselves made it possible for caregivers to accumulate the experience that rendered those means ordinary. To give up the extraordinary flies in the face of the human spirit of struggling to improve the human condition. Moreover, a word like "useful" offers no great gain in clarification over "ordinary." For the minimum done for a patient might well be useless and thereby call for the maximum to be done. For example, doing what was useful in the case of Mr. W (Case 16.7) might have involved putting him in the intensive care unit, which would have been extraordinary. Because "useful" overlaps with "extraordinary," some of the same problems are likely to arise, namely what to do for a given patient when all cannot be helped?

The ethically sensitive and intellectually critical nurse will in any event not be satisfied with any distinction that is not both effective and justifiable in considering what to do or refrain from doing for a given patient. One proposed usage is to drop the distinction altogether and do one's best in every situation. With reference to cardiopulmonary resuscitation, in particular, one tries to make it commonplace, as has occurred with so much in health care. This principle implies that Mr. W be transferred to an intensive care unit, where more resources for resuscitation are available. If he still has a life of quality, his hopes and expectations are unjustifiably ended by a physician who settles for the ordinary.

In the cases of Sandy (Case 16.2), Mr. C (Case 16.6), or Ms. M (Case 16.8), these patients had no hope of recovery and treatment was refused. The appropriate thing to do is for nurses to help these people achieve a good death through compassionate, skilled nursing care. But in the case of the Johns Hopkins infant (Case 16.1) or Mr. W, where something more could have been done to improve life chances, doing more would be the good thing to do. Also, some extraordinary efforts, like those of the "nut" who resuscitated Sandy or the nurse who resuscitated Ms. M, are not good. However, countless ordinary, standard efforts are useful in helping patients.

Despite the difficulties, there are still advantages in using the ordinary/extraordinary distinction on occasion. Use of these terms sharpens one's awareness that the principle of what to do is decided on the basis of doing good and not harm.

The Active/Passive Distinction in Euthanasia

A moral issue that persists is the question whether letting a patient die is morally equivalent to killing, or is omission equivalent to commission? In 1973, the American Medical Association (AMA) House of Delegates adopted the following position on the distinction between active and passive euthanasia:

> The intentional termination of the life of one human being by another—mercy killing—is contrary to that for which the medical profession stands. . . . The cessation of . . . extraordinary means to prolong the life of the body when there is irrefutable evidence that biological death is imminent is the decision of the patient and/or his immediate family.[16]

Killing is wrong, but letting die in the sense of not exercising extraordinary efforts or discontinuing extraordinary efforts is morally permissible, according to the AMA.

Rachels, a philosopher, argued that the distinction between active and passive euthanasia is a distinction without a morally justifiable difference. Whether one drowns someone directly or does nothing to prevent a person from drowning, both the act and the omission are morally equivalent if the intent and result are the same. Rachels cites the example of the case of the Johns Hopkins infant with Down syndrome (Case 16.1) whose parents refused to give consent for surgical repair of a duodenal atresia.[17] The pediatrician mother defended her refusal to consent on the ground that omitting to help is not morally wrong, unlike outright killing. Rachels argues that not saving the infant is equivalent to murder if the intent and the result are the same. If killing a Down syndrome infant is murder, then so is letting it die by refusing to perform minor lifesaving surgery. Rachels compares two hypothetical cases involving the cousins Smith and Jones. Smith stands to gain a large fortune by drowning his 6-year-old cousin in the bathtub. Smith does so and covers his tracks. Jones, too, stands to gain a great deal if his cousin

---

Commonly Accepted Definitions of Euthanasia

- Euthanasia: A good death or an easy death.
- Active euthanasia: Someone other than the patient performs to act to end the person's life; e.g., a lethal injection.
- Passive euthanasia: Omitting an act that allows death to occur; e.g., to remove the ventilator.
- Voluntary euthanasia: The patient consents or requests an act of euthanasia; e.g., refusing life support treatment.
- Involuntary euthanasia: Euthanasia performed without the person's consent.
- Nonvoluntary euthanasia: Euthanasia performed on persons unable to consent, such as comatose patients or anencephalic infants. The decision is made by one's family.
- Suicide: The intended termination of one's life, usually in the form of a lethal medication.
- Physician-assisted suicide: The aid, generally in the form of a lethal medication, that a physician is willing and able to give that enables rational persons who desire to die to terminate their life.

drowns. Jones's cousin slips and falls in the bathtub and drowns while Jones stands by passively. Rachels argues that there is no moral difference between them if the intentions and results are the same.[18]

One may present the counterargument that the Jones cousin died by himself without assistance, and that Jones or the nurse or physician did not actively kill the patient. Rachels's active/passive equivalence may apply to those cases in which the active/passive distinction is used as a pretext for failure to save a life. But there are other types of cases in which there is a morally important difference between killing and letting die.

The case of Sandy (Case 16.2), who was in a irreversible and terminal coma, is an example of the nurse's deliberate shutting off the respirator to end the child's life. Using counterfactual conditional judgments, had she not done so, the child's life would have continued for an indefinite time. Although, in this case, the prognosis was hopeless and irreversible, the saying, "Where there is life, there is hope," has its truth value. In some cases, killing is worse than not interfering with death. To not interfere with death, in contrast to active euthanasia, implies the possibility that a patient might recover, go into a remission, or survive long enough for a new and effective treatment to be discovered. Insulin, for example, has saved the lives of diabetes patients. To not interfere with dying rather than practicing active euthanasia may "buy time" for a patient. That time may be spent in pointless suffering, or it may be a meaningful, enriching experience.

The flaw in Rachels's argument is that the intent and the consequences in either passive or active euthanasia are not always the same. In those cases, like the infant in Case 16.1 for whom refusal to consent is used as a pretext for killing, killing and letting die are identical. Although many patients in cardiopulmonary intensive care units will probably die, such patients are better off if dying is not interfered with, rather if they are killed outright. For not to interfere with dying, rather than killing, may effectively result in letting live. Without the active/passive distinction, one could argue that a dying patient may as well be killed, because not interfering with dying and killing are equivalent. In Case 16.3, for example, involving Jack, the comatose football player, if the nurse refuses to pull the plug, then Jack might be back in school in another 6 months. We do not know; nor does the mother, the nurse, or the physician.

The case of Sandy presents a morally defensible case for preferring killing to not interfering with dying. But whether the nurse had the right to decide to remove Sandy from the respirator is an issue for further careful reflection. Without consulting the family and allied health professionals, such an act may be one of individual arrogance and arbitrariness. Decisions based on reflective dialogue are preferable to decisions made by individuals without consultation. In situations involving unbearable pain and futile prognosis, killing to shorten an unbearably painful dying process may be morally preferable to prolonging dying. Such a case was that of Charles Wertenberger.

> Mr. Wertenberger, upon learning that he was terminally ill, decided to bear the test of pain and live as full a life as possible as long as it was a meaningful one. In the end, he takes his own life in the company of, and assisted by his wife. . . .[19]

Nursing activities are aimed at effective intervention for improving both the quality and the length of life. The processes and goals show that not interfering with dying is, on the whole, morally preferable to killing.

Making omissions morally equivalent to commissions places too heavy a burden on health professionals, one that they cannot possibly carry. Omission may avoid the pain and expense of a useless procedure, because the disease is the murderer, and not the inactive spectator.

Moreover, the use of such words as "allow to die," "permit to die," or "let die" is a dubious linguistic practice. Although these phrases are frequently heard, there is a difference between (a) a health professional who does not interfere with a patient's dying, and (b) a health professional who allows a patient to die by deciding for the patient when life supports are to be terminated (an example of paternalist behavior). There is a distinction between decisions (a) and (b). Choosing (a) demonstrates a health professional's recognition that a patient's life and death are the patient's ultimate right to decide and not a prerogative of health professionals. Choosing (b) implies or suggests that health professionals decide when a patient may die. If patients have any rights at all, they have rights to decide whether life support systems that are likely to be futile may be withdrawn. That decision belongs to the patient, not to the nurse and physician. The person who allows or permits decides. The person who is "allowed" has a privilege, but not a right, therefore, dying patients alone have the right to decide to refuse or to terminate life-sustaining supports of all kinds. The patient does the allowing, or permitting, or letting, not the health professionals. Thus, it is a linguistic mistake to characterize a health care decision not to interfere with a patient's dying as being a case of allowing a patient to die, as if one were giving a dying person permission. The role of health care providers is not to authorize patients to die, but to help enable them to die.

Advance Directives

To offset the problem of health professionals not knowing their patients' wishes regarding life-sustaining treatment, written and updated advance directives are essential to the protection of patients' rights. One model, the *Living Will Declaration* (see Appendix) directs that such life-sustaining procedures as cardiopulmonary resuscitation and support, antibiotics, and artificially administered food and fluids be withheld or withdrawn in case of illness, disease, injury, or mental and physical deterioration that is without hope of recovery or of "regaining a meaningful quality of life."[20] Finally, a federal law, the Patient Self-Determination Act (1991), requires all health care facilities to advise patients upon admission of their rights to accept or reject lifesaving measures if there is no hope of recovery. Patient's wishes are required to be documented and honored. The widespread use of advance directives would reduce health care costs and help patients, family members, and health care providers to set realistic goals and preferences while respecting patients' choices and wishes.

Durable power of attorney statutes exist in all 50 states. These statutes delegate the legal authority to act on the principal's behalf after the principal becomes incapacitated.[21] The power is designated primarily regarding property, but in some states the power may be extended to health care decisions. Appointing a health care agent to make medical decisions when patients cannot speak for themselves is important because that person can interpret and clarify a patient's wishes in specific circumstances.

Each of these advance directives can be used legally to withdraw or withhold artificial feeding if not prohibited by state law. As these restrictions are challenged, there is an emerging consensus that artificial feeding is a life-sustaining treatment that may be refused like any other treatment in accordance with the patient's preference.[22]

Organ Donations

A person's willingness to donate usable organs, as with the woman with the brain tumor who wished to donate her kidneys (Case 16.8), shows how people can help one another. However, views differ on the moral permissibility of organ transplants or of the transfer of any bodily tissue. Jehovah's Witnesses, for example, object to the transfer of any bodily tissue, including blood transfusion, and consider such a transfer as a moral impurity.[23] Some religious and metaphysical views of the organism have held that all the organs naturally belong to a given organism, not to any other.[24] Others compare a person's body with machinery and find nothing wrong with replacing defective parts. Still others, out of respect for donors, impose restrictions on transplants. The patient's right to respect requires free and fully informed consent from the donor or nearest of kin, as with any other intrusion into the body.

A morally favorable attitude toward organ transplants may be found by appealing to utilitarianism, which looks to the greatest happiness of the greatest number. A positive attitude toward organ transplants also consists in appealing to Christian love-based ethics as well as a metaphysical organicist's view, which holds that we are all part of the cosmic process and that nothing is impure. With appropriate safeguards of donors' and recipients' rights, more good than harm is served by favoring organ donations and transplants. The waiting list for transplant applicants has increased tremendously, with the availability in very short supply.

The nurse plays an important role in the altruistic donation of an organ of a brain-dead patient by communicating with appropriate authorities before the organs deteriorate. Moreover, the nurse can be supportive of the family by emphasizing the generosity of this contribution to others as "a gift of life" and a positive experience.

Applying Personhood to "Do Not Resuscitate" Orders: Tracing and Examining Arguments for Appropriate Metaphors and Models

A philosophical move, which may be helpful in deciding what nurses are to do about "do not resuscitate" orders, is to consider a viewpoint and trace it to some acknowledged metaphor, analogy, or comparison on which defense of that viewpoint depends. One may compare a comatose person either to a vegetable or to a spiritual object, such as an angel. One may compare a bedridden 75-year-old man to a piece of useless dead wood or to a wise ruler. One examines the metaphor to determine how it applies or breaks down in practice and in practical discourse. So if one is a vegetable, he or she cannot be a person. A comatose individual who after being "on a respirator for 8 months is now back in school,"[25] to cite a case against "pulling the plug," shows that such an individual is not necessarily or always a vegetable. Such a case refutes the metaphor of a given person being a vegetable, and provides a counterexample to the advisability of "pulling the plug," as Jack's mother wanted the nurse to do in Case 16.3. Thus, one tests an analogy to see if it applies in practical discourse. Questions of truth or falsity arise here. One considers whether supplementary or alternative metaphors or analogies aid in defense of a given viewpoint.

In regard to a comatose or dying patient, one may ask the question, "Does patient X own his or her body?" If X owns her or his body, then X has the right to control what happens in and to her or his body, including, importantly, the right to refuse all treatment such as the right to forego resuscitation. To own property is to have authority over what one owns. If individuals do not own their bodies and lives, and if life is to be taken only by the "one who gives life," then health professionals are obligated not to cause death.

The point is that each metaphor may be examined for its illumination and practical applicability as well as for its implied difficulties. Life, for example, is not always a gift, as the cases of Sandy (Case 16.2) or Mr. C (Case 16.6) amply show. Yet, life was regarded as a gift by Mrs. W (Case 16.7), who spoke on her husband's behalf; and life is regarded for most of us most of the time as a gift, which reveals Aquinas's insight. However, one can also see how Aquinas's metaphor of life as a gift breaks down when it comes up against some hard cases, such as some of those cited here.

On the other hand, human life is not quite like someone's property or factory, with which one can do anything one wishes. A person with a contagious disease can be quarantined, for example. There are dangers in both extremes. Trying to save everyone has counterproductive consequences, because too many malfunctioning or nonfunctioning beings cannot support the growing demands of sustaining life now or in the future. On the other hand, playing God by deciding who has the required quality of life and therefore who lives or dies also reveals a serious moral pitfall of arbitrarily abridging the equal rights of individuals to decide whether to live or die. People's rights to informed consent are crucial to their "rational life plans," whatever else they may want, according to Rawls.

However, let's take a closer look at Ms. M (Case 16.8). The patient asks the nurse not to resuscitate her under certain circumstances. To comply with this patient's right to die requires the nurse—on the view that all life is a gift—to commit murder. But is it murder? It is not, if that life is no longer a gift to that person.[26] In hopelessly terminal cases, if we consult the patients' most fundamental interests as friends, in Aristotle's sense, we might then recognize that because their life prospects are hopeless, were we in our friends' place, we would not consider life a gift. To be a friend in that type of hopeless case is to help, even if it means ending our friend's life, as Freud's physician was willing to do at Freud's request. If a nurse does not resuscitate a terminal patient who has asked not to be resuscitated, we would not think it wrong.[27] The appeal of such rights is not to the older view of option rights, which says, "Don't interfere," but the newer view of rights, which says,

"Help me, care for me." A view of rights that addresses a patient's or nurse's vital, rational interests seems the more adequate at certain key moments in one's life. These deeper rights to live well are associated with a good life and provide the conditions for effectively exercising one's freedom. But if it is not already evident, a defense of such rights comes down on the side of a life of quality, but not without the constraints one finds with well-considered rights, such as the test of other people's retrospective judgments.

To have rights is to have a form of moral standing. With rights, such as one's right to an earned paycheck, one knows where one stands. In health care, a resulting trilogy of patients' rights includes the right to be treated with respect, to receive treatment, and to refuse treatment. These rights are vitally important to one's moral standing as a person, regardless of whether one is a dying patient refusing resuscitation, a nurse, or a physician. Beyond that, rights break down in the recognition that tragedy and stalemate, too, are aspects of the ethical life of persons, which no formalization or objectivity can overcome.

VOLUNTARY AND INVOLUNTARY EUTHANASIA

A related issue to that of active versus passive euthanasia or between killing and letting die is between voluntary and involuntary euthanasia. We all die, but when and under what circumstances is not always known. Some people die suddenly[28]; others die with time to prepare for their death within a finite time frame, ranging from a few days to a few years. In the case of Karen, a 16-year-old adolescent who refused further dialysis, her death involved her decision, consent, and wish. Tragic and terrible as death is for a 16-year-old, respect for her rationality and letting her decide shows that she died with informed consent, and thus illustrates voluntary euthanasia. One cannot apply voluntary euthanasia to a neonate or to a demented person or to a comatose person. One can, however, consider how they would like to be treated. For this purpose, nearest of kin are given the power of proxy consent or what is called "substitute judgment."

The principle of voluntary euthanasia may be stated as follows: Whenever possible, consult the patient's wishes concerning the manner and procedures leading to that patient's death, including the withdrawal or withholding of life-sustaining treatment. Mr. C's wish to terminate treatment and die was ignored (Case 16.6), thus violating the principle of voluntary euthanasia. However, the case of Jack (Case 16.3) leaves us with a dilemma, because the parent wants a course of action taken, namely active euthanasia, that may not express the patient's preferences, and would thus violate the principle of voluntary euthanasia.

An advantage of applying the principle of voluntary euthanasia is that one treats a dying person as a rational being to be honored and respected as a person. Such treatment of a person exerts a moral barrier against other persons, such as family members, health professionals, or officials, who would decide who lives and dies and under what circumstances. In this connection, voluntary euthanasia is said to constitute a necessary condition of a good death.

In those cases in which patients have no opportunity to exercise voluntary euthanasia, one tries to do the next best thing, which is to consider what the patient in a rational frame of mind would want done.

Suicide

Suicide is of particular concern to health professionals, who may be in a position to prevent it. Some cultures, religions, and individuals oppose suicide under all conditions. "Life is a gift," which no one has a right to take, summarizes their position. In the cases cited, Tom (Case 16.5) is morally wrong to attempt suicide, because it is unnatural or contrary to the moral law or to the law of a religion. Suicide, it is said, is evil. One practical argument against suicide is that if everyone who felt like committing suicide acted on such a feeling, there would be no human beings left.[29]

Some cultures, such as the Japanese, and some individuals favor suicide over other negative values, such as dishonor. When Shakespeare's Brutus becomes aware that he will be marched through the streets of Rome in disgrace as a vanquished general, he prefers suicide. Cho-Cho-San in Puccini's opera *Madame Butterfly* prefers suicide to dishonor as a rejected and abandoned woman in 19th-century Japanese culture.

The topic of suicide holds a fascination, partly morbid and partly concern, with fundamental questions of being. Hamlet's question "to be or not to be" affects everyone in this curiously morbid way. Hamlet, who at one time thinks he cannot right the wrong of his father's murder by his uncle, seriously considers suicide. Albert Camus, who thinks all of life is absurd and without hope of a future, does not seem to object to suicide. Other thinkers, such as William James, regard life as worthwhile. Others think that prematurely "cashing in one's chips" is a "failure of nerve," a departure from the robust. Still other thinkers, like Hume, Schopenhauer, and Mill, regard the decision to commit suicide as each person's private business, and immune from moral and legal censure. According to Schopenhauer, to say suicide is wrong is "mere twaddle," for "no one has a greater right over anything in the world than over his own person and life."[30] Schopenhauer additionally thought it ridiculous to pass laws against suicide, because those who make a successful attempt can never be punished.

Is suicide right or wrong? In some types of cases it is wrong. In other types of cases, in which it is regarded as the only alternative to prolonged futile suffering, as in Karen's case (previously mentioned), it does not seem to be wrong. The case of Tom, the 26-year-old with AIDS (Case 16.6) presents a dilemma. . . . with good arguments on both sides of the suicide issue but no conclusively right or wrong answer.

Suicide per se may not be wrong or right; it may be that other conditions accompanying suicide help us to judge whether a given suicide is right or wrong. In this process, it helps to clarify the point that suicide is a self-regarding, self-inflicted death, which occasionally depends on assistance from others.

There are two analogies for a reflective nurse to consider in questions of suicidal patients. One analogy is that human beings are compared to property owners who may dispose of their bodies as they wish. On this view, suicide is morally permissible. More precisely, whether one commits suicide is neither moral nor immoral, but is amoral and up to each person to decide. A second analogy is one in which human bodies are compared to property, only this time belonging to someone else. If life is either a gift or on loan in this sense, one may not do with one's body as one wishes. Instead, one depends on a higher benefactor to decide the time of death. Neither view seems free of difficulties. Surely, one cannot do anything one pleases, even with one's life and body. Airplane hijackers who threaten to blow themselves up along with their hostages provide an example against the individual property view. Secondly, life for some people, like 16-year-old Karen cited in Chapter 11, is no longer a gift, but rather a burden which they do not wish to keep. Suicide, then, has not been shown to be morally right or wrong. It is an issue about which reasonable health professionals and patients may disagree.

Rational Suicide

The right to die, that is intentional self-killing, raises urgent issues. Clinical medicine is contributing to the rise of morbidity by prolonging the lives of the very sick, the disabled, the elderly, and the frail. Moody, an ethicist in geriatrics, holds that "suicide must be recognized as a serious and legitimate answer, and not merely a symptom of individual depression or a failure to provide some needed human services. We need to treat the question with the full seriousness it deserves and assume that suicide can be a rational decision . . . in the sense that it is an intelligible life choice, the outcome of a process of deliberation."[31]

For Prado, important conditions necessary for suicide to be considered rational are unimpaired reasoning, well-grounded personal values, and the consistency of those values and interests with suicide.[32] This view of suicide is in conflict with the beliefs of some mental health professionals who doubt that any suicide can be reasonable. Moody views this position to be plausible if applied to the suicides of young or middle-aged people with external obligations and relationships.[33] Circumstances and conditions that prompt the young and middle-aged toward suicide may be temporary and change. For this group, suicide before old age violently cuts off the natural life span.[34]

Moody views suicide in the elderly as quite a different matter. He asks that if the elderly person has lived a "full life" (assuming that one knows what that means), has fulfilled external obligations, and now faces infirmity and decline, then there should be no the objection to the old person's rational choice of suicide as the form of death.[35] The first argument Moody offers to justify rational suicide by the elderly person is the balance sheet argument, which he defines as the balance of pleasure and pain to be the criterion of a life worth living.[36] Here the losses and gains of living longer are weighed and suicide is justified if the losses outweigh the gains.[37] (This kind of thinking may be the argument that motivates patients with advanced AIDS to commit suicide in preference to the painful and debilitating progression of the infection.) This argument can also be used on altruistic grounds in the dread of being a burden on others. Moody points to the danger of using the utilitarian principle to justify obligatory suicide in old age to maximize the greatest happiness for the greatest number.[38] Yet, Moody's balance sheet argument concerning pain and pleasure is reminiscent of utilitarianism.

CASE 16.10: Rational Physician-Assisted Suicide. Ms. Smith, a woman in her mid-80s and in the terminal stage of cancer, met the Oregon state requirements for assisted suicide. She filled out a one-page form, "Request for medication to end my life in a humane and dignified manner." Two physicians confirmed that she had less than 6 months to live. Lying in her own bed, she took some pills prescribed by her physician, sipped some brandy, lay back in her bed and, surrounded by her family, quietly died. Only 15 people, 8 men and 7 women, were helped to die in 1998, the first year of the law. Thirteen of these were cancer patients and many, their doctors said, "were decisive personalities, or people acting on long-held principles."[39] The Oregon State Health Division found "no run on death, no confusion and no abuse as a result of the law."

Kant (discussed in Chapter 4) rejects this argument as inconsistent with his principle of absolute value that views the human being as "an absolute or unconditional end in itself."[40]

> "But a man is not a thing, that is something which can be used merely as a means but must in all his actions be always considered as an end in himself. I cannot, therefore, dispose in any way of a man in my own person so as to mutilate him, to damage or kill him."[41]

Moody's quality of life argument goes back to the stoics and Socrates discussed in Chapter 3, who, if forced, chose to live well rather than long. When Crito asks Socrates, "Don't you have a duty to save yourself if you can?" Socrates answers "The point, my dear Crito, is not simply to live, but to live well."[42] Aristotle later identified happiness with "living well."[43] Several centuries later, Seneca, another ancient Greek said,

> Mere living is not a good, but living well. Accordingly, the wise man will live as long as he ought, not as long as he can. . . . It is not a question of dying earlier or later, but of dying well or ill. And dying well means escape from the danger of living ill.[44]

The quality of life principle is frequently used to justify refusal or termination of life-sustaining interventions or for the act of suicide itself by the incurably or terminally ill, and some elderly people. Moody offers a counterargument to "rational suicide" couched in the very thinking of the stoics "that only the things within our power are our proper concern. Whatever fate may inflict by way of loss of fortune, bodily ills, or other contingencies, the intrinsic freedom of the mind remains untouched. . . . The good life is entirely a matter of this inner attitude and awareness, not of external circumstances at all."[45]

Moody presents two puzzling sentences about the notion of "rational suicide." (He is not alone in using this phrase.) He says "rational old age suicide is wrong because it violates deep values of community, relationships, solidarity, and indeed an intergenerational ideal of the human life cycle."[46] The second puzzling sentence is, "Rational suicide on grounds of age is less rational than at first it seems to be."[47] Without the qualifier "rational," one could understand both of Moody's sentences and agree or disagree with them. But the word "rational" makes the first of these sentences contradictory. If "rational" means right, then rational suicide cannot be wrong.

Moody holds that suicide on the grounds of age rests on the belief that one can predict the future and its meaning, but old age may present pleasant surprises. Freedom at any age carries risks, but it enables the risk taker "to go on living, to say 'no' to premature closure that would put limits on our understanding of life."[48]

Assisted Suicide

CASE 16.11: A Question of Assisted Suicide.   Louis has an advanced case of AIDS despite receiving all of the useful and experimental drugs available. While he can still exert some control, Louis asks his physician of many years and the nurse of long acquaintance to assist him in committing suicide through a lethal dose of barbiturates. The physician is willing to prescribe the "sleeping medication" and sign the death certificate as AIDS-related, if the nurse is willing to instruct and assist the patient in the proper administration of the drug and provide Louis comfort while he is dying in his home. What should the nurse say and do? What are the nurse's moral grounds and reasoning?

Assisting another human being to end life remains a crime in most states along the courts' repeated conclusion "that termination of life-sustaining treatment is not homicide, suicide, or assisted suicide."[49] Some state courts have held that although persons have a right to die, that right does not extend to the assistance of others in killing themselves.[50] Passive euthanasia has been defined as an act of omission, such as failure to provide food and water through artificial means. Voluntary active euthanasia is to terminate the patient's life by a physician at the patient's request—a commission[51]—such as to remove a patient from a life-sustaining respirator. Assisted suicide is getting some assistance from another person, such as a physician, a nurse, or a layperson, to end life in a merciful and effective way.[52] Clearly, the differentiation among these terms may be arbitrary. Some AIDS advocates hope to make assisted suicide legal for the medical profession.[53]

Since 1972, when a physician helped her mother die at her request and the court refused to impose a prison sentence, the Dutch have allowed voluntary, active, physician-assisted euthanasia. Safeguards require that the patient be conscious and competent, initiate the request, and discuss the decision with family, friends, and advisors. Family members cannot request assisted suicide on behalf of a patient; nor are demented or comatose patients candidates for euthanasia. The patient is required to be without any hope of recovery and in unbearable pain. Two physicians, one of whom has not previously cared for the patient, agree that the case is hopeless. The patient then signs a witnessed authorization for the physician to inject a barbiturate (to induce sleep) combined with curare (to cause death).

CASE 16.12: Death by Choice.   A hospice nurse, writing under a false name, describes a patient who constantly begged his wife to end his misery. The wife was near collapse and the patient in despair. The nurse informed them that the medication the patient was taking kept him from having seizures. Without the medication, he would die. The patient then refused the next dose of his medication and died 12 hours later.[54]

CASE 16.13: An Individual's Choice for Death and Dignity.   Dr. Timothy Quill presents the case of a long-term patient whom he helped through serious illness and finally leukemia. The patient refused any further treatment and requested a prescription for a lethal amount of barbiturates. Dr. Quill wrote the prescription with full knowledge of its intended use, which after various unsuccessful treatments, the patient used to cause her death. Dr. Quill reported acute leukemia as the cause of death. He raised two questions regarding the process of her death: Was it necessary and was it harmful for her to be alone in the last hours of her life?[55]

CASE 16.14: Assisted Suicide by Machine.   Dr. Jack Kevorkian, a retired pathologist, developed a machine designed to deliver a lethal dose of chemicals or poisonous gas to patients who request it. He requires that these patients be conscious, mentally competent, and suffering from an incurable or terminal disease. By 1994, he assisted nearly 20 patients to die with his machines. He was imprisoned for a publicly televised act of "active euthanasia" in which he injected a lethal dose of medication to a person seeking death.

CASE 16.15: Death on Demand.   A still different kind of case was reported in the *Journal of the American Medical Association* (JAMA) in 1988. A gynecology resident was called in the middle of the night by the nurse to attend to Debbie, a 20-year-old patient dying of ovarian cancer, who was unable to rest. She suffered from constant vomiting, required oxygen and intravenous fluids, experienced air hunger, was emaciated, and was unable to eat or sleep for 2 days. She had not responded to chemotherapy and only palliative and supportive care were given. Her only words to the resident physician were "Let's get this over with."[56] Without any further discussion with anyone—not the patient, not the older woman at her side who may have been her mother, or the nurse—the physician concluded that "the patient was tired and needed rest. I could not give her health, but I could give her rest."[57] Thereupon, he instructed the two women to say good-bye since he would now give her something that would let her rest. He injected a lethal dose of morphine that caused Debbie's death within 4 minutes.

The issue of physician-assisted suicide has evoked a furor of controversy both in the media and in the professional literature. We have attempted to summarize the arguments for and against physician-assisted suicide from a wide array of professional, philosophical, and newspaper sources. There is no clear consensus about the difference between active euthanasia, voluntary euthanasia, and physician-assisted suicide, so the terms may be interchangeable at times.

In 1997, a citizen group in Oregon sponsored a ballot initiative permitting "adults to request and obtain prescriptions from doctors to end their life" that became law.[58] The request must come from patients with less than 6 months to live, in writing and witnessed, with a 15-day waiting period. The physician is obligated to ensure that the patient is making an informed and voluntary decision. If there is any suspicion of depression, then the relevant information and the patient are referred to a licensed psychologist or psychiatrist.[59] The Oregon Right to Die Committee frames the issue in terms of the patient's freedom and taking control of the dying process.[60] Wanzer agreed with 11 other physicians that it is not immoral for a physician to assist a rational, terminally ill person to commit suicide.[61] He believes that all dying patients are entitled to a medical environment that optimizes comfort and dignity and that allows a peaceful death.[62] Pain relief is provided, but sometimes all efforts to relieve distress fail, and the patient seeks assistance in ending life. Some physicians view this assistance as the last act in a continuum of care to the hopelessly ill patient.[63] Only 15 people killed themselves in this way in 1998. The law is still legal in Oregon, although it is banned elsewhere by federal law.

Derek Humphrey, author of the book of instructions on suicide, *Final Exit*, writes that there are many reasons why physicians should help suffering terminally ill patients die.[64] Based on their knowledge and training, physicians know best when euthanasia is or is not medically justified, and only they have access to lethal drugs with knowledge of tolerance and interaction possibilities. Patients with cancer of the throat or neurologic disorders may not be able to swallow and need an injected medication to end life. Some patients have outlived family and friends, have unwilling family members, and are fearful of "botching it." When cure is no longer possible and the patient seeks relief through euthanasia, the help of physicians is most appropriate.[65]

Leon Kass, MD, believes that the claim for active euthanasia or assisted suicide based on patient's claims of choice, autonomy, and self-determination, or because of the claims that this quality of life is not worth prolonging, are invalid.[66] Similarly, Kass rejects the contractual model of medicine which he characterizes as "a highly competent hired syringe [who] sells his services on demand restrained only by the law."[67] Kass also rejects the medical model of general benevolence or loving charity: "All acts—including killing the patient—done lovingly are licit, even praiseworthy."[68] Kass uses the argument that all pain can be controlled if the physician is willing to use strong enough doses that induce drowsiness and diminish awareness.[69] But then, he claims, the euthanasia argument shifts from relieving "suffering to ending a life no longer valued by its bearer, or, let us be frank, by the onlookers."[70] From this position, Kass claims, persons in all sorts of degraded conditions, from persistent vegetative states to quadriplegia, from severe depression to Alzheimer's disease, can become candidates for active euthanasia.[71] The patient's free and informed consent is hardly possible under such conditions.

Kass's last argument against euthanasia/assisted suicide is that the expectations of both the public and of physicians for medical miracles lead to the conclusion of medical failure when the technology fails to cure.[72] Because healing has become a largely technical approach, physicians are expected to provide a final technical solution:

> If you cannot cure me, kill me. The last gasp of autonomy or cry for dignity is asserted against a medicalization and institutionalization of the end of life that robs the old and the incurable of most of their autonomy and dignity; intubated and electrified, with bizarre mechanical companions, helpless and regimented, once proud and independent people find themselves cast in the roles of passive, obedient, highly disciplined children.[73]

Beauchamp and Childress ask why competent patients in grim conditions with legal and moral rights to refuse treatment preventing death cannot exercise the same autonomy rights requesting willing physicians help them die.[74] In 1991, the American Medical Association and the American Geriatric Society officially opposed all physician involvement in killing or assisted suicide.[75] This position insists that "practices of killing patients are inconsistent with the roles of nursing, caregiving, and healing, would introduce conflicts of interests into those roles and would taint the roles. . . ."[76]

Bioethicists acknowledge that ethics does not result in algorithms, formulas, rules or codes; yet bioethicists seem to be searching for just such codifications, perhaps to ease the futility of reversing tragic human endings. There are no final formulas. After one consults love-based ethics and other ethical theories in cases involving arguments for and against assisted suicide, one has to decide what is right or wrong and come up against other ethical theories that oppose one's reasoned views.

Nursing ethics is not a science; nor does it need to be. Nursing ethics may draw on guidelines and rules to minimize harm and bad choices that imply harm. But individuals facing tragic choices have in the end to make up their own minds, hopefully using what Spinoza, a philosopher, called "rational intuition" to make the best possible decision for themselves (See Chapter 1 for the role of intuition in ethics). In making up one's mind about assisting in suicide, there are rational safeguards to consider in order to avoid the Nazi's use of people as means only and to avoid the ease with which any person's life can be abusively taken. After carefully considering a given case one decides, in Hamlet's phrase, "to be or not to be."

RELIGIOUS ASPECTS OF THE NURSING CARE OF THE DYING

For some people, religious beliefs are ultimate values that guide and justify the believer's moral conduct in important matters of living and dying. Firmly held religious beliefs influence perceptions of human relationships, religious duties and obligations, and notions of immortality following death. For those patients and families, it is essential that all prescribed religious practices are fulfilled. In contrast, some patients have been inactive in religious matters, but when death is imminent, they confront and reevaluate religious beliefs learned as children. As a consequence, some will request the comfort of appropriate religious ritual. The nurse respects these values regardless of the nurse's own religious beliefs or nonbelief. The nurse offers to contact the appropriate clergy or religious representative and follows through until the patient's religious desires are fulfilled.

On admission, the patient is usually asked to state a religious preference. As part of the assessment process the nurse has the opportunity to elicit the patient's wishes for religious involvement. If the answer is affirmative, then a hospital chaplain of that faith is reached. If the patient's response is negative toward religious involvement, the nurse respects that point of view as well. This view provides the nurse with the singular opportunity to offer expressions of concern and caring as the last human contact while the patient is alive. The dying person's need for human presence emphasizes the concept of personhood until the last breath is drawn.

Some of the major religions have particular rituals and rites for the dying that are required of the faithful, while others do not. Instead, these nonritualistic religions emphasize human attachments, care, and concern throughout life up to the moment of death. These groups have leaders, visitors, or simply members who visit the dying and provide support. Whatever the patient's or nurse's constellation of religious beliefs or nonbeliefs, the nurse has the opportunity to coordinate human support, care, and concern for the dying person in the effort to soften the impersonal, technical, and sometimes disrespectful means of prolonged dying. The nurse accepts the reality of a patient's belief system, whether religion is or is not an important value, as deeply rooted in that person's personality and way of life. The values of an individual facing death are an expression of personal choice and an extension of the person's right to freedom of thought and of speech.

The Role of Religion in Health Care, Society, and Literature

The role of religious beliefs is to give dying patients reassurance that the lives they led were good, rather than useless or evil. Religion, thus conceived, is designed to help overcome the sense of alienation of the individual dying patient in the face of modern societal demands for youth, productivity, and pleasure. Religion increasingly finds a pastoral and therapeutic role, with a message of love, communion, and emotional support. Religions help to strengthen family and community life; to keep families from falling apart; and to counsel those who are suicidal, alcoholic, jobless, undervalued, or diseased and offer them reassurance of their essential worth. Religion means a bringing together. In the fragmented state of society, religion has the role of uniting people through love and wisdom in human relationships. It aims to give individuals reassurance that their lives are meaningful.

People seek trust, love, compassion, character, goodness, and individual security, and they find it by appealing to priestly relationships with health professionals. The force of religion is also expressed through literary works, like Tolstoy's *The Death of Ivan Ilych*. In this novel, the dying man is rejected by his family but is accepted to the end by his servant, who nurses his cancer wounds and cares for him with religious love. Although religions differ in the form of their expression, they seek to unite the true, the good, the faithful, and the beautiful.

A therapeutic perception may be that even though many religions believe in or seek God or a higher power, what they also believe in and seek is some idea of the good in human relations and experience. For the nonbeliever, "God" may be spelled with two O's as another way of interpreting religious experience.[77] Finally, a religious belief or "blik," as Hare has put it, orients and guides one's moral beliefs. We may reason out what is good or bad for the dying patient, but religion helps us to put our hearts into it.

THE ROLE OF THE NURSE IN THE CARE OF THE DYING PATIENT

Helping an individual to die well is to support that person's sense of self-respect, dignity, and choice until the last moment of life. Achievement of this goal requires skilled and compassionate nursing care to minimize suffering and maximize comfort. The nurse provides calm, sensitive, individualized care to each person so that this final human experience is as free from pain and anxiety as possible.[78]

Patients differ enormously in their attitudes toward death. The term "attitude" has affective, cognitive, and behavioral dimensions. These attitudes, along with ethical and religious or humanistic principles, are integral parts of how individuals think and feel about death, and ultimately how they behave when faced with death.[79] Some patients want to know all of the truth as their condition deteriorates. Other patients steadfastly find benign reasons for their symptoms of failing health. The individual's personality, maturity, cultural and ethnic orientations, education, presence or absence of religious belief, age, role, social status, and family relationships are but some of the variables that influence the patient's response to imminent death.

Kübler-Ross's widely recognized work on the attitudes of the dying stresses stage approaches.[80] The author describes five stages through which dying persons move. The first stage is one of denial and isolation, in which the evidence of impending death is rejected and ignored or regarded as false. "No, not me," "It's not true," or "It's just arthritis (not cancer)," are typical denials. In the second stage, outrage and bitter anger and resentment are expressed toward death as unjust and unfair. "Why me?" is a typical response to this stage. The third stage is characterized as a bargaining phase in which the individual promises to reform or to make amends to postpone death until the marriage or birth of a grandchild, for example. "Yes, but after . . ." is a remark typical of this stage. In view of the advancement of the disease process, however, the dying person recognizes the bargaining to be futile and becomes depressed. The fourth stage, depression, is a reaction to the anticipated loss of life and of loved ones. "Yes, I am slipping" is acknowledgment of impending death. The fifth stage is one in which the inevitability of death is accepted. "I have done my best" is one expression of acceptance and resignation.

Kübler-Ross views these stages as normal and adaptive for the individual's progression toward acceptance of death. She views the stage of acceptance of death as the culmination of the necessary work of grieving to be done by the patient. Kübler-Ross sees the role of the health care provider or counselor to facilitate the dying patient's movement through these stages with "minimal regression . . . to denial or anger"[81] after a more advanced stage has been reached. However, she concedes that patients move back and forth between stages and may occupy two stages simultaneously.

Kalish points to the possibility that the stages are so familiar that there is danger of their "becoming a self-fulfilling prophecy . . ."[82] It is difficult to ascertain whether the stages are universal, modal, culture-bound, or even adaptive, because no consistent research findings have been reported, and medical clinicians themselves are in disagreement.[83] Given the lack of research, Kalish identifies the ethical issue as one that questions the practice of intervening with dying persons to help them pass through the five stages.[84]

Other investigations with different questions and different methods have produced other insights. One study by Hinton, who conducted interviews with the dying, demonstrated that dying persons want to understand their prognosis and are aware, especially those with children and with discomfort, of their condition, even without being given an official medical diagnosis.[85] Another investigation conducted with the dying adds an additional category to their awareness of their condition. Weisman calls this "middle knowledge," which lies between open acknowledgment of death and its denial. He warns against trying to set firm categories, because patients appear to know and want to know their condition, yet talk as if they did not want to be reminded of information received.[86] The nursing implication is, "Wait until the patient is ready to discuss his or her condition and to focus the discussion on those questions and issues with which the patient is presently able to cope."

In several studies reported by Kalish, the coping ability of dying patients is enhanced by "good marital relationships, having good interpersonal relationships in general, expressing greater life satisfaction, and maintaining open communication about dying."[87] Competent and sensitive nurses support the coping abilities of dying patients as they struggle to maintain control and equanimity in the face of declining powers.

Another investigation shows that patients who live longer than predicted are likely to have good human relations and maintain intimacy until death. They have the capacity to ask for and receive support in relation to medical care and emotional relationships. They accept the fact of a serious illness, but not the inevitability of death. They are able to express resentment about their illness and treatment, but are seldom deeply depressed.[88]

Thus, another function of the nurse is to regard the anger and resentment of a dying patient as the natural expression of powerlessness without personal animosity. The anger serves the purpose of ventilating negative emotions.

Nursing Interventions

A useful assumption is that fear of death is natural and present in everyone and that attempts at control, attaining power, and relating to the transcendent are ways of reducing that fear. Thus, an important goal of nursing practice is to enhance the patient's right to autonomy as a manifestation of power over self and limits on the interventions of care providers. One way of accomplishing this goal is through involving the individual in the planning and implementation of care as the primary decision maker.[89] If, for example, the dying patient decides that a visit with loved ones is more important than a dressing change or treating a bowel obstruction, that is a priority to be respected. This is a way of lessening the fear of abandonment by significant others and to bolster the sense of control by "making available those experiences that the patient values."[90]

Symptom control is important to the self-esteem of persons in fear of losing control and to those who find pain frightening and burdensome. The prospect of uncontrolled pain is a specter that haunts most patients. Mental dysfunction, nausea, constipation, diarrhea, infections, bedsores, and respiratory problems may be equally distressing. Most of these can be controlled through well-known measures and the remainder through aggressive therapies. Each situation is best considered individually as an effort to control present and anticipated symptoms. Staff and resource shortages, as in the case of Mr. W (Case 16.7), who was not put in an intensive care unit, can result in loss of control of symptoms with resulting death.

Pain can almost always be controlled. Pain-management techniques now give patients direct control over the amount and timing of their pain relief. Causes of pain are expected to be identified and followed by specific interventions, such as prophylactic nailing of pathologic fractures and radiation or chemotherapy for relieving symptoms.[91] The choice of drugs and combinations of drugs to relieve pain, apprehension, and depression are increasing and improving constantly. The recommended administration of narcotics, such as morphine, in small, frequent doses is recommended for the rapid control of pain for patients not previously taking narcotics.[92] Effective control of pain can be maintained, along with alertness, through continual experimentation. For some patients who are close to death, the patient or family may agree to sedation in order to avoid pain. The President's Commission recommends that the administration of narcotics be regularly scheduled so that each new dose takes effect as the last one wanes. Sometimes increased frequency is more effective than increased dose. Orders written as PRN enable the nurse caring for the patient to adjust the dose to prevent pain without excessive sedation. However, respiratory depression and oversedation can be reversed by use of naloxone (Narcan) in prescribed amounts and intervals.[93] The concerns of nurses and other caregivers regarding the "dying patients becoming addicted to narcotics are both mistaken and, in any case, irrelevant. Few patients develop problems because of physical dependence. . . . Furthermore, physical and psychological addiction, when it occurs, is not particularly troubling to a patient who is dying, nor should be to caregivers."[94] This statement is a direct application of Kantian ethics, which treats humans as ends rather than as means only. This statement applies the principle to every dying patient for control of pain and of symptoms that otherwise dehumanize the dying person.

The nurse can effectively use nursing observations of the patient's responses to medications as the basis for recommending changes in drugs, in dose, or in frequency. From systematic nursing assessments of patients' responses to the illness and to the therapeutic regimens, the nurse evaluates the effectiveness of current therapies and raises the issue of change when indicated. Competent nursing care is essential to control of pain and other symptoms, enabling the patient to live as fully as possible for as long as possible. A nurse who promises control of a patient's pain and who demonstrates the truth of that statement eases the patient's fear of and attention to pain. The patient is more able to trust the staff on other matters and is usually more cooperative as a consequence.

The trust that a dying patient is able to invest in skilled and compassionate nursing staff may contribute directly to reducing the patient's fears of abandonment and of losing control of the situation. The family's trust in the competence and concern of the nurse may reduce the family's fears that the patient will be neglected in their absence. Trust among patient, family, and care providers is significant when mental dysfunctions appear as a consequence of the disease or the treatment. Anxiety and depression are expected expressions of behavior in dying patients. Consistently given sympathy and support by the nurse, along with pain and symptom control, comfort measures, mild psychotropic drugs, and attention to the environment, can give relief.

Whatever the symptoms of the dying patient—and some, such as dyspnea, can be quite agonizing—there are relieving measures that can be used. These measures cover a wide range of specific nursing techniques, such as bathing, positioning, suctioning, skin care and care of bedsores, bowel and urinary control, providing an esthetic environment free from noxious smells, and administering analgesics on time and without unnecessary discomfort. The nurse's opportunities to implement the Kantian principle of treating persons as ends are varied and plentiful. The nurse caring for the dying has multiple opportunities and ways to help make this experience deep and meaningful for patient, family, and self. A nurse who is aware of Aquinas's love-based ethics and who is deeply committed and caring may alleviate a patient's torment and suffering by listening and showing care.

The central principle is that the nurse as advocate of the dying person seeks to protect the basic human values of dignity, respect, and autonomy while providing the highest standards of care possible. The nurse's competence and compassion will largely determine how well this last human experience comes to an end. The nurse's concern can be extended to the family through kindnesses and courtesies that show respect for them as well as for the dying person. Family members can be guided in offering nourishment, in wiping the brow, or in holding the patient's hand and lending their presence. In this last phase of relationship, unfinished projects and unresolved tensions can be put aside as family members and significant others, with the help and support of nurses, conduct this last human experience with the sensitivity and consideration that the finality of death warrants.

The Hospice Concept

The hospice movement provides compassionate, skilled care for the dying adult and child that is consistent with the Kantian imperative of treating humans as ends. The term *hospice* is defined as a "lodging for travelers, young persons, or the underprivileged."[95] The term "hospitable," which follows the word "hospice" in the dictionary, is defined as "given to generous and cordial reception of guests."[96] These terms were translated into care of the dying by the founder of the modern hospice movement, Cicely Saunders, MD, a former nurse and director of St. Christopher's Hospital in London. Saunders' conception of the hospice is to provide the dying with a comfortable, cheerful environment with the amenities of a home in which family members, friends, children, and pets are welcomed and given hospitality. Pain and other symptoms are controlled so that the dying process will be a meaningful, enriched, final separation from life and one's loved ones. The patient is cared for skillfully and compassionately until the last breath. Patients feel secure in the skill and concern of their nurses and care providers. Thus, there is less suffering and less anxiety about the control of pain and symptoms and more serenity about imminent death. The topic of dying and death is openly discussed. Emotional support is consistently given by everyone, including patients to one another, because the concept of a sharing, caring community pervades the hospital. At St. Christopher's and elsewhere in England, "Brompton's cocktail," which contains heroin as one of its ingredients, is given orally as often as necessary to keep the patient free from pain and from the anticipation of pain. The patient need never suffer while waiting for the next dose of medication to come due. Addiction does not necessarily happen, but if it does, priority is given to freedom from pain and to helping the patient achieve a "good" death.

In the United States, the hospice concept has undergone variations. Some hospice programs began as home care programs with community health nurses and progressed to include full-time hospice care. In some hospitals, the hospice team, which includes nurses, assumes responsibility for the supervision of the care of dying patients in units throughout the hospital. The team gives care, advocates for the patient's best interests and wishes to the unit staff, counsels the family and staff concerning their feelings about death, and works toward providing a caring environment for the dying patient. Another hospice program involves the family, community, and hospital staff in providing care at home and in the hospital if needed. Hospice staff are on call 24 hours of every day so that no one need feel abandoned.

These and many other programs in the United States not discussed are consistent with the hospice concept. The dying patient is identified and supported as a self-determining human being worthy of respect, care, and affection until the very last moment of life. The traditional isolation of the dying is transformed into inclusion of the individual as a member of the community of the living, fully participating in all of life's joys. The physical suffering of the dying is controlled. The patient need not fear pain or abandonment. Death is treated as the end of life that happens to everyone.

SUMMARY

Death is a tragedy to some individuals; to others not. Death to each person is, as Wittgenstein remarked, "not an event of life. Death is not lived through."[97] Some physicists say that in billions of years, the universe will be a "black hole," and that nothing will be left; that is how some people believe it is for the individual who dies. To those who continue to live, the griefs, troubles, and satisfactions of life continue. For them, the death of others is an event lived through.

The nurse at a dying patient's bedside can give succor and support to that patient, helping the patient through the stages of dying, sharing the patient's grief with compassion, support, and understanding. The nurse with ethical sensitivity, oriented by love-based ethics at a dying patient's last hours, gives as one person to another in the recognition that they have this life and this fate in common. The nurse who can share as a person is aware that she or he, too, will die and that how one ends life, whether well or badly, depends in part on the wisdom and love or lack of it shown by relevant others at this time. In the course of this book, we have accordingly tried to indicate opportunities and limits to the rights to initiate, sustain and terminate life.

Discussion Questions

1. How is the distinction between ordinary and extraordinary useful in deciding whether to treat an HIV-positive patient?

2. What are the moral reasons to support or oppose Rachels's argument concerning the moral equivalence of active and passive euthanasia?
3. What, if anything, is morally wrong with "allowing" rather than "enabling" or assisting someone to die?
4. What strength or difficulty do you find in Schopenhauer's argument against prohibiting suicide?

REFERENCES

1. President's Commission for the Study of Ethical Problems in Medicine and Biomedical and Behavioral Research. *Deciding to forego life-sustaining treatment.* Washington, DC: US Government Printing Office; March 1983:17–18.
2. Guidelines for the Determination of Death. In: *Legal and ethical aspects of treatment for critically and terminally ill patients.* New York: American Society for Law and Medicine and Concern for Dying. 1981;54–63.
3. Black P. Definitions of brain death. In: Beauchamp T, Perlin S (eds). *Ethical issues in death and dying.* Englewood Cliffs, NJ: Prentice-Hall. 1978;9.
4. Heifetz MD, Mangel C. *The right to die.* New York: Berkley. 1975;59–60.
5. Muyskens J. *Moral problems in nursing.* Totowa, NJ: Littlefield, Adams. 1983;92–93.
6. Davis AJ, Aroskar MA. *Ethical dilemmas and nursing practice.* (2nd ed) Norwalk, Conn: Appleton-Century-Crofts. 1983;223.
7. Cross J. Whose life is it anyway? *Empire State Report.* March 1983;25.
8. Muyskens J. *Moral problems in nursing.* Totowa, NJ: Littlefield, Adams. 1983;92.
9. Levine M. Nursing ethics and the ethical nurse. *Am J Nurs* 1977;77(5):843.
10. Carson R, Siegler M. Does "doing everything" include CPR? *Hasting Center Report* 1982;12(5):27.
11. Pope Pius XII. Symposium on anesthesiology. In: Hayes EJ, Hayes PJ, Kelly DE (eds). *Moral principles of nursing.* New York: Macmillan. 1964;131.
12. President's Commission. *Deciding to forego life-sustaining treatment.* March 1983;90.
13. Pope Pius XII. Symposium on anesthesiology. In: Hayes E. J., Hayes PJ, Kelly DE (eds). *Moral principles of nursing:* N.Y. Macmillan. 1964;131.
14. ibid, p. 62. President's Commission #12.
15. ibid, p. 85. President's Commission #12.
16. Rachels J. Active and passive euthanasia. *N Engl J Med* 1975;292(2):78.
17. ibid.
18. ibid.
19. Kohl M. Karen Quinlan: Human rights and wrongful killing. In: Bandman EL, Bandman B (eds). *Bioethics and human rights: A reader for health professionals.* Lanham, Md: University Press of America. 1986;125.
20. Society for the Right to Die. *Living will declaration.* New York; 1985;1–2.
21. Society for the Right to Die. *The physician and the hopelessly ill patient.* New York; 1985;26.
22. ibid, p. 32.
23. Machlin R. Consent, coercion and conflicts of rights. In: Arras J, Hunt R (eds). *Ethical issues in modern medicine.* (2nd ed) Palo Alto, Calif: Mayfield. 1983;231–238.
24. McCormick R. Organ transplants: Ethical principles. In: Reich W (ed). *Encyclopedia of bioethics.* New York: Free Press. 1978;1169–1172.
25. Davis AJ, Aroskar MA. *Ethical dilemmas and nursing practice.* (2nd ed) Norwalk, Conn: Appleton-Century-Crofts. 1993;223.

26. Bandman B, Bandman E. The nurse's role in an interest-based view of patient's rights. In: Spicker S, Gadow S (eds). *Nursing image and ideals.* New York: Springer. 1980; 135–136.

27. ibid.

28. President's Commission. *Deciding to forego life-sustaining treatment.* March 1983;16.

29. Kant I. *Fundamental principles of the metaphysics of morals.* Indianapolis: Bobbs-Merrill. 1949;39.

30. Schopenhauer A. On suicide. In: Beck R, Orr J (eds). *Ethical choice.* New York: Free Press. 1970;78.

31. Moody HR. *Ethics in an aging society.* Baltimore: Johns Hopkins University Press. 1992;73.

32. Prado CG. *The last choice: Preemptive suicide in advanced age.* Westport, Conn: Greenwood Press. 1990;69.

33. Moody HR. *Ethics in an aging society.* Baltimore: Johns Hopkins University Press. 1992;73.

34. ibid.

35. ibid.

36. ibid, p. 74–75.

37. ibid.

38. ibid, p. 77.

39. Editorial, "Assisted Suicide in Practice." *The New York Times.* February 24, 1999;A14.

40. Kant I. *Fundamental principles of the metaphysics of morals.* Abbot TK (trans). New York: Bobbs-Merrill. 1949;39.

41. Kant I. *Fundamental principles of the metaphysics of morals.* In: Moody HR (ed). *Ethics in an aging society.* Baltimore: Johns Hopkins University Press. 1992;73.

42. Edman I (ed). *The philosophy of Plato.* New York: Modern Library. 1928;91–106.

43. Aristotle. *Nicomachean ethics.* Thomson JAK (trans). Aylesbury Bucks, England: Penguin. 1975;66,78.

44. Seneca. *Letters from a stoic.* Campbell R (trans). Baltimore: Penguin;1969.

45. Moody HR. *Ethics in an aging society.* Baltimore: Johns Hopkins University Press. 1992;80.

46. ibid, p. 87.

47. ibid.

48. ibid, p. 88.

49. Moody HR. *Aging: Concepts and controversies.* Thousand Oaks, Calif: Pine Forge Press. 1994;105.

50. Munson R. *Intervention and reflection: Basic issues in medical ethics.* (4th ed) Belmont, Calif: Wadsworth. 1992;144.

51. McCarrick PM. Active euthanasia and assisted suicide. *Kennedy Inst Ethics J* 1992;2(1):79–100.

52. ibid.

53. Munson R. *Intervention and reflection: Basic issues in medical ethics.* (4th ed) Belmont, Calif: Wadsworth. 1992;144.

53. ibid, p. 148.

54. Cate S. Death by choice. *Am J Nurs* 1991;91(7):32–34.

55. Quill TE. Death and dignity: A case of individualized decision making. *N Engl J Med* 1991;324(10):691–694.

56. It's over, Debbie. *JAMA* 1988;259(2):272.

57. ibid.

58. Campbell CS. Oregon's fight over the right to die. *Hastings Center Report* 1994; 24(2):3.

59. ibid.

60. ibid.

61. Wanzer SH et al. The physician's responsibility toward hopelessly ill patients: A second look. *N Engl J Med* 1989;320(13);846–848.

62. ibid.

63. ibid.

64. Humphrey D. *Final exit: The practicalities of self-deliverance and assisted suicide for the dying.* Eugene, Ore: The Hemlock Society and Dell Paperbacks. 1992.

65. ibid.

66. Kass L. Neither for love nor money: Why doctors must not kill. *The Public Interest* 1989;94:26–37, 42–45.

67. ibid.

68. ibid.

69. ibid.

70. ibid.

71. ibid.

72. ibid.

73. ibid.

74. Beauchamp TL, Childress JF. *Principles of biomedical ethics.* (4th ed) New York: Oxford University Press. 1994;226.

75. ibid, p. 227.

76. ibid.

77. Hare RM. Religion and morals. In: Mitchell B (ed). *Faith and logic.* London: Allen & Unwin. 1957;192.

78. American Nurses Association. *Code for nurses with interpretive statements.* Kansas City, Mo; 1976;6.

79. Kalish RA. Death, attitudes toward. In: *Encyclopedia of bioethics.* Vol. 1. 286.

80. Kübler-Ross E. *On death and dying.* New York: Macmillan; 1969.

81. ibid.

82. Kalish. Death, attitudes toward. In: *Encyclopedia of bioethics.* Vol. 1; 287.

83. ibid.

84. ibid.

85. ibid.

86. ibid.

87. ibid, p. 288.

88. ibid.

89. American Nurses Association. *Code for nurses with interpretive statements.* Kansas City, Mo: 1976;4.

90. President's Commission. *Deciding to forego life-sustaining treatment.* 1983;276.

91. ibid, p. 278.

92. ibid, p. 279.

93. ibid, p. 283.

94. ibid, p. 284.

95. *Webster's New Collegiate Dictionary.* Springfield, Mass: Merriam. 1974;553.

96. ibid.

97. Wittgenstein L. *Tractatus logicus philosophicus.* New York: Humanities Press. 1951; 185.

Glossary of Selected Terms

Abortion. Deliberate termination of the life of a fetus. Has resulted in controversy as to whether termination of pregnancy is murder or a woman's right of free choice.

Adolescents. Generally, children from age 12 to 21 years.

Advocacy. Giving support and protection to specific persons in need.

Agapism. Love-based ethics derived from the Greek word *agape* (love).

Ageism. Irrational and unfair discrimination against the aging population.

AIDS. Acquired immunodeficiency disease syndrome; the virtual loss of all immunity against viral and bacterial infections.

Altruism. Showing as much love for others as for oneself. See **Agapism.**

Aquinas, St. Thomas. (1225-1274) Medieval philosopher who developed natural law, altruism (or agapism or love-based ethics), and the doctrine of double effect.

Aristotle. (384-322 BC) Greek philosopher whose ethical theory has had a powerful influence on virtue ethics; a student of Plato.

Assisted suicide. A health professional's deliberate assistance in facilitating a patient's death.

Autonomy. The exercise of a person's rational will as distinct from self-determination, the exercise of one's will. The idea of autonomy was first developed by Immanuel Kant.

Bentham, Jeremy. (1748-1832). British philosopher of law and founder of utilitarian ethics.

Best-interest standard. An objective and desirable health care standard for deciding on patient treatment.

Bioethics. Philosophical ethics applied to biology, medicine, nursing, theology, social work, law, and other fields that deal with health care. Bioethics triangulates between medical cases, laws, and philosophical ethics.

Biological/biographical distinction. Biological functioning is physical and bodily, whereas biographical functioning is the use of one's thinking processes in developing projects.

Care. Sustained concern and devotion to a patient's health care interests (see Chapters 1, 5, 12–14).

Categorical imperative. The statement formulated by Immanuel Kant that one is obligated to act on that principle that everyone else can rationally act on for any given moral situation (see Chapter 4).

Children. Human beings aged 2 to 11 years (see Chapter 10).

Club membership model. Liberty is accorded people to do as they wish within institutional rules, but with indifference to their interests (see Chapter 7).

Code for nurses. The nursing profession's code of conduct (see Chapter 2).

Competence. *Patient competence* is awareness of one's time and space surroundings and the subsequent capacity to make reasonable decisions. *Professional competence* is effective patient treatment (see Chapter 6).

Confidentiality. Respect for a person's or patient's privacy regarding his or her biographical data (see Chapter 12).

Decision-making process. 1) The identification and definition of the ethical problem and the nature of the ethical conflict; 2) identification of the actors involved and their source of authority. Requirements of informed consent are fulfilled; 3) analysis of the proposed actions, the alternatives, and their consequences; 4) justification for the decision in relation to the ethical theories and the common morality discussed in this work.

Descartes, René. (1596-1650) French philosopher, who emphasizes that one's mind is crucial to one's being, especially in his *"cogito ergo sum"* ("I think, therefore I am"). The emphasis on one's capacity to think influenced the definition of brain death.

Egoism. An ethical theory that emphasizes that the individual's interests take precedence over any other (see Chapters 3, 4).

Eudaemonistic ethics. Aristotle's happiness-based ethics (see Chapter 3).

Euthanasia. An easy and painless death, usually one that is actively and voluntarily sought, rather than one over which one has no control (passive euthanasia) or that is involuntary (see Chapter 14).

Existentialism. A philosophy stemming from Kierkegaard based on a doctrine that each individual is responsible for actions and omissions (see Chapters 4, 5).

Fallacy. An error in reasoning. *Abuse of person* fallacy consists in attacking a person, rather than giving reasons for a decision. *Fallacy of accident* is the indiscriminate application of a rule or principle to every situation without regard for "accidental" differences or circumstances. The *appeal to force* fallacy consists in the irrelevant use of force. The *appeal to authority* fallacy assumes that persons with appropriate authority are experts in fields beyond their area of expertise. The fallacy of *appeal to the populace* assumes that because everyone is doing a particular thing, it must be good. The *complex question* fallacy consists in asking a question that depends on an affirmative answer to a previous question. The *slippery slope* fallacy consists in arguing that if one allows one step or concession, then an uncontrollable chain of unwanted events will follow. *Slothful induction* is the refusal to allow any evidence to be presented that contradicts the conclusion of one's argument.

Golden rule. The precept that one should treat others as one wants to be treated; sometimes known as the reciprocity principle.

Greatest happiness principle. Making decisions that bring about happiness for the majority (see Chapter 4).

Harm. Causing death, injury, violence, or abuse.

Informed consent. A decision made by a patient based on data and reasoned evidence, and given only after the patient decides to undergo treatment.

Justice. Fair and equitable distribution of health care resources and services based on reconciliation of competing standards of justice, need, and merit (see Chapters 3–7, 9–16).

Justification. Adequate reasons for a conclusion in ethics and health care and nursing ethics. See also **Paradigm Case Argument** for examples in health care ethics.

Kant, Immanuel. (1724-1804) German philosopher who enunciated the categorical imperative, that one is to treat people as rational people treat one another.

Legal moralism. The view developed by P. Devlin that society is a "seamless web," that all individuals fit together in a society; and that those who do not fit are excluded.

Legal paternalism. Those in authority make decisions for the good of others that accord with conventional moral standards. For example, a lifeguard is given the authority to blow the whistle to try to prevent swimmers from engaging in unsafe swimming behavior.

Libertarianism. Emphasis on individual freedom in deciding how to live; compatible with self-determination.

Love-based ethics. Showing love, caring, and devotion to another person, e.g., selflessly helping AIDS patients (see Chapters 4, 9–16). See also **Altruism.**

Malthus, Thomas. (1766-1834) English economist who traced food production and population expansion and noted inadequacy of the food production to sustain growing populations (see Chapter 8).

Marx, Karl. (1818-1883) German social and political philosopher who argued against exploitation of the poor by the rich. He favored communal property and land and common ownership of the means of production (see Chapter 6).

Metaphor. Comparison, analogy, or model using a word picture (see Chapter 2).

Mill, John Stuart. (1806-1873) Important utilitarian, who developed Bentham's pleasure-pain ethics with concern for quality; authored *On Liberty*, which became the basis of libertarian ethics (see Chapter 4).

Moore, George Edward. (1873-1958) British moral philosopher and critic of utilitarianism, on logical grounds. He exposed the naturalistic fallacy, also known as the is-ought fallacy (see Chapters 5, 6).

Morality. Doing good rather than harm, and giving reasons to justify one's doing good, usually by a formal, dialectical, empirical, inductive, or intuitive approach (see Chapters 1, 3–7; for applications, see Chapters 9–16).

Nursing ethics. The critical-philosophical evaluation and justification of moral decisions in nursing.

Ownership model. A person in a position of power makes decisions affecting others without consulting them or their interests. (see Chapter 9).

Paradigm case argument. Using a morally significant case to rebut a contrary moral presumption, e.g., Tuskegee syphilis experiment showing maltreatment of African Americans in health care (see Chapter 7).

Partnership model. Democratic and shared decision making (see Chapter 9).

Patient's Bill of Rights. American Hospital Association's statement assuring patients of their rights to informed consent, confidentiality, and respect (see Appendix).

Personhood. A human being to whom rational faculties are attributable.

Phenomenology. The philosophical view that consciousness determines reality in space and time (see Chapters 1, 3–7).

Plato. (428-347 BC) Greek philosopher who developed a range of philosophical ideas applicable to health care, including (what we term as) rational paternalism (see Chapters 4–7).

Potentiality principle. The assumption that a being's future possibilities for development of its features justifies treating that being as actually having those features.

Quality of life. Aspects of living such as feelings of pleasure and pain, consciousness, and self-awareness (see Chapter 11).

Quorum feature. The majority features one must have in order to qualify as a person, e.g., consciousness (see Chapters 11–13).

Rawls, John. (1921-) Author of *A Theory of Justice,* a pivotal work for health care and nursing ethics emphasizing justice as fairness—understood through "the veil of ignorance"—and resulting principles for living together with just institutions (see Chapter 7).

Relativism. The view that values change with each person at any time and with each society (see Chapter 3).

Rights. Justified reasons for acting or receiving benefits. *Liberty rights* are rights to freedom of expression and action. *Welfare rights* are rights to assistance (see Chapters 7–16).

Rights-based ethics. An ethical theory that emphasizes the role of rights. One of three kinds of ethics, developed by R. Dworkin; the others are goal-based ethics (utilitarianism) and duty-based ethics (Kantian ethics) (see Chapter 7).

Self-determination principle. Each individual decides how to live and what treatment to accept or refuse.

Situationalism. A form of utilitarianism developed by Joseph Fletcher, which emphasizes one's time and place for making moral decisions (see Chapter 6).

Social contract. Despite different origins, motivations, and philosophical expressions, the emphasis of the social contract is to keep one's agreements whether made by oneself or others (see Chapters 3–7).

Socrates. (470-399 BC) Greek philosopher and teacher who taught that "the un-examined life is not worth living," and became a model philosopher, human being, and teacher for subsequent centuries. He developed a method of systematically questioning fundamental moral assumptions, the Socratic method (see Chapter 4).

Substitute judgment standard. Deciding what a patient would want to have done.

Sufferability principle. Jeremy Bentham's notion that the capacity to suffer among all animals is a more important indicator of their value than intelligence or conscious thinking (see Chapter 5).

Suicide. Personal decision to die owing to a terminal condition, which may be regarded by some people as "rational," and which may call for assistance by other competent health professionals, known as assisted suicide (see Chapter 16).

Tarasoff v. Regents of University of California. Case of a young woman murdered by a suitor who confessed to a psychologist that he intended to kill her. The psychologist failed to warn Ms. Tarasoff (see Chapter 14).

Truth-telling. A principle of ethics formulated by I. Kant and later by S. Bok emphasizing integrity as a rational way for anyone to follow (see Chapter 6).

Tuskeegee syphilis experiment. Federally funded study from 1932–1972 designed to show the terminal phase of 385 African American men with syphilis (see Chapter 7).

Universality principle. Kant's categorical imperative to act only on that principle which everyone else would rationally act upon in a given situation (see Chapter 6).

Universal moral principle. Principle enunciated by I. Kant that applies to everyone without exception, e.g., adultery is wrong for everyone (see Chapter 6).

Utilitarianism. Philosophical view that the good is the greatest happiness of the greatest number (see Chapter 5).

Values. Preferences people have in which they rate one interest ahead of another (see Chapter 7).

Veil of ignorance. J. Rawls's idea that people decide what rules to live by based on their not knowing their own origins and life circumstances, e.g., sex, race, socioeconomic status (see Chapter 7).

Virtue ethics. The belief that the best way to live is to cultivate traditional virtues of honesty, courage, thrift, love, and wisdom (see Chapter 4 and Part 2).

Voluntarism. The view that the will, individual or collective, determines the rationale for social change (see Chapter 6).

Voluntary euthanasia. Personal decision to seek an easy and painless death based on evidence presented to a given person to the effect that a quality life is no longer viable (see Chapter 16).

Appendix

CODE FOR NURSES WITH INTERPRETIVE STATEMENTS*

Preamble

A code of ethics makes explicit the primary goals and values of the profession. When individuals become nurses, they make a moral commitment to uphold the values and special moral obligations expressed in their code. The *Code for Nurses* is based on a belief about the nature of individuals, nursing, health, and society. Nursing encompasses the protection, promotion, and restoration of health; the prevention of illness; and the alleviation of suffering in the care of clients, including individuals, families, groups, and communities. In the context of these functions, nursing is defined as the diagnosis and treatment of human responses to actual or potential health problems.

Since clients themselves are the primary decision makers in matters concerning their own health, treatment, and well-being, the goal of nursing actions is to support and enhance the client's responsibility and self-determination to the greatest extent possible. In this context, health is not necessarily an end in itself, but rather a means to a life that is meaningful from the client's perspective. When making clinical judgments, nurses base their decisions on consideration of consequences and of universal moral principles, both of which prescribe and justify nursing actions. The most fundamental of these principles is respect for persons. Other principles stemming from this basic principle are autonomy (self-determination), beneficence (doing good), nonmaleficence (avoiding harm), veracity (truth-telling), confidentiality (respecting privileged information), fidelity (keeping promises), and justice (treating people fairly).

In brief, then, the statements of the code and their interpretation provide guidance for conduct and relationships in carrying out nursing responsibilities consistent with the ethical obligations of the profession and with high quality in nursing care.

Introduction

A code of ethics indicates a profession's acceptance of the responsibility and trust with which it has been invested by society. Under the terms of the implicit contract between society and the nursing profession, society grants the profession

---

*Reprinted from *Code for Nurses with Interpretive Statements,* © 1985. American Nurses Publishing, American Nurses Foundation/American Nurses Association, Washington, DC.

considerable autonomy and authority to function in the conduct of its affairs. The development of a code of ethics is an essential activity of a profession and provides one means for the exercise of professional self-regulation.

Upon entering the profession, each nurse inherits a measure of both the responsibility and the trust that have accrued to nursing over the years, as well as the corresponding obligation to adhere to the profession's code of conduct and relationships for ethical practice. *The Code for Nurses With Interpretive Statements* is thus more a collective expression of nursing conscience and philosophy than a set of external rules imposed upon an individual practitioner of nursing. Personal and professional integrity can be assured only if an individual is committed to the profession's code of conduct.

A code of ethical conduct offers general principles to guide and evaluate nursing actions. It does not assure the virtues required for professional practice within the character of each nurse. In particular situations, the justification of behavior as ethical must satisfy not only the individual nurse acting as a moral agent but also the standards for professional peer review.

The *Code for Nurses* was adopted by the American Nurses Association in 1950 and has been revised periodically. It serves to inform both the nurse and society of the profession's expectations and requirements in ethical matters. The code and the interpretive statements together provide a framework within which nurses can make ethical decisions and discharge their responsibilities to the public, to other members of the health team, and to the profession.

Although a particular situation by its nature may determine the use of specific moral principles, the basic philosophical values, directives, and suggestions provided here are widely applicable to situations encountered in clinical practice. The *Code for Nurses* is not open to negotiation in employment settings, nor is it permissible for individuals or groups of nurses to adapt or change the language of this code.

The requirements of the code may often exceed those of the law. Violations of the law may subject the nurse to civil or criminal liability. The state nurses associations, in fulfilling the profession's duty to society, may discipline their members for violations of the code. Loss of the respect and confidence of society and of one's colleagues is a serious sanction resulting from violation of the code. In addition, every nurse has a personal obligation to uphold and adhere to the code and to ensure that nursing colleagues do likewise.

Guidance and assistance in applying the code to local situations may be obtained from the American Nurses Association and the constituent state nurses associations.

> 1. *The nurse provides services with respect for human dignity and the uniqueness of the client, unrestricted by considerations of social or economic status, personal attributes, or the nature of health problems.*

1.1 Respect for Human Dignity

The fundamental principle of nursing practice is respect for the inherent dignity and worth of every client. Nurses are morally obligated to respect human existence and the individuality of all persons who are the recipients of nursing actions.

Nurses therefore must take all reasonable means to protect and preserve human life when there is hope of recovery or reasonable hope of benefit from life-prolonging treatment.

Truth telling and the process of reaching informed choice underlie the exercise of self-determination, which is basic to respect for persons. Clients should be as fully involved as possible in the planning and implementation of their own health care. Clients have the moral right to determine what will be done with their own person; to be given accurate information, and all the information necessary for making informed judgments; to be assisted with weighing the benefits and burdens of options in their treatment; to accept, refuse, or terminate treatment without coercion; and to be given necessary emotional support. Each nurse has an obligation to be knowledgeable about the moral and legal rights of all clients and to protect and support those rights. In situations in which the client lacks the capacity to make a decision, a surrogate decision maker should be designated.

Individuals are interdependent members of the community. Taking into account both individual rights and the interdependence of persons in decision making, the nurse recognizes those situations in which individual rights to autonomy in health care may temporarily be overridden to preserve the life of the human community; for example, when a disaster demands triage or when an individual presents a direct danger to others. The many variables involved make it imperative that each case be considered with full awareness of the need to preserve the rights and responsibilities of clients and the demands of justice. The suspension of individual rights must always be considered a deviation to be tolerated as briefly as possible.

1.2 Status and Attributes of Clients

The need for health care is universal, transcending all national, ethnic, racial, religious, cultural, political, educational, economic, developmental, personality, role, and sexual differences. Nursing care is delivered without prejudicial behavior. Individual value systems and lifestyles should be considered in the planning of health care with and for each client. Attributes of clients influence nursing practice to the extent that they represent factors the nurse must understand, consider, and respect in tailoring care to personal needs and in maintaining the individual's self-respect and dignity.

1.3 The Nature of Health Problems

The nurse's respect for the worth and dignity of the individual human being applies, irrespective of the nature of the health problem. It is reflected in care given the person who is disabled as well as one without disability, the person with long-term illness as well as one with acute illness, the recovering patient as well as one in the last phase of life. This respect extends to all who require the services of the nurse for the promotion of health, the prevention of illness, the restoration of health, the alleviation of suffering, and the provision of supportive care of the dying. The nurse does not act deliberately to terminate the life of any person.

The nurse's concern for human dignity and for the provision of high quality nursing care is not limited by personal attitudes or beliefs. If ethically opposed to interventions in a particular case because of the procedures to be used, the nurse is justified in refusing to participate. Such refusal should be made known in advance and in time for other appropriate arrangements to be made for the client's nursing care. If the nurse becomes involved in such a case and the client's life is in jeopardy, the nurse is obliged to provide for the client's safety, to avoid abandonment, and to withdraw only when assured that alternative sources of nursing care are available to the client.

The measures nurses take to care for the dying client and the client's family emphasize human contact. They enable the client to live with as much physical, emotional, and spiritual comfort as possible, and they maximize the values the client has treasured in life. Nursing care is directed toward the prevention and relief of the suffering commonly associated with the dying process. The nurse may provide interventions to relieve symptoms in the dying client even when the interventions entail substantial risks of hastening death.

1.4 The Setting for Health Care

The nurse adheres to the principle of nondiscriminatory, nonprejudicial care in every situation and endeavors to promote its acceptance by others. The setting shall not determine the nurse's readiness to respect clients and to render or obtain needed services.

> 2. *The nurse safeguards the client's right to privacy by judiciously protecting information of a confidential nature.*

2.1 The Client's Right to Privacy

The right to privacy is an inalienable human right. The client trusts the nurse to hold all information in confidence. This trust could be destroyed and the client's welfare jeopardized by injudicious disclosure of information provided in confidence. The duty of confidentiality, however, is not absolute when innocent parties are in direct jeopardy.

2.2 Protection of Information

The rights, well-being, and safety of the individual client should be the determining factors in arriving at any professional judgment concerning the disposition of confidential information received from the client relevant to his or her treatment. The standards of nursing practice and the nursing responsibility to provide high quality health services require that relevant data be shared with members of the health team. Only information pertinent to a client's treatment and welfare is disclosed, and it is disclosed only to those directly concerned with the client's care.

Information documenting the appropriateness, necessity, and quality of care required for the purposes of peer review, third-party payment, and other quality assurance mechanisms must be disclosed only under defined policies, mandates, or protocols. These written guidelines must assure that the rights, well-being, and safety of the client are maintained.

2.3 Access to Records

If in the course of providing care there is a need for the nurse to have access to the records of persons not under the nurse's care, the persons affected should be notified and, whenever possible, permission should be obtained first. Although records belong to the agency where the data are collected, the individual maintains the right of control over the information in the record. Similarly, professionals may exercise the right of control over information they have generated in the course of health care.

If the nurse wishes to use a client's treatment record for research or nonclinical purposes in which anonymity cannot be guaranteed, the client's consent must be obtained first. Ethically, this ensures the client's right to privacy; legally, it protects the client against unlawful invasion of privacy.

3. *The nurse acts to safeguard the client and the public when health care and safety are affected by incompetent, unethical, or illegal practice by any person.*

3.1 Safeguarding the Health and Safety of the Client

The nurse's primary commitment is to the health, welfare, and safety of the client. As an advocate for the client, the nurse must be alert to and take appropriate action regarding any instances of incompetent, unethical, or illegal practice by any member of the health care team or the health care system, or any action on the part of others that places the rights or best interests of the client in jeopardy. To function effectively in this role, nurses must be aware of the employing institution's policies and procedures, nursing standards of practice, the *Code for Nurses*, and laws governing nursing and health care practice with regard to incompetent, unethical, or illegal practice.

3.2 Acting on Questionable Practice

When the nurse is aware of inappropriate or questionable practice in the provision of health care, concern should be expressed to the person carrying out the questionable practice and attention called to the possible detrimental effect upon the client's welfare. When factors in the health care delivery system threaten the welfare of the client, similar action should be directed to the responsible administrative person. If indicated, the practice should then be reported to the appropriate authority within the institution, agency, or larger system.

There should be an established process for the reporting and handling of incompetent, unethical, or illegal practice within the employment setting so that such reporting can go through official channels without causing fear of reprisal. The nurse should be knowledgeable about the process and be prepared to use it if necessary. When questions are raised about the practices of individual practitioners or of health care systems, written documentation of the observed practices or behaviors must be available to the appropriate authorities. State nurses associations should be prepared to provide assistance and support in the development and evaluation of such processes and in reporting procedures.

When incompetent, unethical, or illegal practice on the part of anyone concerned with the client's care is not corrected within the employment setting and continues to jeopardize the client's welfare and safety, the problem should be reported to other appropriate authorities such as practice committees of the pertinent professional organizations or the legally constituted bodies concerned with licensing of specific categories of health workers or professional practitioners. Some situations may warrant the concern and involvement of all such groups. Accurate reporting and documentation undergird all actions.

3.3 Review Mechanisms

The nurse should participate in the planning, establishment, implementation, and evaluation of review mechanisms that serve to safeguard clients, such as duly constituted peer review processes or committees and ethics committees. Such ongoing review mechanisms are based on established criteria, have stated purposes, include a process for making recommendations, and facilitate improved delivery of nursing and other health services to clients wherever nursing services are provided.

> 4. *The nurse assumes responsibility and accountability for individual nursing judgments and actions.*

4.1 Acceptance of Responsibility and Accountability

The recipients of professional nursing services are entitled to high quality nursing care. Individual professional licensure is the protective mechanism legislated by the public to ensure the basic and minimum competencies of the professional nurse. Beyond that, society has accorded to the nursing profession the right to regulate its own practice. The regulation and control of nursing practice by nurses demand that individual practitioners of professional nursing must bear primary responsibility for the nursing care clients receive and must be individually accountable for their own practice.

4.2 Responsibility for Nursing Judgment and Action

Responsibility refers to the carrying out of duties associated with a particular role assumed by the nurse. Nursing obligations are reflected in the ANA publications *Nursing: A Social Policy Statement* and *Standards of Clinical Nursing Practice*. In recognizing the rights of clients, the standards describe a collaborative relationship between the nurse and the client through use of the nursing process. Nursing responsibilities include data collection and assessment of the health status of the client, formation of nursing diagnoses derived from client assessment; development of a nursing care plan that is directed toward designated goals, assists the client in maximizing his or her health capabilities, and provides for the client's participation in promoting, maintaining, and restoring his or her health; evaluation of the effectiveness of nursing care in achieving goals as determined by the client and the nurse; and subsequent reassessment and revision of the nursing care plan as warranted. In the process of assuming these responsibilities, the nurse is held accountable for them.

4.3 Accountability for Nursing Judgment and Action

Accountability refers to being answerable to someone for something one has done. It means providing an explanation or rationale to oneself, to clients, to peers, to the nursing profession, and to society. In order to be accountable, nurses act under a code of ethical conduct that is grounded in the moral principles of fidelity and respect for the dignity, worth, and self-determination of clients.

The nursing profession continues to develop ways to clarify nursing's accountability to society. The contract between the profession and society is made explicit through such mechanisms as (a) the *Code for Nurse,* (b) the standards of nursing practice, (c) the development of nursing theory derived from nursing research in order to guide nursing actions, (d) educational requirements for practice, (e) certification, and (f) mechanisms for evaluating the effectiveness of the nurse's performance of nursing responsibilities.

Nurses are accountable for judgments made and actions taken in the course of nursing practice. Neither physicians' orders nor the employing agency's policies relieve the nurse of accountability for actions taken and judgments made.

5. The nurse maintains competence in nursing.

5.1 Personal Responsibility for Competence

The profession of nursing is obliged to provide adequate and competent nursing care. Therefore, it is the personal responsibility of each nurse to maintain competency in practice. For the client's optimum well-being and for the nurse's own professional development, the care of the client reflects and incorporates new techniques and knowledge in health care as these develop, especially as they relate to the nurse's particular field of practice. The nurse must be aware of the need for continued professional learning and must assume personal responsibility for currency of knowledge and skills.

5.2 Measurement of Competence in Nursing Practice

Evaluation of one's performance by peers is a hallmark of professionalism and a method by which the profession is held accountable to society. Nurses must be willing to have their practice reviewed and evaluated by their peers. Guidelines for evaluating the scope of practice and the appropriateness, effectiveness, and efficiency of nursing practice are found in nursing practice acts, ANA standards of practice, and other quality assurance mechanisms. Each nurse is responsible for participating in the development of objective criteria for evaluation. In addition, the nurse engages in ongoing self-evaluation of clinical competency, decision-making abilities, and professional judgments.

5.3 Intraprofessional Responsibility for Competence in Nursing Care

Nurses share responsibility for high-quality nursing care. Nurses are required to have knowledge relevant to the current scope of nursing practice, changing issues and concerns, and ethical concepts and principles. Since individual competencies

vary, nurses refer clients to and consult with other nurses with expertise and recognized competencies in various fields of practice.

6. *The nurse exercises informed judgment and uses individual competency
   and qualifications as criteria in seeking consultation, accepting responsibilities, and delegating nursing activities.*

6.1 Changing Functions

Nurses are faced with decisions in the context of the increased complexity of
health care, changing patterns in the delivery of health services, and the development of evolving nursing practice in response to the health needs of clients. As the
scope of nursing practice changes, the nurse must exercise judgment in accepting
responsibilities, seeking consultation, and assigning responsibilities to others who
carry out nursing care.

6.2 Accepting Responsibilities

The nurse must not engage in practices prohibited by law or delegate to others activities prohibited by practice acts of other health care personnel or by other laws.
Nurses determine the scope of their practice in light of their education, knowledge, competency, and extent of experience. If the nurse concludes that he or she
lacks competence or is inadequately prepared to carry out a specific function, the
nurse has the responsibility to refuse that work and to seek alternative sources of
care based on concern for the client's welfare. In that refusal, both the client and
the nurse are protected. Inasmuch as the nurse is responsible for the continuous
care of patients in health care settings, the nurse is frequently called upon to carry
out components of care delegated by other health professionals as part of the
client's treatment regimen. The nurse should not accept these interdependent
functions if they are so extensive as to prevent the nurse from fulfilling the responsibility to provide appropriate nursing care to clients.

6.3 Consultation and Collaboration

The provision of health and illness care to clients is a complex process that requires a wide range of knowledge, skills, and collaborative efforts. Nurses must be
aware of their own individual competencies. When the needs of the client are beyond the qualifications and competencies of the nurse, consultation and collaboration must be sought from qualified nurses, other health professionals, or other appropriate sources. Participation on intradisciplinary or interdisciplinary teams is
often an effective approach to the provision of high-quality total health services.

6.4 Delegation of Nursing Activities

Inasmuch as the nurse is accountable for the quality of nursing care rendered to
clients, nurses are accountable for the delegation of nursing care activities to other
health workers. Therefore, the nurse must assess individual competency in assigning selected components of nursing care to other nursing service personnel. The
nurse should not delegate to any member of the nursing team a function for

which that person is not prepared or qualified. Employer policies or directives do not relieve the nurse of accountability for making judgments about the delegation of nursing care activities.

> 7. *The nurse participates in activities that contribute to the ongoing development of the profession's body of knowledge.*

7.1 The Nurse and Development of Knowledge

Every profession must engage in scholarly inquiry to identify, verify, and continually enlarge the body of knowledge that forms the foundation for its practice. A unique body of verified knowledge provides both framework, and direction for the profession in all of its activities and for the practitioner in the provision of nursing care. The accrual of scientific and humanistic knowledge promotes the advancement of practice and the well-being of the profession's clients. Ongoing scholarly activity such as research and the development of theory is indispensable to the full discharge of a profession's obligations to society. Each nurse has a role in this area of professional activity, whether as an investigator in furthering knowledge, as a participant in research, or as a user of theoretical and empirical knowledge.

7.2 Protection of Rights of Human Participants in Research

Individual rights valued by society and by the nursing profession that have particular application in research include the right of adequately informed consent, the right to freedom from risk of injury, and the right of privacy and preservation of dignity. Inherent in these rights is respect for each individual's rights to exercise self-determination, to choose to participate or not, to have full information, and to terminate participation in research without penalty.

It is the duty of the nurse functioning in any research role to maintain vigilance in protecting the life, health, and privacy of human subjects from both anticipated and unanticipated risks and in assuring informed consent. Subjects' integrity, privacy, and rights must be especially safeguarded if the subjects are unable to protect themselves because of incapacity or because they are in a dependent relationship to the investigator. The investigation should be discontinued if its continuance might be harmful to the subject.

7.3 General Guidelines for Participating in Research

Before participating in research conducted by others, the nurse has an obligation to (a) obtain information about the intent and the nature of the research and (b) ascertain that the study proposal is approved by the appropriate bodies, such as institutional review boards.

Research should be conducted and directed by qualified persons. The nurse who participates in research in any capacity should be fully informed about both the nurse's and the client's rights and obligations.

> 8. *The nurse participates in the profession's efforts to implement and improve standards of nursing.*

8.1 Responsibility to the Public for Standards

Nursing is responsible and accountable for admitting to the profession only those individuals who have demonstrated the knowledge, skills, and commitment considered essential to professional practice. Nurse educators have a major responsibility that these competencies and a demonstrated commitment to professional practices have been achieved before the entry of an individual into the practice of professional nursing.

Established standards and guidelines for nursing practice provide guidance for the delivery of professional nursing care and are a means for evaluating care received by the public. The nurse has a personal responsibility and commitment to clients for implementation and maintenance of optimal standards of nursing practice.

8.3 Responsibility to the Profession for Standards

Established standards reflect the practice of nursing grounded in ethical commitments and a body of knowledge. Professional standards or guidelines exist in nursing practice, nursing service, nursing education, and nursing research. The nurse has the responsibility to monitor these standards in daily practice actively in the profession's ongoing efforts to foster optimal standards of practice at the local, regional, state, and national levels of the health care system.

Nurse educators have the additional responsibility to maintain optimal standards of nursing practice and education in nursing education programs and in any other settings where planned learning activities for nursing students take place.

> 9. *The nurse participates in the profession's efforts to establish and maintain conditions of employment conducive to high-quality nursing care.*

9.1 Responsibility for Conditions of Employment

The nurse must be concerned with conditions of employment that (a) enable the nurse to practice in accordance with the standards of nursing practice and (b) provide a care environment that meets the standards of nursing service. The provision of high-quality nursing care is the responsibility of both the individual nurse and the nursing profession. Professional autonomy and self-regulated control of conditions of practice are necessary for implementing nursing standards.

9.2 Maintaining Conditions for High-Quality Nursing Care

Articulation and control of nursing practice can be accomplished through individual agreement and collective action. A nurse may enter into an agreement with individuals or organizations to provide health care. Nurses may participate in collective action such as collective bargaining through their state nurses association to determine the terms and conditions of employment conducive to high-quality nursing care. Such agreements should be consistent with the profession's standards of practice, the state law regulating nursing practice, and the *Code for Nurses*.

> 10. *The nurse participates in the profession's effort to protect the public from misinformation and misrepresentation and to maintain the integrity of nursing.*

10.1 Protection from Misinformation and Misrepresentation

Nurses are responsible for advising clients against the use of products that endanger the clients' safety and welfare. The nurse shall not use any form of public or professional communication to make claims that are false, fraudulent, misleading, deceptive, or unfair.

The nurse does not give or imply endorsement to advertising, promotion, or sale of commercial products or services in a manner that may be interpreted as reflecting the opinion or judgment of the profession as a whole. The nurse may use knowledge of specific services or products in advising an individual client, since this may contribute to the client's health and well-being. In the course of providing information or education to clients or other practitioners about commercial products or services, however, a variety of similar products or services should be offered or described so the client or practitioner can make an informed choice.

10.2 Maintaining the Integrity of Nursing

The use of the title *registered nurse* is granted by state governments for the protection of the public. Use of that title carries with it the responsibility to act in the public interest. The nurse may use the title *R.N.* and symbols of academic degrees or other earned or honorary professional symbols of recognition in all ways that are legal and appropriate. The title and other symbols of the profession should not be used, however, for benefits unrelated to nursing practice or the profession, or used by those who may seek to exploit them for other purposes.

Nurses should refrain from casting a vote in any deliberations involving health care services or facilities where the nurse has business or other interests that could be construed as a conflict of interest.

> 11. *The nurse collaborates with members of the health professions and other citizens in promoting community and national efforts to meet the health needs of the public.*

11.1 Collaboration With Others to Meet Health Needs

The availability and accessibility of high-quality health services to all people require collaborative planning at the local, state, national, and international levels that respects the interdependence of health professionals and clients in health care systems. Nursing care is an integral part of high-quality health care, and nurses have an obligation to promote equitable access to nursing and health care for all people.

11.2 Responsibility to the Public

The nursing profession is committed to promoting the welfare and safety of all people. The goals and values of nursing are essential to effective delivery of health services. For the benefit of the individual client and the public at large, nursing's goals and commitments need adequate representation. Nurses should ensure this representation by active participation in decision making in institutional and political arenas to assure a just distribution of health care and nursing resources.

11.3 Relationships with Other Disciplines

The complexity of health care delivery systems requires a multidisciplinary approach to delivery of services that has the strong support and active participation of all the health professions. Nurses should actively promote the collaborative planning required to ensure the availability and accessibility of high-quality health services to all persons whose health needs are unmet.

AMERICAN MEDICAL ASSOCIATION: *CODE OF MEDICAL ETHICS**

Preamble

The medical profession has long subscribed to a body of ethical statements developed primarily for the benefit of the patient. As a member of this profession, a physician must recognize responsibility not only to patients, but also to society, other health professionals, and to self. The following principles adopted by the American Medical Association are not laws, but standards of conduct which define the essentials of honorable behavior for the physician.

 I. A physician shall be dedicated to providing competent medical service with compassion and respect for human dignity.

 II. A physician shall deal honestly with patients and colleagues, and strive to expose those physicians deficient in character or competence, or who engage in fraud or deception.

 III. A physician shall respect the law and also recognize a responsibility to seek changes in those requirements which are contrary to the best interests of the patient.

 IV. A physician shall respect the rights of patients, of colleagues, and of other health professionals, and shall safeguard patient confidences within the constraints of the law.

 V. A physician shall continue to study, apply and advance scientific knowledge, make relevant information available to patients, colleagues, and the public, obtain consultation, and use the talents of other health professionals when indicated.

 VI. A physician shall, in the provision of appropriate patient care, except in emergencies, be free to choose whom to serve, with whom to associate, and the environment in which to provide medical services.

 VII. A physician shall recognize a responsibility to participate in activities contributing to an improved community.

*Reprinted with permission of the American Medical Association, 515 N St, Chicago, Illinois 60610. Source: Code of Medical Ethics, American Medical Association, copyright 1994.

Fundamental Elements of the Patient-Physician Relationship

From ancient times, physicians have recognized that the health and well-being of patients depends upon a collaborative effort between physician and patient. Patients share with physicians the responsibility for their own health care. The patient-physician relationship is of greatest benefit to patients when they bring medical problems to the attention of their physicians in a timely fashion, provide information about their medical condition to the best of their ability, and work with their physicians in a mutually respectful alliance. Physicians can best contribute to this alliance by serving as their patients' advocate and by fostering these rights:

1. The patient has the right to receive information from physicians and to discuss the benefits, risks, and costs of appropriate treatment alternatives. Patients should receive guidance from their physicians as to the optimal course of action. Patients are also entitled to obtain copies or summaries of their medical records, to have their questions answered, to be advised of potential conflicts of interest that their physicians might have, and to receive independent professional opinions.
2. The patient has the right to make decisions regarding the health care that is recommended by his or her physician. Accordingly, patients may accept or refuse any recommended medical treatment.
3. The patient has the right to courtesy, respect, dignity, responsiveness, and timely attention to his or her needs.
4. The patient has the right to confidentiality. The physician should not reveal confidential communications or information without the consent of the patient, unless provided for by law or by the need to protect the welfare of the individual or the public interest.
5. The patient has the right to continuity of health care. The physician has an obligation to cooperate in the coordination of medically indicated care with other health care providers treating the patient. The physician may not discontinue treatment of a patient as long as further treatment is medically indicated, without giving the patient reasonable assistance and sufficient opportunity to make alternative arrangements for care.
6. The patient has a basic right to have available adequate health care. Physicians, along with the rest of society, should continue to work toward its goal. Fulfillment of this right is dependent on society providing resources so that no patient is deprived of necessary care because of an inability to pay for the care. Physicians should continue their traditional assumption of a part of the responsibility for the medical care of those who cannot afford essential health care. Physicians should advocate for patients in dealing with third parties when appropriate.

Patient Responsibilities

It has long been recognized that successful medical care requires an ongoing collaborative effort between patients and physicians. Physicians and patients are bound in a partnership that requires both individuals to take an active role in the healing process. Such a partnership does not imply that both partners have identical responsibilities or equal power. While physicians have the responsibility to provide health care services to patients to the best of their ability, patients have the responsibility to communicate openly, to participate in decisions about the diagnostic and treatment recommendations, and to comply with the agreed upon treatment program.

Like patients' rights, patients' responsibilities are derived from the principle of autonomy. The principle of patient autonomy holds that an individual's physical-emotional, and psychological integrity should be respected and upheld. This principle also recognizes the human capacity to self-govern and choose a course of action from among different alternative options. Autonomous, competent patients assert some control over the decisions which direct their health care. With exercise of self-governance and free choice comes a number of responsibilities.

1. Good communication is essential to a successful patient-physician relationship. To the extent possible, patients have a responsibility to be truthful and to express their concerns clearly to their physicians.

2. Patients have a responsibility to provide a complete medical history, to the extent possible, including information about past illnesses, medications, hospitalizations, family history of illness, and other matters relating to present health.

3. Patients have a responsibility to request information or clarification about their health status or treatment when they do not fully understand what has been described.

4. Once patients and physicians agree upon the goals of therapy and a treatment plan, patients have a responsibility to cooperate with that treatment plan. Compliance with physician instructions is often essential to public and individual safety. Patients also have a responsibility to disclose whether previously agreed upon treatments are being followed and to indicate when they would like to reconsider the treatment plan.

5. Patients generally have a responsibility to meet their financial obligations with regard to medical care or to discuss financial hardships with their physicians. Patients should be cognizant of the costs associated with using a limited resource like health care and try to use medical resources judiciously.

6. Patients should discuss end-of-life decisions with their physicians and make their wishes known. Such a discussion might also include writing an advance directive.

7. Patients should be committed to health maintenance through health-enhancing behavior. Illness can often be prevented by a healthy lifestyle, and patients should take personal responsibility when they are able to avert the development of disease.

8. Patients should also have an active interest in the effects of their conduct on others and refrain from behavior that unreasonably places the health of others at risk. Patients should inquire as to the means and likelihood of infectious disease transmission and act upon that information which can best prevent further transmission.

9. Patients should discuss organ donation with their physicians and, if donation is desired, make applicable provisions. Patients who are part of an organ allocation system and await a needed transplant should not try to go outside of or manipulate the system. A fair system of allocation should be answered with public trust and an awareness of limited resources.
10. Patients should not initiate or participate in fraudulent health care and should report illegal or unethical behavior by physicians or other providers to the appropriate medical societies, licensing boards, or law enforcement authorities.

AMERICAN HOSPITAL ASSOCIATION: *A PATIENT'S BILL OF RIGHTS**

Introduction

Effective health care requires collaboration between patients and physicians and other health care professionals, open and honest communication, respect for personal and professional values, and sensitivity to differences are integral to optimal patient care. As the setting for the provision of health services, hospitals must provide a foundation for understanding and respecting the rights and responsibilities of patients, their families, physicians, and other caregivers. Hospitals must ensure a health care ethic that respects the role of patients in decision making about treatment choices and other aspects of their care. Hospitals must be sensitive to cultural, racial, linguistic, religious, age, gender, and other differences as well as the needs of persons with disabilities.

The American Hospital Association presents *A Patient's Bill of Rights* with the expectation that it will contribute to more effective patient care and be supported by the hospital on behalf of the institution, its medical staff, employees, and patients. The American Hospital Association encourages health care institutions to tailor this bill of rights to their patient community by translating and/or simplifying the language of this bill of rights as may be necessary to ensure that patients and their families understand their rights and responsibilities.

---

*These rights can be exercised on the patient's behalf by a designated surrogate or proxy decision maker if the patient lacks decision-making capacity, is legally incompetent, or is a minor.

A Patient's Bill of Rights was first adopted by the American Hospital Association in 1971. This revision was approved by the Board of Trustees on October 21, 1992. Reprinted with permission of the American Hospital Association, copyright 1992.

Bill of Rights

1. The patient has the right to considerate and respectful care.
2. The patient has the right to and is encouraged to obtain from physicians and other direct caregivers relevant, current, and understandable information concerning diagnosis, treatment, and prognosis.

Except in emergencies when the patient lacks decision-making capacity and the need for treatment is urgent, the patient is entitled to the opportunity to discuss and request information related to the specific procedures and/or treatments, the risks involved, the possible length of recuperation, and the medically reasonable alternatives and their accompanying risks and benefits.

Patients have the right to know the identity of physicians, nurses, and others involved in their care, as well as when those involved are students, residents, or other trainees. The patient also has the right to know the immediate and long-term financial implications of treatment choices, insofar as they are known.

3. The patient has the right to make decisions about the plan of care prior to and during the course of treatment and to refuse a recommended treatment or plan of care to the extent permitted by law and hospital policy and to be informed of the medical consequences of this action. In the case of such refusal, the patient is entitled to other appropriate care and services that the hospital provides or transfer to another hospital. The hospital should notify patients of any policy that might affect patient choice within the institution.
4. The patient has the right to have an advance directive (such as a living will, health care proxy, or durable power of attorney for health care) concerning treatment or designating a surrogate decision maker with the expectation that the hospital will honor the intent of that directive to the extent permitted by law and hospital policy.

Health care institutions must advise patients of their rights under state law and hospital policy to make informed medical choices, ask if the patient has an advance directive, and include that information in patient records. The patient has the right to timely information about hospital policy that may limit its ability to implement fully a legally valid advance directive.

5. The patient has the right to every consideration of privacy. Case discussion, consultation, examination, and treatment should be conducted so as to protect each patient's privacy.
6. The patient has the right to expect that all communications and records pertaining to his/her care will be treated as confidential by the hospital, except in cases such as suspected abuse and public health hazards when reporting is permitted or required by law. The patient has the right to expect that the hospital will emphasize the confidentiality of this information

when it releases it to any other parties entitled to review information in these records.

7. The patient has the right to review the records pertaining to his/her medical care and to have the information explained or interpreted as necessary, except when restricted by law.

8. The patient has the right to expect that, within its capacity and policies, a hospital will make reasonable response to the request of a patient for appropriate and medically indicated care and services. The hospital must provide evaluation, service, and/or referral as indicated by the urgency of the case. When medically appropriate and legally permissible, or when a patient has so requested, a patient may be transferred to another facility. The institution to which the patient is to be transferred must first have accepted the patient for transfer. The patient must also have the benefit of complete information and explanation concerning the need for, risks, benefits, and alternatives to such a transfer.

9. The patient has the right to ask and be informed of the existence of business relationships among the hospital, educational institutions, other health care providers, or payers that may influence the patient's treatment and care.

10. The patient has the right to consent to or decline to participate in proposed research studies or human experimentation affecting care and treatment or requiring direct patient involvement, and to have those studies fully explained prior to consent. A patient who declines to participate in research or experimentation is entitled to the most effective care that the hospital can otherwise provide.

11. The patient has the right to expect reasonable continuity of care when appropriate and to be informed by physicians and other caregivers of available and realistic patient care options when hospital care is no longer appropriate.

12. The patient has the right to be informed of hospital policies and practices that relate to patient care, treatment, and responsibilities. The patient has the right to he informed of available resources for resolving disputes, grievances, and conflicts, such as ethics committees, patient representatives, or other mechanisms available in the institution. The patient has the right to be informed of the hospital's charges for services and available payment methods.

The collaborative nature of health care requires that patients, or their families-surrogates, participate in their care. The effectiveness of care and patient satisfaction with the course of treatment depend, in part, on the patient fulfilling certain responsibilities. Patients are responsible for providing information about past illnesses, hospitalizations, medications, and other matters related to health status to participate effectively in decision making, patients must be encouraged to take responsibility for requesting additional information or clarification about their health status or treatment when they do not fully understand information and instructions. Patients are also responsible for ensuring that the health care institution has a copy of their written advance directive if they have one. Patients are responsible for informing their physicians and other caregivers if they anticipate problems in following prescribed treatment.

Patients should also be aware of the hospital's obligation to be reasonably efficient and equitable in providing care to other patients and the community. The hospital's rules and regulations are designed to help the hospital meet this obligation. Patients and their families are responsible for making reasonable accommodations to the needs of the hospital, other patients, medical staff, and hospital employees. Patients are responsible for providing necessary information for insurance claims and for working with the hospital to make payment arrangements, when necessary.

A person's health depends on much more than health care services. Patients are responsible for recognizing the impact of their lifestyle on their personal health.

Conclusion

Hospitals have many functions to perform, including the enhancement of health status, health promotion, and the prevention and treatment of injury and disease; the immediate and ongoing care and rehabilitation of patients; the education of health professionals, patients, and the community; and research. All these activities must be conducted with overriding concern for the values and dignity of patients.

CHOICE IN DYING LIVING WILL*

I, _____ being of sound mind, make this statement as a directive to be followed if I become permanently unable to participate in decisions regarding my medical care. These instructions reflect my firm and settled commitment to decline medical treatment under the circumstances indicated below:

I direct my attending physician to withhold or withdraw treatment that merely prolongs my dying, if I should be in an incurable or irreversible mental or physical condition with no reasonable expectation of recovery, including but not limited to: (a) a terminal condition, (b) a permanently unconscious condition; or (c) a minimally conscious condition in which I am permanently unable to make decisions or express my wishes, I direct that treatment be limited to measures to keep me comfortable and to relieve pain, including any pain that might occur by withholding or withdrawing treatment.

*Courtesy of Choice in Dying Inc. Reprinted by permission of Partnership For Caring, 1035 30th St NW, Washington, DC 20007; 800-989-9455.

While I understand that I am not legally required to be specific about future treatments, if I am in the conditions described above, I feel especially strongly about the following forms of treatment:

I do not want cardiac resuscitation. I do not want mechanical respiration. I do not want tube feeding. I do not want antibiotics. However, I do want maximum pain relief, even if it may hasten my death.

Add personal instructions, if any:

These directions express my legal right to refuse treatment under federal and state law. I intend my instructions to be carried out, unless I have revoked them in a new writing or by clearly indicating that I have changed my mind.

Signed: _____ Date: _____

Address: (please print): _____

_____

Witnessing Procedure

I declare that the person who signed this document appeared to execute the living will willingly and free from duress. He or she signed (or asked another to sign for him or her) this document in my presence.

Witness No. 1: _____

Address: _____

_____

Witness No. 2: _____

Address: _____

_____

Index

A

Abnormal infant, issue of treatment for, 161

Abortion
  birth of very premature as result of spontaneous or induced, 163
  nursing ethics and problem of, 141–59
    ethical and religious issues in, 146–53
    legal status of, 142–44
    reproductive technology and, 144–46
    role of nurse in, 153–56
  pro-choice versus pro-life debate over, 8
  Thomson's argument on, 89

Abrams, N., 24

Absolutism, 55
  rational antidote to, 43

Abuse
  battered women and, 125
  child, 178
  circumstantial, 110
  of elderly patient, 250–51
  exposure of incest and, 180–81
  family, 124–25
  of the person, 110–11
  reporting, 181
  rights as form of moral standing against arbitrary, 90
  sexual, 196

Accident, fallacy of, 112

Acquired immunodeficiency syndrome (AIDS), 6, 124. *See also* HIV/AIDS
  right to bear children and, 127–28
  spread of, 197

Active euthanasia, 262–63, 268

Active-passive euthanasia, 262, 267–70

Adams, Barry, 25

Adolescents, ethical issues in nursing care of, 194–205
  biological/biographical social/cognitive distinction applied to, 203–4

controversy between parental authority and autonomy of, 200–201
developmental highlights for, 194–96
eating disorders and disturbances in body concept, 196
health care issues for, 196–97
life and death of, 197–99
life-saving treatment for
  right of to, 198
  right to exercise autonomy by refusing, 197–98
parental refusal to consent to tonsillectomies of, 199
pregnancies of, 196
in quality-of-life cases, 199
in relationship with nurses, parents, and, 202–3
role of nurse in care of, 199–201
sexual abuse, 196
surgery for, versus parental refusal of consent, 199

Adults, ethical issues in nursing care of, 208–30
  allocation of scarce resources, 211
  confidentiality in, 214–15, 220
  deception in, 211–12, 216–17
  development of, 208–10
  informed consent in, 212–13, 215, 217–18
  nurse's role with, 225–29
  prevention of harm, 211, 215
  privacy in, 214–15, 220
  in receiving and refusing treatment, 213–14, 218–19
  truth-telling in, 211–12, 216–17

Advance directives, 98, 270–71

Advanced old age, 235

Advocacy. *See also* Patient advocacy
  importance of, 23–24
  levels of, 200

Agapistic ethics, 2, 62

Alpha-fetoprotein screening, 145

Altruism, 46
  Christian, 62–63
  social contract and, 55

Alzheimer's disease, 124
American Academy of Pediatrics (AAP)
  Task Force on Pediatric
  Research, Informed Consent,
  and Medical Ethics, Statement
  on Consent by, 179
American Hospital Association (AHA)
  A Patient's Bill of Rights, 229–30,
  253
  Technical Panel on Biomedical
  Ethics, 9
American Medical Association (AMA)
  Code of Ethics, 36
  on distinction between active and
  passive euthanasia, 268
American Nurses Association (ANA),
  Code for Nurses, 10, 26–33, 40,
  45, 87, 97–98, 166–67
  description of nurse in, 184
  harmful conditions of patient care
  and, 45
  patient advocate in, 166–67, 253
  specific provisions of, 26–33
  universal moral principles in, 10,
  15, 40
Americans with Disabilities Act (ADA)
  (1990), 168
Amniocentesis, 141, 145
Anemia, screening program
  for iron-deficiency, 179–80
  for sickle-cell, 133, 135
Anoxia, 180
Anti-equality argument, 244
Anti-freeloader argument, 244
Anti-semitism, 43
Appeal, philosophical sources of, in ethics
  of caring, 14
Appeal to force, fallacy of, 110
Arbitrary abuses, rights as form of moral
  standing against, 90
Aristotle, 7, 14, 41, 54, 173
  conception of ethics applied to
  nursing, happiness through self-
  realization, 58–61
Aroskar, Mila Ann, 15
Artificial insemination, 129
Assisted suicide, 238, 277–80
  by machine, 278
  physician, 268, 276–77

Attribution, appropriate, of rights, 91
Authority, appeal to inappropriate, 111
Autonomy
  adolescent's right to exercise, by
  refusing life-saving treatment,
  197–98
  patient, 21

B
Battered women, 125
Beal v. *Doe,* 142
Becker, L., 90–91
Begging the question, 153
Beneficence principle, 162
Benign ownership view, 119–20
Benn, Stanley, 170
Benner, P., 92, 93
Bentham, Jeremy, 47, 68–70, 85
Berlin, Iasiah, 78, 87–88
Best interest standard, 178
  versus substitute judgment, 103–4
Bettelheim, Bruno, 63
Bioethics, 58
Biographical life, conception of, 187
Biological/biographical distinction
  for children, 187–88
  in utilitarianism, 71
Biological/biographical social/cognitive
  distinction applied to
  adolescents, 203–4
Blood transfusions, refusal of Jehovah's
  Witnesses to accept
  transfusions, 87, 103, 203
Body concept, 196
Bradley, F. H., 88
Brain damage, nurse's decision on
  treatment and, 180
Brain-death definition, 180, 261–62
Brandt, Karl, 89
Brody. B., 151–52
Brompton's cocktail, 285–86
Buber, M., 78
Burgess, E. W., 118, 119
Busy ethic, 234–35

C
Camus, Albert, 274
Cancer, 124
Canterbury v. *Spence,* 218

Cardiac repair, use of embryonic tissue and, 146

Caring. *See also* Nursing
in context of feminist framework, 13–14
in nursing ethics, 13–14, 93
philosophical sources of appeal in ethics of, 14

Carnegie, Elizabeth, 88

Categorical imperatives, 75
comparison to golden rule, 76

Catholic Church
on abortion, 146
on artificial insemination, 129

Catlin, A. J., 162–65

Cephalus, 12

Child abuse, 178

Children, ethical issues in nursing care of, 176–91. *See also* Infants
for children with HIV/AIDS, 181–83
developmental highlights, 176–77
disagreement with parents over treatment, 179
helping express fears, 186
on informed consent, 177–81, 189
exposure of incest, 180–81
on issues of life or death, 180
to kidney donation, 180
mass screening program for children based on mother coercion, 179–80
withholding life-saving drugs, 178–79
moral implications in nursing care of, 183–86
nurses as advocates of, 185
rights of handicapped, 177
right to bear
AIDS and, 127–28
despite consequences, 132–34
treatment of deformed, 184
values reflected in rearing practices, 176–77

Chorionic villus sampling, 145

Christian altruism, 62–63

Christian Scientists, 10

Circumstantial abuse, fallacy of, 110

Civil-disobedience model, 24

Civil law, 61

Clark, Barney, 90

Clark, Brian, 57

Classical utilitarianism in nursing ethics, 68–71

Club membership model of family and marriage, 120–21, 177

Code for Nurses, 87
description of nurse in, 184
harmful conditions of patient care and, 45
patient advocate in, 166–67, 253
specific provisions of, 26–33
universal moral principles in, 10, 15, 40

Codes of ethics. *See also Code for Nurses; Ethics*
American Medical Association, 36
evaluation of professional, 36
function of, for nurses, 34–36
for International Council for Nurses, 33–34
moral implications in, 26

Collectivism, 47, 77

Competence
patient's right to refuse and, 239
rights of elderly patients and, 247–49

Complementary models of patient advocacy, 190–91

Complex question, fallacy of, 112

Condoms, spread of AIDS and, 197

Confidentiality, right to, 214–15, 220

Conflict of rights, 239

Consciousness, 187

Consent. *See also* Informed consent
parental refusal
for adolescents' tonsillectomies, 199
for surgery for adolescents on grounds of religious beliefs, 199

Consequentialist ethics, 66–72. *See also* Utilitarianism
Kant's answer to, 75

Consumer model of physician-patient relationship, 20

Contracted clinician, nurse as, 22

Control versus freedom, 8

Conventional reasoning, 11

Counseling, nurse's role in genetic, 136–37

Courage, 14
Creationism, 10
Cystic fibrosis, genetic screening and, 135

D

Darling, Kenneth, 204
*Darling v. Charleston Community
    Memorial Hospital,* 55, 89
Death and dying, ethical issues in nursing
        care
    active euthanasia, 262–63
    active/passive euthanasia, 262, 267–70
    for adolescents, 197–99
    adult's right to, 263–64
    advance directives, 270–71
    definitions of, 261–62
    "Do not resuscitate" orders, 264,
        271–73
    ethical issues in nursing care of,
        260–89
    hospice concept in, 285–86
    nurse's decision on issue of, 180
    organ donations, 271
    paternalism versus libertarianism, 264
    patient's right to know the truth, 263
    quality versus length of life, 265–66
    relief of individual suffering versus
        principle of double effect, 266
    religious aspects of nursing care of,
        280–81
    rights of patients, 265
    right to suicide, 263
    role of nurse in care of patient, 281–86
    unplugging respirator, 263
    voluntary and involuntary euthanasia,
        273–80
The Death of Ivan Ilych, 281
Deception, 211–12
    avoidance of, 216–17
    versus veracity, 9
Decision making. *See also* Ethical
        decision making in nursing
    in families, 127
    nursing dilemmas in, 49–50
    rational
        patient capacity to make, 101–2
        patient incapacity to make, 102–3
    shared
        guidelines for, 108–9
        values supportive of, 97–98

values and principles underlying
        reasonable process of, 97–98
Declaration of Helsinki (1975), 89
Declaration of the Rights of the Child
        (United Nations, 1959), 177,
        195–196
Deformed children, treatment of, 184
Deformed infants, arguments for and
        against saving, 162–65
Deliberative model of physician-patient
        relationship, 20
Dementia, 235–36
Dependency, 189
    in adolescence, 195
Descartes, René, 53, 72, 261–62
Diagnostically related groupings, 243
Dialectical reasoning, 12
Dilemma, defined, 6
Distributive justice
    problem of providing, in health care,
        245
    values in, 85–86
Divine law, 61
Divorce, 125–26
Doe v. Bolton, 142
"Do no harm" principle, 4, 167, 178
"Do not resuscitate" orders, 264, 271–73
Dostoevsky, 60
Double effect, doctrine of, 32, 266
Down syndrome, 145, 161, 164
Drugs, parents' decision to withhold life-
        saving, 178–79
Durable power of attorney, 98, 270–71
Duties, distinguishing between perfect
        and imperfect, 76–77
Duty-based ethics, 74–82, 203
Dworkin, Ronald, 87
Dying. *See* Death and dying

E

Eating disorders and disturbances, 196
Ego integrity, 236
Egoism, 41, 42, 46
Elderly patients, ethical issues in care of,
        233–59
    abuse of, 250–51
    advanced old age, 235
    allocating health care to, 238,
        240–46
    assisted suicide and, 238, 277–80

competence and patient's right to refuse treatment, 239
competence and rights of, 247–49
conflict of rights, 239
dementia, 235–36
developmental highlights, 233–36
frail, 235
freedom versus control and prevention of harm, 250
granny pregnancies and, 130
informed consent, 246–47, 253–54
justice between generations, 249–50
nurse as patient advocate, 240
patient's rights, 246–47
    to decide, 239
prejudice against, 237
problems and prospects for, 236–38
resources for, allocation of, 238, 240–41
retirement, 234–35
role of patient advocate, 252–53
sanctity of life versus quality of life, 255–56
truth-telling, 240, 246, 255–56
Elders, Jocelyn, 128
Electroconvulsive therapy, right of nurses' to refuse to administer, 89–90
Emanuel, E. J., 20–21
Emanuel, L. L., 20–21
Embryonic tissue, use of, 146
Empirical knowledge versus personal belief, 10
Empiric approach to ethics, 11
Engels, F., 78
Engineering model of physician-patient relationship, 20
Epictetus, view of ethics, 60–61
Equal consideration, principle of, 245–46
Equality, 87
    principle of, 244–45
Equity, principle of, 101
Erikson, E. H., 236, 249
Essential information, patient access to, 105–8
Eternal law, 61
Ethical decision making in nursing, 96–113. *See also* Decision making; Nursing ethics
assessment of patient capacity and competence, 101–8

fallacies in, 109–12
guidelines for shared decision making, 108–9
Patient Self-Determination Act (1990) in, 98–101
values supportive of shared health care decisions, 97–98
Ethical issues. *See* Nursing ethics
Ethical justification, 12
Ethical-philosophical approaches to nurse-child-parent relationships, 187–91
Ethical theory, major differences between scientific theory and, 3–4
Ethics. *See also* Codes of ethics; Health care ethics; Nursing ethics
agapistic, 2, 62
Aquinas's view of, 61–63
of caring, 93
consequentialist or utilitarian, 66–72
conventional approach to, 11
defined, 6
deontological, 171
dialectal, 12
duty-based, 74–82
Epictetus's view of, 60–61
function of nursing, 4–6
happiness-based, 14, 58–60
interdisciplinary role of nurse in, 15–16
of Jesus, 70
justice as basis for, 85–86
rights-based, 84–94, 156
role of nurse in, 14–15
science and, 2–4
virtue, in nursing, 53–64
Ethics Rounds, 16
Eudaimonism, 58–60
Euthanasia, 268
    active, 262–63, 268
    active/passive, 262, 267–70
    involuntary, 268, 273–80
    nonvoluntary, 268
    passive, 268
    voluntary, 268, 273–80
Existentialism, 47–48, 48–49, 78
Experience, 59

F
Facts, relation of, to values, 67
Fagin, Claire, 89

Fair equality of opportunity principle, 85
Faith healing cases, 204
Fallacies, 109–12
  abuse of the person, 110–11
  of accident, 112
  appeal to force, 110
  appeal to inappropriate authority,
    111
  complex question, 112
  is-ought, 11, 67–68, 70, 109–10, 242,
    244
  slippery-slope, 111–12, 147
  slothful induction, 112
Families
  club membership model of, 120–21,
    177
  definition of, 118
  dynamics of, 118–19, 123–26
  family planning and socioeconomic
    differences in, 177
  functions of, 118–19
  nursing ethics in procreative,
    117–38
  ownership model of, 119–20, 176
  partnership model of, 121–23, 177,
    185–86
  role of nurse in hierarchies in, 120
  values of, 118–19, 123–26
Family caregiving, 124
Family communes, 121
Family ethical issues, role of nurse in,
  126–27
Family planning, 128–29
  contraception and, 127–28
  family socioeconomic differences and,
    177
Family sovereign, 119–20
Fears, helping children express, 186
Feinberg, Joel, 170
Feminist framework, care in context of,
  13–14
Fetal reduction, 146
Fetal therapy, 130–31
Fetoscopy, 130
Final Exit (Humphrey), 279
Fletcher, John, 146
Fletcher, Joseph, 53, 71, 129, 187
Forced labor, 151
Foreman, C. H., 128
Formal deduction, 10–11

Fourteenth Amendment, 142, 197
Frail elderly, 235
Frankena, William, 62
Freedom, moral value of, 87
Freedom of Access to Clinic Entrance
  Act (1994), 144
Freedom versus control, 8
Freud, S., 60
Freund, Paul, 76
Friendship, 14, 59–60
Fromer, Margot, 187

G
Gadow, Sally, 22
Gaylin, Willard, 141
Genetics, 132–34
  role of nurse in counseling, 136–37
Genetic screening
  for cystic fibrosis, 135
  ethical issues in, 130–31
  for Huntington's disease, 135
  mandatory versus voluntary,
    134–36
  for muscular dystrophy, 135
  for phenylketonuria (PKU), 135
  for retinoblastoma, 133–34, 135
  for sickle-cell anemia, 133, 135
  for Tay-Sachs disease, 130–31, 132,
    135
Genovese, Kitty, 49, 149, 150
Gershkovich, Arkadey, 62
Gilligan, C., 92
Glaucon, 44
Goal-based ethics, handicapped infants
  and, 172
Golden rule, 41, 54
  comparison to categorical imperative,
    76
Golding, M. P., 61
Goldman, A., 119
Good, identification of, 6, 78
Good life
  defined, 7
  health as goal of, 7
Goodman, Paul, 36
Goodnow, Minnie, 23
Good Samaritan, 149
Granny pregnancies, 130
Greatest benefit principle, 85
Greatest-happiness criterion, 76

Green, Chad, 10, 178–79, 204
Greene, Rita, 9–10
Greenlaw, Jane, 106
Griswold v. *Connecticut,* 142
Group confrontational model, 190
Guidance-cooperation model, 204

H
Handicapped child, rights of, 177
Handicapped infants, application of
    philosophical moves to, 171–73
Happiness
    meaning of, 60
    through self-realization, 58–61
Happiness-based ethics, 14, 58–60
Harding, G. J., 124
Harm
    identification of, 6
    prevention of, 211, 215–16, 250
Health as goal of good life, 7
Health care
    allocating, to elderly, 241–46
    issues for adolescents, 196–97
    paradigm case arguments in, 88
    rationing, 7–8
    rights in and to, HIV/AIDS, 222–25
Health care ethics. *See also* Ethics;
    Nursing ethics
    argument for rights in, 88–89
    moral importance of human rights in,
    91
Health teaching and counseling, nursing
    practices of, 226
Heart-death definition, 261
Hedonism, 41
Hegel, 78
Heifitz, Milton, 164–65
Henderson, Virginia, 78
Herodotus, 11
HIV/AIDS. *See also* Acquired
    immunodeficiency syndrome
    (AIDS)
    ethical issues in care of children with,
    181–83
    moral-philosophical responses to,
    224–25
    rights in and to health care and,
    222–25
    testing newborns for, 165–66
Hobbes, Thomas, 44

Hoffman, Paul, 9–10
Holmes method, 241–42
Homicide, 196
Hospice concept, 285–86
Human Genome Project, 132
Humankind, meaning of nursing in
    history of, 1–2
Human law, 61
Human rights, moral importance of, in
    health care ethics, 91
Hume, David, 14, 66–68, 274
Humphrey, Derek, 279
Huntington's disease, 134
    genetic screening for, 135
Hydrocephalus, 145
Hyperactive child and prescription drugs
    for, 178
Hypothetical imperatives, 75

I
If-then judgments, 75
Imperatives
    categorical, 75, 76
    hypothetical, 75
Imperfect duties, distinguishing from
    perfect duties, 76–77
Incest, exposure of, by nurse, 180–81
Individual confrontation model of patient
    advocacy, 191
Individualism, 77, 78
    in relation to collectivism,
    existentialism, and
    phenomenology, 47–49
Individual suffering, relief of, versus
    principle of double effect, 266
Induction, slothful, 112
Inductive reasoning, 11, 68
Infants, ethical issues in nursing care of,
    160–75. *See also* Children
    arguments for and against saving
    deformed, 162–65
    arguments for and against saving
    premature, 162–65
    developmental highlights, 160–62
    ethical and philosophical
    considerations, 169–73
    ethical considerations in nursing care
    of, 166–69
    evaluating viability of, 161
    handicaps in, 171–73

Infants, (*cont.*)
   HIV testing, 165–66
   issue of treatment for abnormal, 161
   potentiality-actuality distinction,
      170–71
   quorum features, 169
Information, patient access to essential,
      105–8
Informative model of physician-patient
      relationship, 20, 21
Informed consent, 253–54. *See also*
      Consent
   elderly patient's right to, 246–47,
      253–54
   in nursing care of adults, 212–13, 215,
      217–18
   in nursing care of children, 177–81, 189
      exposure of incest, 180–81
      on issues of life or death, 180
      to kidney donation, 180
      mass screening program for
         children based on mother
         coercion, 179–80
      withholding life-saving drugs,
         178–79
Integrity, 236
Interdisciplinary role of the nurse in
      ethics, 15–16
International Council for Nurses, *Code of
      Ethics,* 33–34
Interpretive model of physician-patient
      relationship, 20
Intuition in moral reasoning, 11–12
In vitro fertilization and implantation,
      130
Involuntary euthanasia, 268, 273–80
Iron-deficiency anemia, mass screening
      program for, 179–80
Is-ought fallacy, 11, 67–68, 70, 109–10,
      242, 244
I-Thou relation, 78

J
Jaggar, A., 152
James, William, 118, 274
Jazelik, Beverly, 155
Jehovah's Witnesses
   organ donations and, 271
   refusal to accept blood transfusions,
      87, 103, 203

Jesus, ethics of, 70
John Paul II (Pope) on abortion, 146
Joint Commission on Accreditation of
      Healthcare Organizations
      (JCAHO) criteria, 15–16
Judgment, best interest versus substitute,
      103–4
Justice, ethics based on, 85–86
Justice-based model, 122
Justification of rights, 92
Just savings principle, 85

K
Kalish, R. A., 282
Kant, Immanuel, 7, 49, 54, 126, 249–50,
      276
   deontological ethics and, 171
   difficulties of ethics, 77
   on duty-based ethics, 118–19, 182
   principle of treating persons, 285
   principles of universality, 74–76
   strengths of ethics of, 76–77
   substantive principle, 242
   voluntarism and, 77–78
Kass, Leon, 279–80
Kevorkian, Jack, 278
Kidney donation, informed consent
      to, 180
Kierkergaard, Soren, 47, 78
King, Martin Luther, Jr., 12, 61
Kohlberg, Lawrence, 15
   stages of morality of, 79–80
Kübler-Ross, E., 60, 282

L
Ladd, John, 77
Laetrile, 178
Lappe, M., 136–37
Law
   civil, 61
   divine, 61
   eternal, 61
   human, 61
Legal moralism, 136
Legal paternalism, 136
Length of life versus quality of, 265–66
Lenon, J. L., 130
Leukemia, withholding of life-saving
      drugs and, 178–79

Libertarianism, 86–87, 136
  paternalism versus and, 264
Lidz. T., 236
Life
  defining the good, 7
  health as goal of the good, 7
  nurse's decision on issue of, 180
  quantity versus quality of, 7–8
Lifeboat method, 241–42
Life-saving drugs, parents' decision to
      withhold, 178–79
Life-saving treatment, adolescent's right
      to, 198
  exercise autonomy by refusing, 197–98
Limited resources
  allocation of, 237–38
  distribution of, 9–10
Listening, importance of, to children, 186
Living will, 98, 270
Lottery method, 243–44
Love as form of family interaction,
      117–18
Love-based ethics, 62, 203–4

M

Machine, assisted suicide by, 278
MacIntyre, A., 92
Madison, James, 122
Madsen v. *Women's Health Center,* 144
Maher v. *Roe,* 142–43
Majority rule, 76
Malthus, Thomas, 152–53
Manipulation, forms of, 105
Marriage
  club membership model of, 120–21,
      177
  ownership model of, 119–20, 176
  partnership model of, 121–23, 177,
      185–86
Marx, Karl, 47, 78
Marxism, 77, 78
Mass screening program for iron-
      deficiency anemia, 179–80
Master-slave dominance-submission
      relationship, 119
McCormick, Richard, 146
Mean, doctrine of, 59
Memorial Hospital v. *Darling,* 35. *See also*
      Darling
Mental retardation, 145

Middle age, 210
Mifepristone, 144–45
Mill, John Stuart, 23–24, 46, 68, 70, 86,
      122, 274
  version of utilitarianism, 242
Mind-body problem, brain-death
      definition and, 262
Minimally Decent Samaritan, 149–50
Minor premise, 153
Models
  civil-disobedience, 24
  club membership, of family and
      marriage, 120–21, 177
  complementary, of patient advocacy,
      190–91
  consumer, of physician-patient
      relationship, 20
  defined, 19
  deliberative, of physician-patient
      relationship, 20
  engineering, of physician-patient
      relationship, 20
  group confrontational, 190
  guidance-cooperation, 204
  individual confrontation, of patient
      advocacy, 191
  informative, of physician-patient
      relationship, 20, 21
  Interpretive, of physician-patient
      relationship, 20
  justice-based, 122
  of moral value, 3
  mutual participation, 204
  nursing, 21–22
  ownership, of family and marriage,
      119–20, 176
  parental, 20
  of parent-child relations, 176–77
  partnership, of family and marriage,
      121–23, 177, 185–86
  paternalistic, 20
  patient advocate, 24–25
  of physician-patient relationships,
      20–21
  priestly, of physician-patient
      relationship, 20
  of professional relationships, 19–37
  scientific, of physician-patient
      relationship, 20
Moore, G. E., 41, 49, 88

Moral importance of human rights in health care ethics, 91
Morality
  Kohlberg's stages of, 79–80
  self-interest, 40–51
Moral-philosophical responses to HIV/AIDS, 224–25
Moral problems in nursing, 40
Moral reasoning
  intuition in, 11–12
  methods of, 10–12
Moral relations, 123
Moral significance
  in codes of ethics, 26
  of nursing, 1–17
  in nursing care of children, 183–86
Moral standing, rights as form of, against arbitrary abuses, 90
Moral value
  of freedom, 87
  models of, 3
Mothers, mass screening program of children based on coercion of, 179–80
Mother Theresa, 265
Multiple pregnancies, fetal reduction and, 146
Muscular dystrophy, genetic screening and, 135
Mutuality and reciprocity, 249
Mutual participation model, 204
Myelomeningocele, 161

N
Natural law, 61–62
Nazi experiments, 89
Nazism, 43, 78
Neural tube defects, 145
Newborns. See Infants
New York Task Force on Life and the Law, 131
Nietzsche, Friedrich, 47, 53, 78, 80
Nightingale, Florence, 78
Nihilism, 41, 42
  social contract and, 56
Noddings, N., 14, 92
Nonmaleficence principle, 162, 178
Nonvoluntary euthanasia, 268
Nozick, Robert, 86, 150–51

Nurse
  as contracted clinician, 22
  decision of, on issues of life and death for children, 180
  in ethics, 14–15
  exposure of incest by, 180–81
  in family ethical issues, 126–27
  in family hierarchies, 120
  functions of code for, 34–36
  in genetic counseling, 136–37
  interdisciplinary role of, in ethics, 15–16
  as patient advocate, 22–23, 240, 252–53
    arguments for and against, 25–26
    for elderly, 239
  reporting of abuse by, 181
  in reproductive technology, 132
  rights of, 89–90
  secular, 2
  self-regulation in, 2
  as technician, 21
  virtue ethics in, 53–64
Nurse-child-parent relationships
  concept of rights applied to, 188–89
  ethical-philosophical approaches to, 187–91
Nurse-patient-child shared decision making, process of, 186
Nurse-patient relationships, values expressed in, 97
Nursing
  in abortion, 153–56
  in adolescent care, 199–201
  with adults, 225–29
  allocation of resources, 240–41
  in care of dying patient, 281–86
  ethical decision making in, 49–50, 96–113
    assessment of patient capacity and competence, 101–8
    fallacies in, 109–12
    guidelines for shared decision making, 108–9
    Patient Self-Determination Act (1990) in, 98–101
    values supportive of shared health care decisions, 97–98
  meaning of, in history of humankind, 1–2
  moral significance of, 1–17, 40

Nursing ethics, 7–10. *See also* Ethics
  abortion and, 141–59
    birth of very premature as result of
      spontaneous or induced, 163
    ethical and religious issues in,
      146–53
    legal status of, 142–44
    reproductive technology and,
      144–46
    role of nurse in, 153–56
  in care of adolescents, 194–205
    adolescent-nurse-parent
      relationship in, 202–3
    biological/biographical
      social/cognitive distinction
      applied to, 203–4
    controversy between parental
      authority and autonomy of,
      200–201
    developmental highlights for,
      194–96
    eating disorders and disturbances
      in body concept, 196
    health care issues for, 196–97
    life and death of, 197–99
    life-saving treatment for,
      197–98
    parental refusal to consent to
      tonsillectomies of, 199
    pregnancies of, 196
    in quality-of-life cases, 199
    in relationship with nurses,
      parents, and, 202–3
    role of nurse in care of, 199–201
    sexual abuse, 196
    surgery for versus parental refusal
      of consent, 199
  in care of adults, 208–30
    allocation of scarce resources, 211
    confidentiality, 214–15, 220
    deception, 211–12, 216–17
    deception in, 211–12, 216–17
    development of, 208–10
    informed consent in, 212–13, 215,
      217–18
    nurse's role with, 225–29
    prevention of harm, 211, 215
    privacy, 214–15, 220
    receiving and refusing treatment,
      213–14, 218–19

    right to receive and refuse
      treatment, 213–14, 218–19
    truth-telling in, 211–12, 216–17
  in care of children, 176–91
    for children with HIV/AIDS,
      181–83
    developmental highlights, 176–77
    disagreement with parents over
      treatment, 179
    helping express fears, 186
    with HIV/AIDS, 181–83
    on informed consent, 177–81, 189
      exposure of incest, 180–81
      on issues of life or death, 180
      to kidney donation, 180
      mass screening program for
        children based on mother
        coercion, 179–80
      withholding life-saving drugs,
        178–79
    moral implications in nursing care
      of, 183–86
    nurses as advocates of, 185
    rights of handicapped, 177
    right to bear
      AIDS and, 127–28
      despite consequences, 132–34
    treatment of deformed, 184
    values reflected in rearing
      practices, 176–77
  in care of elderly, 233–59
    abuse of, 250–51
    advanced old age, 235
    allocating health care to, 238,
      240–46
    assisted suicide and, 238, 277–80
    competence and patient's right to
      refuse treatment, 239
    competence and rights of, 247–49
    conflict of rights, 239
    dementia, 235–36
    developmental highlights, 233–36
    frail, 235
    freedom versus control and
      prevention of harm, 250
    granny pregnancies and, 130
    informed consent, 246–47, 253–54
    justice between generations,
      249–50
    nurse as patient advocate, 240

Nursing ethics, (*cont.*)
  patient's rights, 246–47
    to decide, 239
  prejudice against, 237
  problems and prospects for,
    236–38
  resources for, allocation of, 238,
    240–41
  retirement, 234–35
  role of patient advocate, 252–53
  sanctity of life versus quality of life,
    255–56
  truth-telling, 240, 246, 255–56
  in care of infants, 160–75, 166–69
    arguments for and against saving
      deformed, 162–65
    arguments for and against saving
      premature, 162–65
    developmental highlights, 160–62
    ethical and philosophical
      considerations, 169–73
    ethical considerations in nursing
      care of, 166–69
    evaluating viability of, 161
    handicaps in, 171–73
    HIV testing, 165–66
    issue of treatment for abnormal,
      161
    potentiality-actuality distinction,
      170–71
    quorum features, 169
  classical utilitarianism in, 68–71
  in death and dying
    active euthanasia, 262–63
    active/passive euthanasia, 262,
      267–70
    for adolescents, 197–99
    adult's right to, 263–64
    advance directives, 270–71
    definitions of, 261–62
    "Do not resuscitate" orders, 264,
      271–73
    ethical issues in nursing care of,
      260–89
    hospice concept in, 285–86
    nurse's decision on issue of, 180
    organ donations, 271
    paternalism versus libertarianism,
      264
      patient's right to know the truth,
        263
      quality versus length of life, 265–66
      relief of individual suffering versus
        principle of double effect,
        266
      religious aspects of nursing care of,
        280–81
      rights of patients, 265
      right to suicide, 263
      role of nurse in care of patient,
        281–86
      unplugging respirator, 263
      voluntary and involuntary
        euthanasia, 273–80
  defined, 6
  distribution of limited resources in,
    9–10
  empirical knowledge versus personal
    belief in, 10
  freedom versus control in, 8
  function of, 4–6
  in genetic screening, mandatory versus
    voluntary, 134–36
  important issues in, 7–10
  perennial issues in, 41–44
  pro-choice versus pro-life in, 8
  in procreative family, 117–38
    club membership model of,
      120–21, 177
    family functions, dynamics, and
      values in, 118–19, 123–26
    genetic screening in, 134–36
    genetics in, 132–34
    nurse's role in ethical issues,
      126–27
    nurse's role in genetic counseling,
      136–37
    ownership model of family and
      marriage, 119–20, 176
    partnership model of, 121–23, 177,
      185–86
    reproductive technology in, 127–32
  in quality-of-life cases of adolescents,
    199
  quantity versus quality of life in, 7–8
  in reproductive technology, 127–32
  role of care in, 13–14
  role of rights and virtue in, 92–93

Socratic method in, 56
veracity versus deception in, 9
Nursing homes
elder abuse in, 251
quality of health care and human
services given in, 236
Nursing models, 21–22

O

Objectivism, 41, 42
social contract and, 55
Old age, advanced, 235
One person one vote principle, 85
Openness, 215
Oregon Right to Die Committee, 278–79
Orem, Dorothy, 78
Organ donations, 271
Orwell, George, 121
Ownership model of family and marriage,
119–20, 176

P

Parental attachment in adolescence, 195
Parental authority, controversy between
adolescent autonomy and,
200–201
Parental model, 20
Parental refusal of consent
versus adolescent's surgery, 199
to adolescents' tonsillectomies, 199
Parent-child relations, models of, 176–77
Parents
decision of, to withhold life-saving
drugs, 178–79
refusal to consent to surgery for
adolescent on grounds of
religious beliefs, 199
Parkinson's disease, use of embryonic
tissue and, 146
Participation, strategies for maximizing,
108–9
Partnership model of family and
marriage, 121–23, 177, 185–86
Passive euthanasia, 268
Paternalism, 20, 22, 189–90
versus libertarianism and, 264
rational, 44, 54, 190
Patient advocacy. *See also* Advocacy
expression of, 166–67

models of, 24–25, 190–91
nurse as, 22–23
with adults, 225–26
with elderly, 240, 252–53
Patients
access to essential information, 105–8
autonomy of, 21, 124
capacity to make rational decisions,
101–2
incapacity to make rational decisions,
102–3
right to decide, 239
voluntariness, 104–5
A Patient's Bill of Rights, 217, 225
Patient Self-Determination Act, 98–101,
270
Peer values, acceptance of, 200
Peplau, Hildegard, 78, 89
Perfect duties, distinguishing from
imperfect duties, 76–77
Personal belief versus empirical
knowledge, 10
Personhood
applying to "Do Not Resuscitate"
orders, 271–73
reason and freedom as marks of,
220–22
Phenomenology, 48–49, 78
Phenylketonuria (PKU), genetic
screening and, 135
Physician-assisted suicide, 268, 276–77
Physician-patient relationships, models
of, 20–21
Pius XII (Pope), 266
on abortion, 146
Planned Parenthood v. *Casey,* 143–44,
154
Plato, 44, 46, 49–50, 54, 56, 190, 247
response to perennial issues, 57–58
Populace, appeal to, 111
Population control, economic aid and, 129
Potentiality-actuality distinction, 170–71
Practical syllogism, 59
Pregnancy
adolescent, 196
in AIDS patient, 127–28, 165–66
case of unintended, 153–55
granny, 130
multiple, and fetal reduction, 146

Prejudice against elderly, 237
Premature infants, arguments for and against saving, 162–65
Prenatal tests
    benefits, harms, and risks of, 145
    of fetal health, 145
President's Commission for the Study of Ethical Problems in Medicine and Biomedical and Behavioral Research, 266
Priestly model of physician-patient relationship, 20
Prima facie values, 78–79
Privacy, right to, 214–15, 220
Pro-choice versus pro-life, 8
Procreative family, nursing ethics in, 117–38
    club membership model of, 120–21, 177
    family functions, dynamics, and values in, 118–19, 123–26
    genetic screening in, 134–36
    genetics in, 132–34
    nurse's role in ethical issues, 126–27
    nurse's role in genetic counseling, 136–37
    ownership model of family and marriage, 119–20, 176
    partnership model of, 121–23, 177, 185–86
    reproductive technology in, 127–32
Professional relationships, models of, 19–37
Pro-life versus pro-choice, 8
Prudence, 14
Psychiatric patients, right of, to refuse treatment, 228
Puccini, 274

Q
Quality of life, 72
    argument on, 162, 167, 168
    ethical issues in, for adolescents, 199
    versus length of life, 265–66
    versus quantity of life, 7–8
    versus sanctity of life and, 255–56
Quantity of life versus quality of life, 7–8

R
Rachels, 187
Racism, 43
Rational decisions
    patient capacity to make, 101–2
    patient incapacity to make, 102–3
Rational intuition, 280
Rational paternalism, 44, 54, 119–20, 190
    response to perennial issues and to self-interest ethics, 57–58
Rational suicide, 275–77
Rationing, of health care, 7–8
Rawls, John, 45, 187
    ethics based on justice, 85–86
    justice-based model, 122
    responses to social contract view, 86–87
Reasoning
    conventional, 11
    dialectical, 12
    fallacies as pitfalls of, 109–12
    inductive, 11, 68
    intuition in moral, 11–12
    methods of moral, 10–12
Reciprocity, rule of, 41
Redlich, F. C., 89
Reductio ad absurdum, 55–56
Rehabilitation Act (1973), 168, 172
Relativism, 41–42, 42–43
    pros and cons of, 43–44
Religious beliefs, 10
    abortion and, 146–53
    nursing care of dying and, 280–81
    parent's refusal to consent to surgery for adolescent on grounds of, 199
Renaissance, 54
Reproductive technology
    abortion and, 144–46
    AIDS as issue in, 127–28
    alpha-fetoprotein screening in, 145
    amniocentesis in, 141, 145
    artificial insemination and, 129
    benefits, harms, and risks of prenatal tests, 145
    chorionic villus sampling in, 145
    ethical issues in, 127–32
    family planning and contraception and, 127–29
    fetal reduction in, 146

fetal therapy, 130–31
   granny pregnancies and, 130
   in vitro fertilization and implantation,
      130
   prenatal tests of fetal health in, 145
   role of nurse in, 132
   surrogate motherhood and, 131–32
   use of embryonic tissue, 146
Republic (Plato), 56
Resource allocation, 9–10
   for adults, 211
   for elderly, 237–38, 239
   HIV/AIDS and, 223–25
   lifeboat method, 241–42
   lottery method, 243–44
   principle of equal consideration,
      245–46
   principle of equality, 244–45
   utilitarian method, 71, 242–43
Respect, elderly patient's right to, 246
Respirator, unplugging, 263
Restraints, 250
Retinoblastoma, genetic screening and,
   133–34, 135
Retirement, 234–35
Rights
   appropriate attribution of, 91
   argument for, in health care ethics,
      88–89
   concept of, applied to nurse-child-
      parent relationships, 188–89
   justification of, 92
   meaning and importance of, 90–91
   of nurses, 89–90
   role of, in nursing ethics, 92–93
   and virtues, 93
Rights-based ethics, 84–94, 156
   appropriate attribution of rights,
      91
   argument for rights in health care
      ethics, 88–89
   justification of rights in, 92
   meaning and importance of rights,
      90–91
   moral importance of human rights in
      health care ethics, 91
   paradigm case arguments in health
      care and, 88
   rights as form of moral standing
      against arbitrary abuses, 90

Rights in trust, 189
Right to bear children, acquired
      immunodeficiency syndrome
      (AIDS) and, 127–28
The Ring of Gyges (Plato), 44
Roe v. Wade, 8, 142, 143, 154
Ross, W. D., 78–79
Rousseau, Jean Jacques, 137
RU-486 (mifepristone), 8, 144–45
Ruddick, W., 187

S
Sade, Robert, 86
St. Augustine, 11–12, 85
St. Christopher's Hospital in London,
   285
St. Francis of Assisi, 62
St. Thomas Aquinas, 2, 13, 14, 54, 141,
   150, 170
   view of ethics, 61–63
Sanctity of life, 162, 165
   versus quality of life, 255–56
Sartre, Jean-Paul, 48, 187
Saunders, Cicely, 285
Scanlon, Thomas, 72
Scarce resources
   allocation of, 211, 239
   competition for, 71
Schopenhauer, A., 78, 274
Science, ethics and, 2–4
Scientific model of physician-patient
   relationship, 20
Scientific theory, major differences
      between ethical theory and,
      3–4
Secular nursing, 2
Self-aggrandizement, 120
Self-corrective feedback, 215
Self-determination, principle of, 77, 97,
   217
Self-interest morality, 40–51
   collectivism and, 47
   existentialism and, 47–48, 48–49
   nursing dilemmas in decision making,
      49–50
   phenomenology and, 48–49
   in relation to alternative theories,
      41–44
   social contract and, 44–46

Self-interest theories of ethics, 53
  rational paternalism and, 57–58
  in relation to alternative theories,
    41–44
Self-love, 42
Self-realization, 58–61, 59
  happiness through, 58–61
Self-regulation in nursing profession, 2
Sexism, 43
Sexual abuse, 196
Shakespeare, W., 274
Shared decision making, 122
  guidelines for, 108–9
  values supportive of, 97–98
Sherwin, S., 153
Sickle-cell anemia, genetic screening
    and, 133, 135
Singer, P., 91
Situationalism, 71
Skepticism, 41, 42
  social contract and, 55–56
Slippery-slope fallacy, 111–12, 147
Slothful induction, 112
Smith, Adam, 75
Social contract
  altruism and, 55
  defined, 44, 54
  nihilism and, 56
  objectivism and, 55
  responses to Rawl's view of, 86–87
  skepticism and, 55–56
  views of, 44, 54–56
Social deterioration in adolescence,
    196–97
Sociological approach to ethics, 11
Socrates, 12, 42, 44, 46, 49, 53–54, 58,
    247, 276
Socratic method, use of, in nursing ethics,
    56
Spina bifida, 145
Spinoza, 280
Stoicism, 41, 60–61
Subjectivism, 41, 42
  pros and cons of, 43–44
Substitute judgment, best interest versus,
    103–4
Sufferability, principle of, 69
Suicide, 268, 274–75
  assisted, 238, 277–80

  physician-assisted, 268, 276–77
  rational, 275–77
  right to, 263
Surrogate motherhood, 131–32
Syllogism, practical, 59

T
Tarasoff v. *Regents of University of
    California,* 220
Tay-Sachs disease, genetic screening and,
    130–31, 132, 135, 145
Technician, nurse as, 21
Teenagers. *See* Adolescents
Temperance, 14
Thomson, Judith, 49, 89, 97, 147–50
Thrasymachus, 42, 54, 80
Tolstoy, Leo, 60, 123–24, 137, 281
Toulmin, Stephen, 15, 92, 123
Treatment
  elderly patient's rights
    to receive appropriate, 247
    to terminate or refuse, 247
  ordinary versus extraordinary, 266–67
  right to receive and to refuse, 213–14,
    218–19, 227–28
Trisomy 18 syndrome, 161, 164
Truth-telling
  and ethical issues of death and dying,
    263
  in nursing care of adults, 211–12,
    216–17
  in nursing care of elderly, 240, 246,
    255–56
Tuma, Jolene, 34, 55
Tuskeegee experiment, 88–89

U
Universality, Kant's principles of, 74–76
Universalizability principle, 76
Utilitarian ethics, 66–72
Utilitarianism, 14, 41, 66–68, 74
  classical, in nursing ethics, 68–70
  competition for scarce resources and,
    71, 242–43
  handicapped infants and, 172
  recent formulations and applications,
    71–72

V

Values
  in conflict, 87–88
  in distributive justice, 85–86
  expressed in nurse-patient
      relationships, 97
  prima facie, 78–79
  relation of facts to, 67
  supportive of shared health care
      decisions, 97–98
Veil of ignorance, 242
Veracity versus deception, 9
Virtue, role of, in nursing ethics, 92–93
Virtue ethics, 92, 123–24
  in nursing, 53–64
Virtues, rights and, 93
Voluntariness, patient, 104–5
Voluntarism, 77–78
Voluntary euthanasia, 268, 273–80

W

Warren, M. A., 153
Wasserstrom, Richard, 69
Well-being, principle of, 100
Whitehead, Mary Beth, 131
Whose Life Is It Anyway?, 8
Wilder, Mary, 144
Will, weakness of, 60
Wisdom, 14
Women, battered, 125
Women's rights movement, 89
Work ethic, 234
Wrubel, J., 92, 93

Y

Young adulthood, 209
Youth, 209. *See also* Adolescents